Comparative Effectiveness Review
Number 139

Core Needle and Open Surgical Biopsy for Diagnosis of Breast Lesions:
An Update to the 2009 Report

Prepared for:
Agency for Healthcare Research and Quality
U.S. Department of Health and Human Services
540 Gaither Road
Rockville, MD 20850
www.ahrq.gov

Contract No. 290-2012-00012 -I

Prepared by:
Brown Evidence-Based Practice Center
Providence, RI

Investigators:
Issa J. Dahabreh, M.D., M.S.
Lisa Susan Wieland, Ph.D.
Gaelen P. Adam, M.L.I.S.
Christopher Halladay, B.A., M.S.
Joseph Lau, M.D.
Thomas A. Trikalinos, M.D.

AHRQ Publication No. 14-EHC040-EF
September 2014

This report is based on research conducted by Brown Evidence-based Practice Center (EPC) under contract to the Agency for Healthcare Research and Quality (AHRQ), Rockville, MD (Contract No. 290-2012-00012-I). The findings and conclusions in this document are those of the authors, who are responsible for its contents; the findings and conclusions do not necessarily represent the views of AHRQ. Therefore, no statement in this report should be construed as an official position of AHRQ or of the U.S. Department of Health and Human Services.

The information in this report is intended to help health care decisionmakers—patients and clinicians, health system leaders, and policymakers, among others—make well-informed decisions and thereby improve the quality of health care services. This report is not intended to be a substitute for the application of clinical judgment. Anyone who makes decisions concerning the provision of clinical care should consider this report in the same way as any medical reference and in conjunction with all other pertinent information, i.e., in the context of available resources and circumstances presented by individual patients.

This report may be used, in whole or in part, as the basis for development of clinical practice guidelines and other quality enhancement tools, or as a basis for reimbursement and coverage policies. AHRQ or U.S. Department of Health and Human Services endorsement of such derivative products may not be stated or implied.

This report may periodically be assessed for the urgency to update. If an assessment is done, the resulting surveillance report describing the methodology and findings will be found on the Effective Health Care Program Web site at: www.effectivehealthcare.ahrq.gov. Search on the title of the report.

This document is in the public domain and may be used and reprinted without permission except those copyrighted materials that are clearly noted in the document. Further reproduction of those copyrighted materials is prohibited without the specific permission of copyright holders.

Persons using assistive technology may not be able to fully access information in this report. For assistance contact EffectiveHealthCare@ahrq.hhs.gov.

None of the investigators have any affiliations or financial involvement that conflicts with the material presented in this report.

Suggested citation: Dahabreh IJ, Wieland LS, Adam GP, Halladay C, Lau J, Trikalinos TA. Core Needle and Open Surgical Biopsy for Diagnosis of Breast Lesions: An Update to the 2009 Report. Comparative Effectiveness Review No. 139. (Prepared by the Brown Evidence-based Practice Center under Contract 290-2012-00012-I.) AHRQ Publication No. 14-EHC040-EF. Rockville, MD: Agency for Healthcare Research and Quality. September 2014. www.effectivehealthcare.ahrq.gov/reports/final.cfm.

Preface

The Agency for Healthcare Research and Quality (AHRQ), through its Evidence-based Practice Centers (EPCs), sponsors the development of systematic reviews to assist public- and private-sector organizations in their efforts to improve the quality of health care in the United States. These reviews provide comprehensive, science-based information on common, costly medical conditions, and new health care technologies and strategies.

Systematic reviews are the building blocks underlying evidence-based practice; they focus attention on the strength and limits of evidence from research studies about the effectiveness and safety of a clinical intervention. In the context of developing recommendations for practice, systematic reviews can help clarify whether assertions about the value of the intervention are based on strong evidence from clinical studies. For more information about AHRQ EPC systematic reviews, see www.effectivehealthcare.ahrq.gov/reference/purpose.cfm.

AHRQ expects that these systematic reviews will be helpful to health plans, providers, purchasers, government programs, and the health care system as a whole. Transparency and stakeholder input are essential to the Effective Health Care Program. Please visit the Web site (www.effectivehealthcare.ahrq.gov) to see draft research questions and reports or to join an e-mail list to learn about new program products and opportunities for input.

We welcome comments on this systematic review. They may be sent by mail to the Task Order Officer named below at: Agency for Healthcare Research and Quality, 540 Gaither Road, Rockville, MD 20850, or by email to epc@ahrq.hhs.gov.

Richard Kronick, Ph.D.
Director
Agency for Healthcare Research and Quality

Yen-Pin Chiang, Ph.D.
Acting Deputy Director
Center for Evidence and Practice Improvement
Agency for Healthcare Research and Quality

Stephanie Chang, M.D., M.P.H.
Director
Evidence-based Practice Program
Center for Evidence and Practice Improvement
Agency for Healthcare Research and Quality

Elisabeth Kato, M.D., M.R.P.
Task Order Officer
Center for Evidence and Practice Improvement
Agency for Healthcare Research and Quality

Technical Expert Panel

In designing the study questions and methodology at the outset of this report, the EPC consulted several technical and content experts. Broad expertise and perspectives were sought. Divergent and conflicting opinions are common and perceived as healthy scientific discourse that results in a thoughtful, relevant systematic review. Therefore, in the end, study questions, design, methodologic approaches, and/or conclusions do not necessarily represent the views of individual technical and content experts.

Technical Experts must disclose any financial conflicts of interest greater than $10,000 and any other relevant business or professional conflicts of interest. Because of their unique clinical or content expertise, individuals with potential conflicts may be retained. The TOO and the EPC work to balance, manage, or mitigate any potential conflicts of interest identified.

One Technical Expert was a patient and remains anonymous. The list of the remaining Technical Experts who participated in developing this report follows:

Patricia Carney, Ph.D.
Oregon Health and Science University
Portland, OR

Joanne Elmore, M.D., M.P.H.
University of Washington
School of Public Health
Seattle, WA

Richard E. Fine, M.D.
Department of Surgery
Department of Surgical Oncology
University of Tennessee College of Medicine
The West Clinic Comprehensive Breast Center
Memphis, TN

Mark A. Helvie, M.D.
University of Michigan Health System
Ann Arbor, MI

Carol Lee, M.D.
Memorial Sloan Kettering Cancer Center
New York City, NY

Barabara Monsees, M.D.
Evens Professor of Women's Health
Department of Radiology
Washington University School of Medicine
St. Louis, MO

Liane Philpotts, M.D.
Yale University School of Medicine
New Haven, CT

Melissa Pilewskie, M.D.
Memorial Sloan-Kettering Cancer Center
Evelyn H. Lauder Breast Center
New York City, NY

Peer Reviewers

Prior to publication of the final evidence report, EPCs sought input from independent Peer Reviewers without financial conflicts of interest. However, the conclusions and synthesis of the scientific literature presented in this report does not necessarily represent the views of individual reviewers.

Peer Reviewers must disclose any financial conflicts of interest greater than $10,000 and any other relevant business or professional conflicts of interest. Because of their unique clinical or content expertise, individuals with potential non-financial conflicts may be retained. The TOO and the EPC work to balance, manage, or mitigate any potential non-financial conflicts of interest identified.

The list of Peer Reviewers follows:

Binita Ashar, M.D.
Center for Devices and Radiological Health
U.S. Food and Drug Administration
Baltimore, MD

Ira J. Bleiweiss, M.D.
Icahn School of Medicine at Mount Sinai
New York City, NY

Edi Brogi, M.D.
Memorial Sloan-Kettering Cancer Center
New York City, NY

Laurie L. Fajardo, M.D.
University of Iowa Health Care
Iowa City, IA

Seema Khan, M.D.
Feinberg School of Medicine
Northwestern University
Chicago, IL

Tracy Lively, Ph.D.
Cancer Diagnosis Program
National Cancer Institute
Bethesda, MD

Robert A. Smith, Ph.D.
American Cancer Society
Atlanta, GA

Core Needle and Open Surgical Biopsy for Diagnosis of Breast Lesions: An Update to the 2009 Report

Structured Abstract

Objective. Core needle biopsy and open surgical biopsy are the most frequently used procedures for diagnosis of suspicious breast lesions. An AHRQ evidence report on the comparative effectiveness and adverse events of breast biopsy methods was completed in 2009. The availability of additional studies and the uncertainties surrounding newer biopsy techniques prompted an update of that report.

Study eligibility criteria. We searched nine electronic databases (last search on December 16, 2013) for English-language full-text reports of prospective or retrospective cohort studies of women not previously diagnosed with breast cancer who were undergoing biopsy for diagnosis of a breast lesion.

Study appraisal and synthesis methods. A single investigator extracted quantitative and qualitative data from each study; a second reviewer verified extracted data. We assessed the strength and applicability of the evidence. We performed Bayesian meta-analyses to estimate summary test performance and performed indirect comparisons to assess the relative effectiveness of alternative core needle biopsy methods. Statistical models accounted for between-study heterogeneity.

Results. One hundred and sixty studies of moderate to high risk of bias provided information on the test performance of alternative core needle biopsy techniques. We found one new study investigating the test performance of open biopsy. For women at average risk of cancer, both ultrasound- and stereotactically guided biopsies had average sensitivities higher than 0.97 and average specificities ranging from 0.92 to 0.99; freehand biopsy methods had average sensitivity of 0.91 and specificity of 0.98. However, evidence on the test performance of magnetic resonance imaging (MRI)-guided biopsy (6 studies) was insufficient to draw conclusions. Test performance did not differ between women at average and high baseline risk of cancer, but results were imprecise. Test performance of automated and vacuum-assisted devices (when using the same imaging guidance) was fairly similar (absolute differences in sensitivity and specificity ≤ 0.1). One hundred and forty-one studies contributed information on potential harms of different core needle biopsy techniques. Overall, core needle biopsy had a lower risk of complications than open surgical biopsy; however information on the latter was sparse. The absolute incidence of adverse events was low and the incidence of severe complications was less than 1 percent for all techniques. Vacuum-assisted procedures appeared to be associated with increased bleeding and hematoma formation; biopsies performed with patients seated upright appeared to be associated with increased risk of vasovagal reactions. Harms were reported inconsistently, raising concerns about selective outcome reporting. We found 10 case reports of patients developing tumors at the site of prior core needle biopsies. We found information on only a few patient-relevant and resource-related outcomes. Based on 42 studies, core needle biopsy obviated the need for surgical procedures in about 75 percent of women. Meta-analysis of

10 studies reporting the number of surgical procedures required after biopsy suggested that the odds of requiring only one procedure were almost 15 times as high among women receiving core needle biopsy, as compared to those receiving open surgical biopsy. However, this result may be confounded by indication.

Limitations. Patient-level data were unavailable and information about study- or population-level characteristics was too limited to allow the identification of modifiers of test performance, adverse events, or clinical outcomes. Studies reported adverse events incompletely, and did not provide details of their outcome ascertainment methods.

Conclusions. A large body of evidence suggests that ultrasound and stereotactically guided core needle biopsy procedures have sensitivity and specificity close to that of open biopsy procedures, and are associated with fewer adverse events. The strength of the evidence on the test performance of these methods is deemed moderate because studies are at medium to high risk of bias, but provide precise and fairly consistent results. Freehand procedures have lower sensitivity than imaging-guided methods. The strength of evidence on the comparative test performance of automated and vacuum-assisted devices (when using the same imaging guidance) is deemed low, because of concerns about the risk of bias of included studies and the reliance on indirect comparisons. There were insufficient data to draw conclusions for MRI-guided biopsy or women at high baseline risk of cancer. There is low strength of evidence that vacuum-assisted procedures have a higher risk of bleeding than automated methods. There is moderate strength of evidence that women diagnosed with breast cancer by core needle biopsy are more likely to have their cancer treated with a single surgical procedure, compared with women diagnosed by open surgical biopsy.

Contents

Executive Summary ES-1

Background 1
   Breast Cancer Epidemiology and Clinical Diagnosis 1
   Original Evidence Report and Rationale for the Update 2
   Key Questions 2

Methods 4
   AHRQ Task Order Officer 4
   External Stakeholder Input 4
   Key Questions 4
   Analytic Framework 4
   Scope of the Review 5
      Populations and Conditions of Interest 5
      Interventions 5
      Comparators (Index and Reference Standard Tests) 5
      Outcomes 6
      Timing 6
      Setting 7
      Study Design and Additional Criteria 7
   Literature Search and Abstract Screening 8
   Study Selection and Eligibility Criteria 9
   Data Abstraction and Management 9
   Assessment of the Risk of Bias of Individual Studies 10
   Data Synthesis 10
   Grading the Strength of Evidence 12
   Assessing Applicability 12
   Peer Review 13

Results 14
   Included Studies 16
   Test Performance for Breast Cancer Diagnosis 16
      Test Performance of Open Surgical Biopsy 16
      Test Performance of Core Needle Biopsy Methods 16
   Contextualizing the Results of Test Performance Meta-Analyses 22
   Comparative Test Performance 24
   Factors That Affect Test Performance 25
      Within-Study Evidence 25
      Meta-Regression Analyses 29
   Risk Of Bias Assessment for Studies Addressing Key Question 1 30
   Adverse Events of Open Biopsy 30
   Adverse Events of Core Needle Biopsy 31
   Hematomas and Bleeding 31

Infections 33
Pain and Use of Pain Medications 34
Vasovagal Reactions 34
Impact of Biopsy Procedure on Usual Activities and Time to Recovery 35
Impact of Biopsy Procedure on Subsequent Mammographic Procedures 35
Miscellaneous Reported Adverse Events 36
Dissemination and Displacement of Cancerous Cells During the Biopsy Procedure 36
Factors That Modify the Association of Biopsy Procedures With Adverse Events 37
Anxiety and Distress 40
Procedure Preference 41
Surgical Procedures Avoided 41
Cosmetic Results 41
Resource Utilization and Costs 42
Physician Experience 42
Availability of a Qualified Pathologist 43
Availability of Equipment/Utilization 43
Procedure Duration Time 43
Time to Complete Tumor Removal 44
Wait Time for Test Results 44
Recurrence Rates 45

Discussion 46
Key Findings and Assessment of the Strength of Evidence 46
Test Performance and Comparative Test Performance 46
Underestimation Rates 47
Adverse Events and Additional Surgeries After Biopsy 48
Limitations of the Evidence Base 49
Strengths and Limitations of This Review 50
Applicability of Review Findings 51
Evidence Gaps and Ongoing Research 51
Future Research Needs 52
Conclusions 53
Abbreviations 54
References 55

Tables

Table A. Definitions of diagnostic groups based on index and reference standard test results ES-4
Table B. Summary estimates of test performance for alternative core needle biopsy methods—women at average risk of cancer ES-9
Table C. Summary estimates of test performance for alternative core needle biopsy methods—women at high risk of cancer ES-9
Table D. Summary estimates of underestimation rates for alternative core needle biopsy methods—women at average risk of cancer ES-10
Table E. Differences in sensitivity between pairs of biopsy methods (meta-regression based indirect comparisons) ES-11

Table F. Strength of evidence about comparative test performance in women at average risk of breast cancer ES-16
Table G. Strength of evidence for underestimation rates in women at average risk of cancer ES-17
Table H. Strength of evidence assessment for adverse events of breast biopsy ES-18
Table 1. Definitions of diagnostic groups based on index and reference standard test results 7
Table 2. Summary of new evidence evaluated in this update 15
Table 3. Summary estimates of test performance for alternative core needle biopsy methods – women at average risk of cancer 18
Table 4. Summary estimates of test performance for alternative core needle biopsy methods – women at high risk of cancer 18
Table 5. Differences in sensitivity between pairs of biopsy methods (meta-regression based indirect comparisons) 25
Table 6. Studies evaluating factors that may affect test performance (20 studies, reporting on multiple factors each) 26
Table 7. Meta-regression analysis for test performance outcomes... 29
Table 8. Adverse events associated with core needle biopsy for breast cancer diagnosis............ 31
Table 9. Core needle biopsy procedures and rates of hematoma formation and bleeding 33
Table 10. Core needle biopsy procedures and rates of infectious complications 34
Table 11. Core needle biopsy procedures and rates of vasovagal reactions................................. 35
Table 12. Studies evaluating factors that may affect the incidence of adverse events 38
Table 13. Strength of evidence about comparative test performance in women at average risk of breast cancer 47
Table 14. Strength of evidence for underestimation rates in women at average risk of cancer ... 48
Table 15. Strength of evidence assessment for adverse events of biopsy 49
Table 16. Evidence gaps for biopsy methods for the diagnosis of breast cancer 51

Figures
Figure A. Outcomes of testing in a hypothetical cohort of 1,000 women ES-13
Figure 1. Analytic framework... 5
Figure 2. Flow chart of included studies... 14
Figure 3. Scatterplot of results in the receiver operating characteristic space and summary receiver operating characteristic curves of alternative core needle biopsy methods for the diagnosis of breast cancer 19
Figure 4. Outcomes of testing in a hypothetical cohort of 1,000 women 23
Figure 5. Positive predictive value of alternative biopsy methods 24

Appendix
Appendix A. Search Strategy
Appendix B. Excluded Studies
Appendix C. Sensitivity Analysis to the Exclusion of High Risk Lesions on Core Needle Biopsy That Were Confirmed to be High Risk Lesions in Subsequent Open Biopsy or Surgical Excision
Appendix D. Assessment of the Strength of Evidence

Executive Summary

Background

Approximately one in eight U.S. women will develop breast cancer during her lifetime.[1] Because the earliest stages of breast cancer are asymptomatic, the process of breast cancer diagnosis is often initiated by detecting an abnormality through self-examination, physical examination by a clinician, or screening mammography. If the initial assessment suggests that the abnormality could be breast cancer, the woman is likely to be referred for a biopsy—a sampling of cells or tissue from the suspicious lesion. Among women screened annually for 10 years, approximately 50 percent will need additional imaging, and 5–7 percent will have biopsies.[2,3]

Three techniques for obtaining samples from suspicious breast lesions are available: fine-needle aspiration, biopsy with a hollow core needle, or open surgical retrieval of tissue. Fine-needle aspiration samples cells and does not assess tissue architecture, is generally considered less sensitive than core needle and open biopsy methods,[4] and is used less frequently. Core-needle biopsy, which retrieves a sample of tissue, and open surgical procedures are the most frequently used biopsy methods. Lesion samples obtained by core needle or surgical biopsy are evaluated by pathologists and classified into histological categories with the primary goal of determining whether the lesion is benign or malignant. Because core needle biopsy samples only part of the breast abnormality, a risk exists that a lesion will be classified as benign, high risk, or noninvasive when invasive cancer is in fact present in unsampled areas. Open surgical biopsy samples most or all of the lesion, and is therefore considered to have a smaller risk of misdiagnosis. However, open procedures may carry a higher risk of complications, such as bleeding or infection, compared to core needle biopsy procedures.[5] Therefore, if core needle biopsy is also highly accurate, women and their clinicians may prefer some type of core needle biopsy to open surgical biopsy.

Alternative core needle biopsy methods differ with respect to the use of imaging (e.g., stereotactic mammography; ultrasound; or magnetic resonance imaging [MRI]), the use of vacuum to assist in tissue acquisition, the use of needles of varying diameter, and the numbers of samples taken. These and other factors may affect test performance and the rate of complications. For example, some biopsy procedures may retrieve larger amounts of tissue, improving test performance, but the retrieval of larger amounts of tissue may also result in more complications, such as bleeding. Imaging methods may also influence the performance of open surgical biopsies because the majority of such biopsies are preceded by an image-guided wire localization procedure. In general, the impact of various aspects of biopsy technique and patient or lesion characteristics on test performance and safety is not clear.

In 2009, the ECRI Evidence-based Practice Center (EPC) conducted a comparative effectiveness review for core needle versus open surgical biopsy commissioned by the Agency for Health Care Research and Quality (AHRQ).[6,7] That evidence report assessed the diagnostic test performance and adverse events of core needle biopsy techniques compared to open surgical biopsy and evaluated differences between open biopsy and core needle biopsy with regards to patient preferences, costs, availability, and other factors. The authors concluded that core needle biopsies were almost as accurate as open surgical biopsies, had a lower risk of severe complications, and were associated with fewer subsequent surgical procedures.[7]

The publication of additional studies and changes in practice raised the concern that the conclusions of the original report may be out of date, particularly for the underestimation rate of ductal carcinoma in situ (DCIS) with stereotactically guided vacuum-assisted core needle biopsy, the performance of MRI-guided core needle biopsy, and the performance of freehand automated device core needle technology. New studies may also provide additional information allowing the exploration of heterogeneity for test performance and safety outcomes. Therefore, an updated review of the published literature was considered necessary to synthesize all evidence on currently available methods for core needle and open surgical breast lesion biopsy.

Key Questions

On the basis of input from clinical experts during the development of our protocol, we made minor revisions to the Key Questions and study eligibility criteria to clarify the focus of the updated review. We specified the following three Key Questions to guide the conduct of the update:

Key Question 1: In women with a palpable or nonpalpable breast abnormality, what is the test performance of different types of core needle breast biopsy compared with open biopsy for diagnosis?

- What factors associated with the patient and her breast abnormality influence the test performance of different types of core needle breast biopsy compared with open biopsy for diagnosis of a breast abnormality?
- What factors associated with the procedure itself influence the test performance of different types of core needle breast biopsy compared with open biopsy for diagnosis of a breast abnormality?
- What clinician and facility factors influence the test performance of core needle breast biopsy compared with open biopsy for diagnosis of a breast abnormality?

Key Question 2: In women with a palpable or nonpalpable breast abnormality, what are the adverse events (harms) associated with different types of core needle breast biopsy compared with open biopsy for diagnosis?

- What factors associated with the patient and her breast abnormality influence the adverse events of core needle breast biopsy compared with the open biopsy technique in the diagnosis of a breast abnormality?
- What factors associated with the procedure itself influence the adverse events of core needle breast biopsy compared with the open biopsy technique in the diagnosis of a breast abnormality?
- What clinician and facility factors influence the adverse events of core needle breast biopsy compared with the open biopsy technique in the diagnosis of a breast abnormality?

Key Question 3: How do open biopsy and various core needle techniques differ in terms of patient preference, availability, costs, availability of qualified pathologist interpretations, and other factors that may influence choice of a particular technique?

Methods

We performed a systematic review of the published scientific literature using methodologies outlined in the AHRQ "Methods Guide for Comparative Effectiveness Reviews,"[8] hereafter referred to as the Methods Guide. We followed the reporting requirements of the "Preferred Reporting Items for Systematic Reviews and Meta-analyses" (PRISMA) statement.[9] A full description of all review steps is included in the full report and the study protocol (PROSPERO registration number CRD42013005690).

External Stakeholder Input

We convened a nine-member Technical Expert Panel (TEP), including representatives of professional societies, experts in the diagnosis and treatment of breast cancer (including radiologists and surgeons), and a patient representative. The TEP provided input to help further refine the Key Questions and protocol, identify important issues, and define the parameters for the evidence review.

Study Eligibility Criteria

We included only English-language full-text articles. Studies included for the assessment of diagnostic test performance (Key Question 1) met the following inclusion criteria: (1) enrolled women not previously diagnosed with breast cancer who received core needle or open biopsy for initial diagnosis of possible breast cancer; (2) compared diagnoses on core needle biopsy to a reference standard of open surgery or followup by clinical examination or imaging of at least 6 months; (3) reported or allowed the calculation of sensitivity, specificity, positive or negative predictive value; (4) were prospective or retrospective cohort studies (including randomized controlled trials); and (5) enrolled 10 or more patients and followed at least 50 percent of them to the completion of the study. In contrast to the original report, we did not restrict eligibility to studies including only women at average risk for breast cancer, because MRI-guided biopsy, which was identified as a topic of interest for this update, is used mainly in women at a higher-than-average risk for breast cancer. Of note, studies often do not provide information on the risk of cancer among included patients. Thus we grouped studies into two categories: (1) studies that explicitly reported that more than 15 percent of included patients were at high risk of cancer; (2) studies that reported that fewer than 15 percent of included patients were at high risk of cancer, or did not provide information on baseline risk. Throughout this review, we refer to the latter group as "studies of women at average risk of cancer"; however, we acknowledge that this group may include studies enrolling patients at higher-than-average cancer risk.

Studies included for the assessment of possible adverse events of core needle biopsy (Key Question 2) or the assessment of patient-relevant outcomes, resource use and logistics, and availability of technology and relevant expertise (Key Question 3) were not required to compare diagnoses on core needle biopsy to a reference standard of open surgery or clinical followup, or to contain extractable information on diagnostic test performance. Furthermore, for Key

Question 2 we included any primary research articles, regardless of design, that addressed the dissemination or displacement of cancer cells by the biopsy procedure (e.g., seeding).

Literature Search and Study Selection

We searched MEDLINE®, Embase®, the Cochrane Central Register of Controlled Trials, the Cochrane Database of Systematic Reviews, the Database of Abstracts of Reviews of Effects, the Health Technology Assessment Database, the U.K. National Health Service Economic Evaluation Database, the U.S. National Guideline Clearinghouse, and CINAHL. Appendix A describes our search strategy, which is based on an expansion of the search strategy used in the original report. We did not use a search filter for studies of diagnostic tests to increase search sensitivity.[10, 11] We also searched for systematic reviews on the topic and used their lists of included studies to validate our search strategy and to make sure we identified all relevant studies.

To identify studies excluded from the original evidence report because they enrolled women at high risk for cancer, we rescreened both the set of abstracts screened for the original report and the full text of studies excluded from the original report because they included women at high risk for cancer. Titles and abstracts were manually screened in duplicate. A single reviewer screened each potentially eligible article in full text to determine eligibility and a second reviewer examined all articles deemed relevant. Disagreements regarding article eligibility were resolved by consensus involving a third reviewer.

Data Abstraction and Management

Data were extracted using electronic forms and entered into the Systematic Review Data Repository (SRDR; http://srdr.ahrq.gov/). We pilot-tested the forms on several studies extracted by multiple team members to ensure consistency in operational definitions. A single reviewer extracted data from each eligible study. A second reviewer verified extracted data and discrepancies were resolved by consensus including a third reviewer. We contacted authors to clarify information reported in their papers and to verify suspected overlap between study populations in publications from the same group of investigators.

Definitions of Test Performance Outcomes and Underestimation Rates

Table A illustrates how index and reference standard results were used to construct 2×2 tables for Key Question 1 (test performance outcomes).

Table A. Definitions of diagnostic groups based on index and reference standard test results

		Reference Standard Results (open surgery or followup)	
		Malignant (invasive or in situ)	Benign
Core Needle Biopsy Results (index test)	Malignant (invasive or in situ)	considered TP	considered TP*
	High risk lesion (e.g., ADH)	considered TP	considered FP
	Benign	considered FN	considered TN

*Some study authors specifically stated that diagnoses of malignancy on core needle biopsy were assumed to be correct, whether or not a tumor was observed upon surgical excision. The original version of this review also classified all diagnoses of malignancy on core needle biopsy as true positives.
ADH = atypical ductal hyperplasia; FN = false negative; FP = false positive; TN = true negative; TP = true positive.

Two issues related to the definition of diagnostic test categories merit additional description. First, occasionally core needle biopsy removes the entire target lesion that is being biopsied, rendering subsequent surgical biopsies unable to confirm the findings of the index test procedure. In such cases of core needle diagnoses of malignancy, we considered the core needle results to be true positive. This operational definition was adopted by several of the primary studies we reviewed and the original ECRI report. Second, in our primary analysis (and consistent with the 2009 ECRI report) core needle biopsy identified high risk lesions that on subsequent surgery (or followup) are not found to be associated with malignant disease were considered false positive. To assess the impact of this operational definition on our findings we performed a sensitivity analysis where high risk lesions on index core needle biopsy found to be nonmalignant (high risk or benign) on subsequent open biopsy or surgical excision were excluded from the analyses.

We defined the underestimation rate for high risk lesions (most often atypical ductal hyperplasia, [ADH]) as the proportion of core needle biopsy findings of high risk lesions that are found to be malignant according to the reference standard). We defined the underestimation rate for ductal carcinoma in situ (DCIS) as the proportion of core needle biopsy findings of DCIS that are found to be invasive according to the reference standard.

Assessment of Risk of Bias

We assessed the risk of bias for each individual study following the Methods Guide. We used elements from the Quality Assessment for Diagnostic Accuracy Studies instrument (QUADAS version 2), to assess risk of bias for studies of diagnostic test accuracy.[12-15] The tool assesses four domains of risk of bias related to patient selection (e.g., consecutive or random selection), index test (e.g., blinding of index test assessors to reference standard results), reference standard test (e.g., blinding of reference standard assessors to the index test results), and patient flow and timing (e.g. differential and partial verification). We used items from the Newcastle-Ottawa scale,[16] the Cochrane Risk of Bias tool,[17] and the checklist proposed by Drummond et al.,[18] to assess nonrandomized cohort studies, randomized controlled trials, and studies of resource utilization and costs, respectively.

Data Synthesis

We summarized included studies qualitatively and presented important features of the study populations, designs, tests used, outcomes, and results in summary tables. Statistical analyses were conducted using methods currently recommend for use in Comparative Effectiveness Reviews of diagnostic tests.[19, 20]

For Key Question 1 we performed meta-analyses when studies were deemed sufficiently similar with respect to included populations, and the core needle biopsy and reference standard tests they employed.

We used a mixed effects binomial-bivariate normal regression model that accounted for different imaging guidance methods, the use of automated or vacuum-assisted devices, and the baseline of risk of cancer of included patients. This model allowed us to estimate the test performance of alternative diagnostic tests, and to perform indirect comparisons among them.[21] Furthermore, it allowed us to derive summary receiver operating characteristic (ROC) curves.[22,23] A univariate mixed effects logistic regression model was used for the meta-analysis of rates of DCIS and high risk lesion underestimation.[24] We used meta-regression methods to evaluate the impact of risk of bias items and other study-level characteristics.[25, 26]

For Key Question 2, we found that adverse events were inconsistently reported across studies and that the methods for ascertaining their occurrence were often not presented in adequate detail. For this reason we refrained from performing meta-analyses for these outcomes. Instead, we calculated descriptive statistics (medians, 25th and 75th percentiles, minimum and maximum values) across all studies and for specific test types.

For Key Question 3, because of the heterogeneity of research designs and outcomes assessed, we were only able to perform a meta-analysis comparing core needle and open surgical biopsies with respect to the number of patients who required one versus more than one surgical procedure for treatment, after the establishment of breast cancer diagnosis. This analysis used a univariate normal random effects model with binomial within-study distribution.

All statistical analyses were performed using Bayesian methods; models were fit using Markov Chain Monte Carlo methods and non-informative prior distributions. Theory and empirical work suggest that, when the number of studies is large, this approach produces results similar to those of maximum likelihood methods (which do not require the specification of priors).[27] Results were summarized as medians of posterior distributions with associated 95 percent central credible intervals (CrIs). A CrI denotes a range of values within which the parameter value is expected to fall with 95 percent probability.

Grading the Strength of Evidence

We followed the Methods Guide[8] to evaluate the strength of the body of evidence for each Key Question with respect to the following domains: risk of bias, consistency, directness, precision, and reporting bias.[8, 28] Generally, strength of evidence was downgraded when risk of bias was not low, in the presence of inconsistency, when evidence was indirect or imprecise, or when we suspected that results were affected by selective analysis or reporting.

We determined risk of bias (low, medium, or high) on the basis of the study design and the methodological quality. We assessed consistency on the basis of the direction and magnitude of results across studies. We considered the evidence to be indirect when we had to rely on comparisons of biopsy methods across different studies (i.e., indirect comparisons). We considered studies to be precise if the CrI was narrow enough for a clinically useful conclusion, and imprecise if the CrI was wide enough to include clinically distinct conclusions. The potential for reporting bias ("suspected" vs. "not suspected") was evaluated with respect to publication and selective outcome and analysis reporting. We made qualitative dispositions rather than perform formal statistical tests to evaluate differences in the effect sizes between more precise (larger) and less precise (smaller) studies because such tests cannot distinguish between "true" heterogeneity between smaller and larger studies, other biases, and chance.[29, 30] Therefore, instead of relying on statistical tests, we evaluated the reported results across studies qualitatively, on the basis of completeness of reporting, number of enrolled patients, and numbers of observed events. Judgment on the potential for selective outcome reporting bias was based on reporting patterns for each outcome of interest across studies. We acknowledge that both types of reporting bias are difficult to reliably detect on the basis of data available in published research studies. We believe that our searches (across multiple databases), combined with our plan for contacting test manufacturers (for additional data) and the authors of published studies (for data clarification) limited the impact of reporting and publication bias on our results, to the extent possible.

Finally, we rated the body of evidence using four strength of evidence levels: high, moderate, low, and insufficient.[8] These describe our level of confidence that the evidence reflects the true effect for the major comparisons of interest.

We qualitatively evaluated similarities and differences in study populations, diagnostic methods, and outcomes among study designs. We used these comparisons to inform our judgments on applicability of study findings to clinical practice.

Results

Our literature searches identified 8,637 potentially relevant citations (including 1,127 rescreened from the original ECRI evidence report). The full-length articles of 2,480 of these studies were obtained and examined in full text. Finally, 128 new studies were considered eligible for inclusion in the updated review (54, 70, and 59 new studies for Key Questions 1, 2, and 3 respectively), for a total of 316 included studies.

Key Question 1: In women with a palpable or nonpalpable breast abnormality, what is the diagnostic test performance of different types of core needle breast biopsy compared with open biopsy or with each other?

One hundred and sixty studies, published between 1990 and 2013, provided information on test performance outcomes of core needle biopsy (54 new studies and 106 studies included in the original evidence report; another study included in the original report overlapped with one of the newer studies and was excluded). Fifty studies were prospectively designed, and 58 were conducted in the United States. Ten studies provided outcome information on more than one group of patients (typically undergoing biopsy with a different biopsy device). In statistical analyses, these groups were treated separately, leading to a total of 171 independent patient groups with information on 69,804 breast lesions.

Test Performance of Open Surgical Biopsy

Published information on the test performance of open surgical biopsy was limited. However, research studies of needle biopsy methods and technical experts generally suggested that open surgical biopsy could be considered a "gold" standard test (i.e., a test without measurement error). One study included in the ECRI report stated that open surgical biopsy may miss one to two percent of breast cancers (i.e., sensitivity of 98% or greater). The original evidence report did not identify any information on underestimation rates for open surgical biopsy. We found a single study that reported underestimation in 16.7 percent of ADH lesions (1 of 6) and 7.1 percent of DCIS lesions (1 of 14) diagnosed thorough open biopsy. The small number of lesions in this study precludes reliable conclusions. Because open surgical biopsy samples the entire target lesion or a large part of it, in theory underestimation rates can be reduced to zero.

Test Performance of Core Needle Biopsy Methods

A total of 160 studies contributed information to analyses of test performance of core needle biopsy methods; 154 enrolled women at average risk and only 6 enrolled women specified to be at high risk of cancer. Studies varied by type of imaging guidance (stereotactic guidance, ultrasound guidance, MRI guidance, other guidance, or freehand), how the biopsy sample was extracted (automated or vacuum), and other factors (e.g., needle size). If studies included multiple cohorts of patients undergoing biopsy by different methods (e.g., some patients were biopsied with vacuum-assistance and others were not) but the study did not report the test performance of each method, these groups were treated together as 'multiple methods' in statistical analyses for that factor. One hundred and thirty-one study groups reported the use of a single form of imaging guidance (83 stereotactic; 41 ultrasound; 6 MRI; 1 grid), whereas 10 used freehand methods, 29 used multiple methods, and one did not report adequate details. Sixty study arms used vacuum-assisted methods to obtain the biopsy sample; 80 used automated methods; 30 used multiple methods; and 1 did not report adequate details. Needle gauge also varied across studies: 57 used 14G needles, 9 used smaller needles, 46 used larger bores, and 48 studies did not report relevant information, or used a range of needle sizes. Reference standard tests also differed across studies: 26 used open biopsy on all included patients; 94 used mean or median followup of between 6 and 24 months for test negative patients, and 40 used mean or median followup of 24 months or more for test negative cases. Additional study details are available in the SRDR. Consistent with the findings of the original report, the risk of bias for this body of evidence was considered moderate to high, mainly due to concerns about spectrum bias, retrospective data collection, differential verification, and lack of information regarding the blinding of reference standard test assessors to the index test results.

The frequency of malignant disease (invasive cancer or DCIS, at the lesion level) ranged from 1 percent to 94 percent, with a median of 34 percent. The proportion of correct diagnoses ranged from 68 percent to 100 percent, with a median of 96 percent. Table B summarizes meta-analysis results for alternative diagnostic biopsy methods, together with information on the number of lesions evaluated with each method, for women at average risk of cancer. Sensitivity estimates were higher than 0.90 and specificity estimates were higher than 0.91 for all methods. CrIs, particularly for ultrasound- and stereotactically-guided biopsy methods, were fairly precise, reflecting the large number of studies reporting information on the test performance of these methods. In contrast, results for MRI-guided methods were based on only three studies and were imprecise, particularly for sensitivity. Table C summarizes the same information for women deemed to be at high risk for cancer (e.g., due to genetic factors or strong family history). Information for this subgroup was limited (6 studies) and we did not find evidence to suggest that the test performance of breast biopsy methods was different between women at average and high risk of cancer. However, there was substantial uncertainty around the relative test performance estimates of the two groups. Table D summarizes the results of analyses of underestimation rates for women at average risk of breast cancer. Results were rather imprecise (e.g., CrI widths were often wider than 0.1) for all estimates except the underestimation rate for stereotactically guided, vacuum-assisted biopsy methods. Analyses of underestimation rates were not possible for women at high risk of cancer because of lack of data.

Table B. Summary estimates of test performance for alternative core needle biopsy methods—women at average risk of cancer

Biopsy Method or Device	N Studies [N biopsies] for Sensitivity & Specificity	Sensitivity	Specificity
Freehand, automated	10 [786]	0.91 (0.80 to 0.96)	0.98 (0.95 to 1.00)
US-guided, automated	27 [16287]	0.99 (0.98 to 0.99)	0.97 (0.95 to 0.98)
US-guided, vacuum-assisted	12 [1543]	0.97 (0.92 to 0.99)	0.98 (0.96 to 0.99)
Stereotactically guided, automated	37 [9535]	0.97 (0.95 to 0.98)	0.97 (0.96 to 0.98)
Stereotactically guided, vacuum-assisted	43 [14667]	0.99 (0.98 to 0.99)	0.92 (0.89 to 0.94)
MRI-guided, automated	2 [89]	0.90 (0.57 to 0.99)	0.99 (0.91 to 1.00)
MRI-guided, vacuum-assisted	1 [10]	1.00 (0.98 to 1.00)	0.91 (0.54 to 0.99)
Multiple methods/other	33 [26028]	0.99 (0.98 to 0.99)	0.96 (0.93 to 0.97)

All numbers are medians with 95% CrIs, unless otherwise stated. 'Other' denotes one study using grid guidance and one study that did not report information on the use of vacuum assistance.
CrI = credible interval; DCIS = ductal carcinoma in situ; MRI = magnetic resonance imaging; N = number; NA = not applicable; US = ultrasound.

Table C. Summary estimates of test performance for alternative core needle biopsy methods—women at high risk of cancer

Biopsy Method or Device	N Studies (N biopsies) for Sensitivity and Specificity	Sensitivity (95% CrI)	Specificity (95% CrI)
Stereotactically guided, automated	1 [416]	0.97 (0.82 to 1.00)	0.97 (0.91 to 0.99)
Stereotactically guided, vacuum-assisted	2 [311]	0.99 (0.93 to 1.00)	0.93 (0.79 to 0.98)
MRI-guided, automated	2 [56]	0.90 (0.58 to 0.98)	0.99 (0.92 to 1.00)
MRI-guided, vacuum-assisted	1 [76]	1.00 (0.98 to 1.00)	0.92 (0.61 to 0.99)

No studies provided information on the test performance of freehand or US-guided biopsy methods, or the use of multiple methods in populations of women at high risk of cancer. Results are based on the model with risk group as a covariate.
CrI = credible interval; DCIS = ductal carcinoma in situ; MRI = magnetic resonance imaging; N = number; US = ultrasound.

Table D. Summary estimates of underestimation rates for alternative core needle biopsy methods—women at average risk of cancer

Biopsy Method or Device	N Studies [N biopsies] for DCIS Under-estimation	DCIS Underestimation Probability	N Studies [N biopsies] for High Risk Lesion Underestimation	High Risk Lesion Under-estimation Probability
Freehand, automated	0 [0]	NA	1 [6]	0.88 (0.32 to 1.00)
US-guided, automated	14 [307]	0.38 (0.26 to 0.51)	21 [601]	0.25 (0.16 to 0.36)
US-guided, vacuum-assisted	5 [48]	0.09 (0.02 to 0.26)	9 [20]	0.11 (0.02 to 0.33)
Stereotactically guided, automated	18 [664]	0.26 (0.19 to 0.36)	29 [357]	0.47 (0.37 to 0.58)
Stereotactically guided, vacuum-assisted	34 [1899]	0.11 (0.08 to 0.14)	40 [1002]	0.18 (0.13 to 0.24)
MRI-guided, automated	0 [0]	NA	1 [1]	0.49 (0.02 to 0.97)
MRI-guided, vacuum-assisted	1 [1]	0.00 (0.00 to 0.38)	0 [0]	NA
Multiple methods/other	18 [628]	0.22 (0.15 to 0.30)	25 [866]	0.32 (0.23 to 0.41)

Analyses for underestimation were not possible for high risk women due to sparse data.
CrI = credible interval; DCIS = ductal carcinoma in situ; MRI = magnetic resonance imaging; N = number; NA = not applicable; US = ultrasound.

Comparative Test Performance

To compare test performance across different biopsy methods we used indirect (meta-regression-based) comparisons. Table E presents comparisons between pairs of biopsy methods using the same imaging guidance for sensitivity and specificity. We only examined comparisons between biopsy methods using the same imaging modality because lesion characteristics (e.g., palpability, ability to visualize a lesions) strongly influence the choice of imaging modality. In general, differences among tests were relatively small: for example, differences in sensitivity or specificity never exceeded 0.1 (i.e., 10% absolute difference). Stereotactically guided automated biopsy had a specificity that was higher by 0.05 compared to vacuum-assisted biopsy methods, and a sensitivity that was 0.02 lower. Comparisons among MRI-guided biopsy methods were imprecise, reflecting the small number of available studies.

Table E. Differences in sensitivity between pairs of biopsy methods (meta-regression based indirect comparisons)

Biopsy Methods Compared	Difference in Sensitivity (95% CrI)	Difference in Specificity (95% CrI)
US-guided, automated vs. vacuum-assisted	0.01 (-0.01, 0.06)	-0.01 (-0.03, 0.01)
Stereotactically guided, automated vs. vacuum-assisted	**-0.02 (-0.04, -0.01)**	**0.05 (0.02, 0.08)**
MRI-guided, automated vs. vacuum assisted	**-0.10 (-0.43, -0.01)**	0.07 (-0.03, 0.43)

CrI = credible interval; MRI = magnetic resonance imaging; US = ultrasound.
All results are shown as medians of differences (95% CrI). Positive values denote that the first-listed biopsy method has higher performance that the comparator (second listed method). CrIs that do not include the null value (0) are highlighted in bold. CrI = credible interval; MRI = magnetic resonance imaging.

Factors That Affect Test Performance

We considered evidence on the impact of patient or study level-factors on test performance from two complementary sources: (1) within-study evidence (i.e., comparisons of test performance over levels of a factor within the patient population enrolled in a study) and (2) evidence from meta-regression analyses (that combine information across studies). Ideally, all studies would consistently report comparisons of test performance across well-defined subgroups (e.g., by patient, or lesion characteristics). Such within-study comparisons are more informative than comparisons across studies: factors related to study setting are common for all patients within the same study and other patient differences can be addressed (at least to some extent) by appropriate analytic methods (e.g., regression adjustment). In the absence of such information, one has to rely on indirect (across-study) comparisons that are generally less convincing because they cannot account for all differences across included studies.

Twenty studies provided information that allowed an evaluation of the impact of any factor on test performance. Specifically, 16 studies provided information on patient and lesion-related factors, 10 on procedural factors, and 3 on clinician and facility factors (some studies provided information on multiple factors). Of note, the majority of studies (140 of 160) did not allow investigation of the impact of any factors on test performance, raising concerns about selective analysis or reporting of results on modifiers of test performance. Among the 20 studies reporting relevant results, factors were coded inconsistently and details that would allow formal statistical testing were not available. Because of these reasons, within-study comparisons could not support conclusions regarding possible modifiers of test performance.

Meta-regression analyses were possible for the following factors: needle gauge, choice of reference standard, proportion of lesions that were palpable, country where the study was performed, whether multiple centers contributed patients to a study, study design, and risk of bias. In general, test performance was not affected by the factors examined (i.e., CrIs included the null value), with the exception of higher sensitivity in studies conducted in the United States (vs. any other country), and higher specificity in studies using followup of 6 to 24 months (as compared to studies using surgical pathology results for all patients) and studies with a prospective design (as compared to studies with a retrospective design). These results must be interpreted with caution given that they reflect indirect comparisons across studies, which cannot be adjusted for other factors that vary across studies.

Overall, within-study analyses and meta-regression analyses were insufficient to confirm (or exclude) any single factor as a modifier of test performance.

Contextualizing the Results of Test Performance Meta-Analyses

To contextualize the results of the test performance meta-analyses presented in the preceding sections we evaluated the impact of testing in a hypothetical cohort of 1,000 women, under alternative scenarios for disease prevalence. Because delayed diagnosis on the basis of biopsy results is the most important (adverse) outcome related to testing we highlight here results based on false negative biopsies (and their complement, true positive biopsies) in Figure A. In populations with low cancer prevalence, the number of cases where treatment may be delayed on the basis of biopsy results (i.e., false negative biopsies) is expected to be small (e.g., for all ultrasound or stereotactically guided biopsy methods less than 5 out of 1,000 women, if prevalence is 10 percent or less). As prevalence increases the number of false negative results increases for all biopsy methods, but more rapidly for MRI-guided automated and freehand methods, which had the lowest sensitivity. However, results for MRI-guided automated methods were based on only six studies. Figure A also presents numerical results for a prevalence of 25 percent, which is approximately the prevalence of breast cancer among women referred for breast biopsy in the United States. All stereotactically and ultrasound-guided methods, and MRI-guided vacuum assisted methods are expected to have fewer than 10 false negative results (for every 1,000 women undergoing biopsy), even when prevalence is as high as 0.30.

Figure A. Outcomes of testing in a hypothetical cohort of 1,000 women

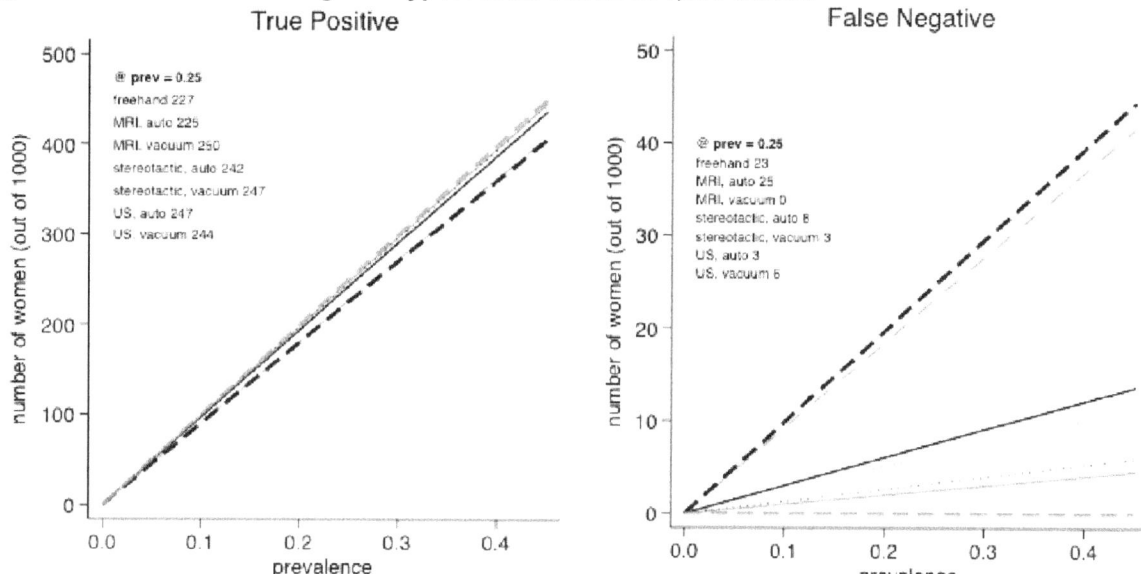

Lines correspond to different test modalities: grey dashed-dotted = freehand; black solid = stereotactically guided, automated; grey solid = stereotactically guided, vacuum-assisted; black dotted = US-guided, automated; grey dotted = US-guided, vacuum-assisted; black dashed = MRI-guided, automated; grey dashed = MRI-guided, vacuum assisted.

Key Question 2: In women with a palpable or nonpalpable breast abnormality, what are the adverse events (harms) associated with different types of core needle breast biopsy compared with open biopsy for diagnosis?

We synthesized information on adverse events from a total of 144 studies (70 new studies and 74 from the original evidence report) reporting on at least one of the outcomes relevant to Key Question 2. Overall, studies were considered to be of moderate to high risk of bias. Selective outcome reporting was considered likely for all adverse events examined, because of the large proportion of studies with unclear or missing data.

Adverse Events of Open Biopsy

Very few studies reported information about complications occurring in association with open surgical biopsy procedures. One study reported that 10.2 percent of wire-localized open biopsy procedures were complicated by vasovagal reactions. A narrative review reported that 2 to 10 percent of breast surgeries are complicated by hematoma formation, and that 3.8 are complicated by infection. Another study reported that 6.3 percent of open surgical biopsies were complicated by infections. One study reported low levels of pain with open biopsy when local lidocaine was used. A fifth study reported that 2.1 percent of open biopsy procedures were complicated by the development of an abscess, but zero abscesses complicated 234 ultrasound-guided vacuum-assisted core needle procedures. A sixth study reported that 4 of 100 surgical biopsies required repeat biopsy, compared to 2 of 100 vacuum-assisted core needle biopsies.

Adverse Events of Core Needle Biopsy

We identified 141 studies reporting information on at least one of the adverse events of interest following core needle biopsy (26 reported information related to the displacement of cancerous cells during biopsy). Overall, core needle biopsy appeared to have a lower risk of complications than open surgical biopsy; however, direct comparative information was sparse. The incidence of severe complications with core needle biopsy was less than 1 percent. The incidence of all adverse events was low: in more than 50 percent of studies reporting information on hematomas, bleeding, vasovagal reactions, and infections, the percentage of patients experiencing each of the aforementioned outcomes was less than 1.5 percent; in 75 percent of studies the event rate was less than 1 percent for infections, less than 5 percent for bleeding and vasovagal reactions, and less than 9 percent for hematoma formation. Overall, 47 studies provided information on bleeding events that required additional treatment; more than half of the studies reported than no bleeding events requiring treatment were observed and the rate was lower than 0.14 percent in 75 percent of the studies. Use of vacuum assistance was associated with a greater rate of bleeding and hematoma formation.

Of 14 studies that used histopathology to demonstrate displacement of cells by core needle biopsy procedures (9 cohort and 5 case series or case reports), the percentage of needle tracks reported to contain displaced cancerous cells ranged from 0 to 69 percent. The clinical significance of these findings is unclear; tumor development on the biopsy needle track is extremely rare.

Factors That Affect the Development of Adverse Events

Five studies provided information on patient and lesion-related factors, eight studies provided information on procedural factors, and one study provided information on clinician and facility factors. The vast majority of studies reporting on adverse events from core needle biopsy did not allow investigation of the impact of factors on adverse events and no individual factor was evaluated by more than five of the total included studies, raising concerns regarding selective outcome and analysis reporting. No studies reported information on factors that affect the development of adverse events from open biopsy. We did not perform meta-regression analyses because studies reported information on adverse events inconsistently and because data were missing from more than half of the studies for all adverse events. Studies suggested that vacuum-assisted biopsy methods led to increased bleeding and performing biopsies with patients seated upright was associated with increased incidence of vasovagal reactions; however, results were reported in a way that precluded quantitation of the relative risk.

Key Question 3: How do open biopsy and various core needle techniques differ in terms of patient preference, availability, costs, availability of qualified pathologist interpretations, and other factors that may influence choice of a particular technique?

We a reviewed a total of 143 studies for Key Question 3 (59 new studies and 84 studies from the original report). Generally, the evidence supported the conclusions of the original report that core needle biopsy costs less than open surgical biopsy, consumes fewer resources, and is preferred by patients. In addition, utilization of core needle biopsy has grown consistently since the mid-1990s. Studies reported that women were generally satisfied with the cosmetic results of core needle procedures. Transient intense anxiety just before and during the procedure may be common, and may be partially ameliorated with the use of medication, relaxation and empathy techniques, or hypnosis. Based on 42 studies providing relevant information, core needle biopsy obviated the need for surgical procedures in about 75 percent of women. Ten studies reported comparisons against open surgical biopsy with respect to the number of patients requiring only one surgical procedure (vs. more than one) after cancer diagnosis. Meta-analysis of these studies suggested that the odds of requiring only one surgical procedure were almost 15 times higher among women receiving core needle biopsy; odds ratio = 14.8 (95% CrI, 7.2 to 50.2). This result should be interpreted with caution because confounding by indication is likely.

Discussion

Key Findings and Assessment of the Strength of Evidence

In this update of the 2009 Comparative Effectiveness Review on breast biopsy methods we synthesized evidence from a total of 316 studies (128 new studies and 188 from the original report). We found few studies providing information on the test performance of open surgical biopsy. In contrast, the evidence base on core needle biopsy methods now includes a large number of studies reporting on almost 70,000 breast lesions. This allowed us to assess the comparative performance of tests (when using the same type of imaging guidance), in addition to updating the 2009 report's evaluation of the performance of individual biopsy methods. Tables F-H summarize our assessment of the strength of evidence. Following the original evidence report, and in view of the paucity of evidence on open surgical biopsy, we refrained from rating the strength of evidence for this technique for all Key Questions. For Key Questions 1 and 2, we assessed the strength of evidence by integrating our (subjective) judgments on the risk of bias of included studies, the consistency of their findings, the directness of the available data, and the precision of quantitative results. For Key Question 3 we only rated the strength of evidence for the outcome of additional surgical procedures required after biopsy. We did not rate the strength of evidence for other Key Question 3 outcomes because of the diversity of designs employed and outcomes addressed (see the Methods section for our approach to rating the strength of evidence).

Test Performance and Comparative Test Performance

Among women at average risk of cancer, core needle biopsy using ultrasound or stereotactic guidance had average sensitivities ranging from 0.97 to 0.99 and average specificities ranging from 0.92 to 0.98. Freehand biopsy methods appeared to have lower average sensitivity (0.91) compared to other methods, but similar specificity. Stereotactically guided automated techniques were associated with lower sensitivity and higher specificity compared to stereotactically guided vacuum-assisted methods. Although these results were fairly precise, they were derived from indirect comparisons across studies of moderate to high risk of bias. MRI-guided biopsies were evaluated in only six studies with small sample sizes, leading to substantial uncertainty around estimates of test performance. Table F summarizes our assessment of the strength of evidence for alternative biopsy methods in women at average risk of cancer and for comparisons among biopsy methods using the same imaging guidance modality.

We did not find a difference in test performance between women at low and high risk of breast cancer. Because the number of studies of women at high risk of cancer was small, comparisons of test performance between low and high risk women had substantial uncertainty and results were not sufficient to support definitive conclusions. Evidence on modifiers of test performance was also sparse for all biopsy methods, raising concerns about selective outcome and analysis reporting.

Table F. Strength of evidence about comparative test performance in women at average risk of breast cancer

Outcome	Comparison or Biopsy Method	Overall Rating	Key Findings and Comments
Test performance of individual biopsy methods	Freehand	Low	– Sensitivity: 0.91 (0.80 to 0.96) – Specificity: 0.98 (0.95 to 1.00)
	Ultrasound, automated	Moderate	– Sensitivity: 0.99 (0.98 to 0.99) – Specificity: 0.97 (0.95 to 0.98)
	Ultrasound, vacuum-assisted	Moderate	– Sensitivity: 0.97 (0.92 to 0.99) – Specificity: 0.98 (0.96 to 0.99)
	Stereotactically guided, automated	Moderate	– Sensitivity: 0.97 (0.95 to 0.98) – Specificity: 0.97 (0.96 to 0.98)
	Stereotactically guided, vacuum-assisted	Moderate	– Sensitivity: 0.99 (0.98 to 0.99) – Specificity: 0.92 (0.89 to 0.94)
	MRI-guided, automated	Insufficient	– Sensitivity: 0.90 (0.57 to 0.99) – Specificity: 0.99 (0.91 to 1.00)
	MRI-guided, vacuum-assisted	Insufficient	– Sensitivity: 1.00 (0.98 to 1.00) – Specificity: 0.91 (0.54 to 0.99)
Comparison of test performance among alternative biopsy methods	Ultrasound-guided, automated vs. vacuum-assisted	Low	– Difference in sensitivity: 0.01 (-0.01 to 0.06) [no difference] – Difference in specificity: -0.01 (-0.03 to 0.01) [no difference]
	Stereotactically guided, automated vs. vacuum-assisted	Low	– Difference in sensitivity: -0.02 (-0.04 to -0.01) [vacuum-assisted is better] – Difference in specificity: 0.05 (0.02 to 0.08) [automated is better]
	MRI-guided, automated vs. vacuum-assisted	Insufficient	– Difference in sensitivity: -0.10 (-0.43 to -0.01) [vacuum-assisted is better] – Difference in specificity: 0.07 (-0.03 to 0.43) [no difference]
Modifiers of test performance for women at average and high risk of breast cancer	All biopsy methods	Insufficient	– Few studies provided within-sample information for each modifier of interest; meta-regression results rely on cross-study comparisons so consistency of effects cannot be assessed – Within-study (direct) evidence was sparse; between study evidence relied on indirect comparisons across studies – In meta-regression analyses CrIs were wide; extreme odds ratio values were often observed because sensitivity and specificity for all tests were very close to 1 (see Results)

CrI = credible interval; MRI = magnetic resonance imaging.

Underestimation Rates

Underestimation rates varied among alternative biopsy methods and were often imprecisely estimated because of the relatively small number of lesions contributing data for these analyses. In general, underestimation was less common with stereotactically guided vacuum-assisted biopsy methods, as compared to stereotactically or ultrasound-guided automated methods. Our assessment of the strength of evidence for this outcome is summarized in Table G.

Table G. Strength of evidence for underestimation rates in women at average risk of cancer

Outcome	Comparison or Biopsy Method	Overall Rating	Key Findings and Comments
DCIS underestimation	Ultrasound-guided, automated	Low	– Average underestimation probability: 0.38 (0.26 to 0.51) [14 studies]
	Ultrasound-guided, vacuum-assisted	Low	– Average underestimation probability: 0.09 (0.02 to 0.26) [5 studies]
	Stereotactically guided, automated	Low	– Average underestimation probability: 0.26 (0.19 to 0.36) [18 studies]
	Stereotactically guided, vacuum-assisted	Low	– Average underestimation probability: 0.11 (0.08 to 0.14) [34 studies]
	Other biopsy methods	Insufficient	No available studies or few studies with small numbers of lesions
High risk lesion underestimation rate	Ultrasound-guided, automated	Low	– Average underestimation probability: 0.25 (0.16 to 0.36) [21 studies]
	Ultrasound-guided, vacuum-assisted	Low	– Average underestimation probability: 0.11 (0.02 to 0.33) [9 studies]
	Stereotactically guided, automated	Low	– Average underestimation probability: 0.47 (0.37 to 0.58) [29 studies]
	Stereotactically guided, vacuum-assisted	Low	– Average underestimation probability: 0.18 (0.13 to 0.24) [40 studies]
	Other biopsy methods	Insufficient	No available studies or few studies with small numbers of lesions

DCIS = ductal carcinoma in situ.

Adverse Events and Additional Surgeries After Biopsy

In general, adverse events were reported inconsistently, raising concerns about selective outcome and analysis reporting. Few studies provided information on the harms of open surgical biopsy. Core needle biopsy was only infrequently associated with serious adverse events. Comparisons between open and core needle biopsy are based on indirect comparisons and expert opinion, with limited empirical evidence. Open biopsy appeared to be associated with an increased incidence of adverse events (including serious adverse events) compared to core needle biopsy. Our assessment of the strength of evidence for adverse events is summarized in Table H.

Among core needle biopsy methods, vacuum-assisted methods appeared to be associated with increased bleeding. Sitting upright during the biopsy procedure was associated with more vasovagal reactions. Information about the dissemination or displacement of cancer cells during the biopsy procedure was provided by a small number of studies with various designs. Studies reported that women were generally satisfied with the cosmetic results of core needle procedures.

Women diagnosed with breast cancer by core needle biopsy were able to have their cancer treated with a single surgical procedure more often than women diagnosed by open surgical biopsy. Although the magnitude of this association was large (the ratio of the odds was approximately 15), women and their physicians are likely to choose biopsy methods on the basis of factors (e.g., lesion location, or characteristics of the lesion on imaging) that may also be associated with the need for additional surgeries. Thus, confounding by indication is likely, and we rated the strength of evidence for this association as moderate. A difference in the rate of additional surgeries among women diagnosed with alternative biopsy methods is likely, but we have less confidence that it is an effect of the biopsy methods per se or that the magnitude of the difference is known.

Table H. Strength of evidence assessment for adverse events of breast biopsy

Outcomes	Test or Comparison	Overall Rating	Key Findings
Bleeding (any severity)	Alternative core needle biopsy methods	Low	– Median %: 1.21 (25th perc. = 0.33; 75th perc = 3.97) – Selective outcome and analysis reporting likely – Few studies reported bleeding requiring treatment; the event rate was low (<0.40 perc.) in those studies
Bleeding events that require treatment	Comparisons among alternative core needle biopsy methods	Low	– Median %: 0 (25th perc. = 0; 75th perc = 0.14) – Selective outcome and analysis reporting likely – Few studies reported bleeding requiring treatment; the event rate was low
Hematoma formation	Alternative core needle biopsy methods	Low	– Median %: 1.44 (25th perc. = 0.25; 75th perc = 8.57) – Selective outcome and analysis reporting likely
Infectious complications	Alternative core needle biopsy methods	Low	– Median %: 0 (25th perc. = 0; 75th perc = 0.33) – Selective outcome and analysis reporting likely
Vasovagal reactions:	Alternative core needle biopsy methods	Low	– Median %: 1.27 (25th perc. = 0.37; 75th perc = 3.88) – Potential for selective outcome and analysis reporting
Pain and severe pain	Alternative core needle biopsy methods	Low	25 studies of a wide variety of biopsy methods reported information about patient pain during the procedure (pain was assessed heterogeneously across studies)
Other adverse events	Alternative core needle biopsy methods	Insufficient	– Most events were reported by a single study precluding assessment of consistency – Individual studies did not provide adequate information for precise estimation of the event rate) – Only informal indirect comparisons among biopsy methods were possible – Selective outcome and analysis reporting likely
Modifiers of adverse events – vasovagal reactions	Sitting upright during the biopsy procedure	Low	– Vasovagal reactions were more common among patients sitting during the biopsy procedure – Results were reported in few studies (11 studies; 8 from the original evidence report and 3 from this update) – Selective outcome and analysis reporting likely
Modifiers of adverse events – bleeding	Vacuum-assisted versus non-vacuum assisted biopsy methods	Low	– Vacuum-assisted procedures were generally associated with increased rates of bleeding and hematoma formation – Bleeding events were generally uncommon – Comparisons among biopsy methods were based on informal indirect comparisons (across studies) – Selective outcome and analysis reporting likely
All other modifiers of adverse events	Comparisons among alternative core needle biopsy methods	Insufficient	– Most factors assessed by a single study limiting our ability to assess consistency – Selective outcome and analysis reporting likely – Within-study comparisons provided direct evidence

perc. = percentile

Applicability of Review Findings

The existing evidence base on core needle biopsy of breast lesions in women at average risk of cancer appears to be applicable to clinical practice in the United States. The average age was similar to that of women undergoing breast biopsy in the United States, and the indications were similar to the prevalent indications in clinical practice (i.e. mammographic findings of suspicious lesions). Almost all studies were carried out in either the United States or in industrialized European or Asian countries where core-biopsy methods are likely sufficiently similar to those used in the United States. The applicability of our findings to women at high risk of breast cancer is uncertain because we found few studies explicitly reporting on groups of patients at high baseline risk of breast cancer and comparisons of test performance between subgroups of women produced imprecise results.

Limitations of the Evidence Base

We believe that the evidence regarding the performance of core needle biopsy for diagnosis of breast lesions is limited in the following ways: (1) published evidence on the test performance and adverse events of open surgical biopsy was sparse; (2) available studies were at moderate to high risk of bias and information on patient selection criteria, patient or lesion characteristics, adverse events, or patient-relevant outcomes was often missing or inconsistently reported, and pathology results were not reported with adequate granularity; (3) studies typically used lesions (or biopsy procedures) as the unit of analysis, instead of patients, reporting results in a way that did not allow for the correlation to be accounted for in our statistical analyses; (4) studies provided limited information to assess the impact of various patient-, lesion-, procedure-, or system- related factors on the outcomes of breast biopsy; (5) the number of studies on MRI-guided biopsy for women at average or high risk of cancer was small; (6) limited information existed on the comparative effectiveness of alternative biopsy methods on patient-relevant outcomes, resource use and logistics, and availability of technology and expertise for different core needle biopsy techniques.

Limitations of This Review

Our work has several limitations, which—to a large extent—reflect the limitations of the underlying evidence base. Because of selective, incomplete, or no reporting of necessary information, our ability to explore between-study heterogeneity was limited. Further, because we relied on published information, we were unable to evaluate the impact of patient- or lesion-level factors on outcomes of interest. We did not include studies published in languages other than English; however, given the very large number of studies from diverse geographic locations included in the review, we believe that the addition of non-English language studies would not affect our conclusions.

The reference standard in the reviewed studies was a combination of clinical followup and pathologic confirmation. We assumed that these diagnostic methods have negligible measurement error (i.e., that they represent a "gold" standard). It is unlikely that this assumption is exactly true. However, we believe that the error rate of the reference standard is low enough that its influence on our estimates is unlikely to be substantial.

Future Research Needs

There is now a large body of evidence indicating that stereotactic and ultrasound guided core needle techniques have comparable sensitivity to each other and to open biopsy. The next focus of research should be biopsy under MRI guidance, which is a new technique that is likely to come into wider use. The data is not yet adequate to define its advantages or disadvantages of MRI guided biopsy compared with alternative techniques. Studies should be powered to achieve adequate precision (i.e., produce confidence intervals or CrIs that are narrow enough to allow clinically meaningful conclusions), have a prospective design, enroll patients across multiple centers, and use standardized histological classification systems for pathological classification.[31, 32] For all biopsy methods, additional well-designed and fully reported prospective cohort studies are needed, primarily for addressing questions about the impact of patient-, lesion-, procedure-, or system-level factors on test performance, adverse events, and patient-relevant outcomes. This would help resolve uncertainties regarding effect modification (e.g., over patient and lesion factors) that cannot be resolved with the currently available data. Such studies could be conducted at relatively low cost, and large-scale databases of prospectively-collected observational data on breast biopsy procedures and outcomes could be used to evaluate the comparative effectiveness of alternative biopsy methods with respect to short and long term outcomes, and potential modifying factors. In all future studies, baseline risk of cancer development should be characterized using consistent and widely accepted criteria to allow appropriate subgroup analyses. We believe that a randomized comparison of alternative biopsy methods would not be fruitful because existing studies indicate that biopsy procedures have sensitivities and specificities that are fairly similar and also close to 1. Additional information is also needed to identify factors that may influence the rate of adverse events of specific biopsy methods. Future research needs to be reported in accordance with recent reporting guidelines (e.g., STAndards for the Reporting of Diagnostic accuracy studies; www.stard-statement.org/), for progress to be made on these questions.[33]

Conclusions

A large body of evidence indicates that ultrasound- and stereotactically-guided core needle biopsy procedures have sensitivity and specificity close to that of open biopsy procedures, and are associated with fewer adverse events. The strength of the evidence on the test performance of these methods is deemed moderate because studies are at medium to high risk of bias, but provide precise results and exhibit low heterogeneity. Freehand procedures have lower sensitivity than imaging-guided methods. The strength of conclusions about the comparative test performance of automated and vacuum-assisted devices (when using the same imaging guidance) is deemed low, because of concerns about the risk of bias of included studies and the reliance on indirect comparisons. There were insufficient data to draw conclusions for MRI-guided biopsy or women at high baseline risk of cancer. Harms were reported inconsistently, raising concerns about selective outcome and analysis reporting. There is low strength of evidence that vacuum-assisted procedures appear to have a higher risk of bleeding than automated methods. There is moderate strength of evidence that women diagnosed with breast cancer by core needle biopsy were more likely to have their cancer treated with a single surgical procedure, compared with women diagnosed by open surgical biopsy.

References

1. American Cancer Society. Breast Cancer Facts & Figures 2013-2014. Atlanta, GA: American Cancer Society; 2013. www.cancer.org/acs/groups/content/@research/documents/document/acspc-042725.pdf. Accessed March 26, 2014.

2. Hubbard RA, Kerlikowske K, Flowers CI, et al. Cumulative probability of false-positive recall or biopsy recommendation after 10 years of screening mammography: a cohort study. Ann Intern Med. 2011 Oct 18;155(8):481-92. PMID: 22007042.

3. Elmore JG, Barton MB, Moceri VM, et al. Ten-year risk of false positive screening mammograms and clinical breast examinations. N Engl J Med. 1998 Apr 16;338(16):1089-96. PMID: 9545356.

4. Yu YH, Wei W, Liu JL. Diagnostic value of fine-needle aspiration biopsy for breast mass: a systematic review and meta-analysis. BMC Cancer. 2012;12:41. PMID: 22277164.

5. Bernardi D, Borsato G, Pellegrini M, et al. On the diagnostic accuracy of stereotactic vacuum-assisted biopsy of nonpalpable breast abnormalities. Results in a consecutive series of 769 procedures performed at the Trento Department of Breast Diagnosis. Tumori. 2012 Jan-Feb;98(1):113-8. PMID: 22495711.

6. Bruening W, Schoelles K, Treadwell J, et al. Comparative Effectiveness of Core-Needle and Open Surgical Biopsy for the Diagnosis of Breast Lesions. Comparative Effectiveness Review No. 19 (Prepared by the ECRI Institute Evidence-based Practice Center under Contract No. 290-02-0019). AHRQ Publication No. 10-EHC007-EF. Rockville, MD: Agency for Healthcare Research and Quality; December 2009. www.ncbi.nlm.nih.gov/books/NBK45220/pdf/TOC/pdf. Accessed April 25, 2013.

7. Bruening W, Fontanarosa J, Tipton K, et al. Systematic review: comparative effectiveness of core-needle and open surgical biopsy to diagnose breast lesions. Ann Intern Med. 2010 Feb 16;152(4):238-46. PMID: 20008742.

8. Agency for Healthcare Research and Quality. Methods Guide for Effectiveness and Comparative Effectiveness Reviews. Rockville, MD: Agency for Healthcare Research and Quality; April 2012. www.effectivehealthcare.ahrq.gov/ehc/products/60/318/MethodsGuide_Prepublication-Draft_20120523.pdf. Accessed April 25, 2013.

9. Moher D, Liberati A, Tetzlaff J, et al. Preferred reporting items for systematic reviews and meta-analyses: the PRISMA statement. Int J Surg. 2010;8(5):336-41. PMID: 20171303.

10. Leeflang MM, Scholten RJ, Rutjes AW, et al. Use of methodological search filters to identify diagnostic accuracy studies can lead to the omission of relevant studies. J Clin Epidemiol. 2006 Mar;59(3):234-40. PMID: 16488353.

11. Whiting P, Westwood M, Burke M, et al. Systematic reviews of test accuracy should search a range of databases to identify primary studies. J Clin Epidemiol. 2008 Apr;61(4):357-64. PMID: 18313560.

12. Whiting PF, Rutjes AW, Westwood ME, et al. QUADAS-2: a revised tool for the quality assessment of diagnostic accuracy studies. Ann Intern Med. 2011 Oct 18;155(8):529-36. PMID: 22007046.

13. Whiting P, Rutjes AW, Reitsma JB, et al. The development of QUADAS: a tool for the quality assessment of studies of diagnostic accuracy included in systematic reviews. BMC Med Res Methodol. 2003 Nov 10;3:25. PMID: 14606960.

14. Whiting P, Rutjes AW, Dinnes J, et al. Development and validation of methods for assessing the quality of diagnostic accuracy studies. Health Technol Assess. 2004 Jun;8(25):iii, 1-234. PMID: 15193208.

15. Whiting PF, Weswood ME, Rutjes AW, et al. Evaluation of QUADAS, a tool for the quality assessment of diagnostic accuracy studies. BMC Med Res Methodol. 2006 Mar 6;6:9. PMID: 16519814.

16. Wells G, Shea B, O'Connell D, et al. The Newcastle-Ottawa Scale (NOS) for assessing the quality of nonrandomised studies in meta-analyses. www.ohri.ca/programs/clinical_epidemiology/oxford.asp. Accessed 29 April 2013.

17. Higgins JP, Altman DG, Gotzsche PC, et al; Cochrane Bias Methods Group/Cochrane Statistical Methods Group. The Cochrane Collaboration's tool for assessing risk of bias in randomised trials. BMJ. 2011 Oct 18;343:d5928. PMID: 22008217.

18. Drummond MF, Jefferson TO. Guidelines for authors and peer reviewers of economic submissions to the BMJ. The BMJ Economic Evaluation Working Party. BMJ. 1996 Aug 3;313(7052):275-83. PMID: 8704542.

19. Trikalinos TA, Balion CM, Coleman CI, et al. Chapter 8: meta-analysis of test performance when there is a "gold standard". J Gen Intern Med. 2012 Jun;27 Suppl 1:S56-66. PMID: 22648676.

20. Trikalinos TA, Balion CM. Chapter 9: options for summarizing medical test performance in the absence of a "gold standard." J Gen Intern Med. 2012 Jun;27 Suppl 1:S67-75. PMID: 22648677.

21. Hamza TH, van Houwelingen HC, Stijnen T. The binomial distribution of meta-analysis was preferred to model within-study variability. J Clin Epidemiol. 2008 Jan;61(1):41-51. PMID: 18083461.

22. Rutter CM, Gatsonis CA. A hierarchical regression approach to meta-analysis of diagnostic test accuracy evaluations. Stat Med. 2001 Oct 15;20(19):2865-84. PMID: 11568945.

23. Arends LR, Hamza TH, van Houwelingen JC, et al. Bivariate random effects meta-analysis of ROC curves. Med Decis Making. 2008 Sep-Oct;28(5):621-38. PMID: 18591542.

24. Stijnen T, Hamza TH, Ozdemir P. Random effects meta-analysis of event outcome in the framework of the generalized linear mixed model with applications in sparse data. Stat Med. 2010 Dec 20;29(29):3046-67. PMID: 20827667.

25. Hamza TH, van Houwelingen HC, Heijenbrok-Kal MH, et al. Associating explanatory variables with summary receiver operating characteristic curves in diagnostic meta-analysis. J Clin Epidemiol. 2009 Dec;62(12):1284-91. PMID: 19398297.

26. van Houwelingen HC, Arends LR, Stijnen T. Advanced methods in meta-analysis: multivariate approach and meta-regression. Stat Med. 2002 Feb 28;21(4):589-624. PMID: 11836738.

27. Dahabreh IJ, Trikalinos TA, Lau J, et al. An Empirical Assessment of Bivariate Methods for Meta-Analysis of Test Accuracy. Rockville (MD); 2012.

28. Singh S, Chang SM, Matchar DB, et al. Grading a body of evidence on diagnostic tests. In: Chang SMM, D. B. Smetana, G. W. Umscheid, C. A., ed Methods Guide for Medical Test Reviews. AHRQ Publication No. 12-EHC017. Rockville, MD: Agency for Healthcare Research and Quality; June 2012:chapter 7. www.ncbi.nlm.nih.gov/books/NBK98241/ Accessed April 25, 2013.

29. Lau J, Ioannidis JP, Terrin N, et al. The case of the misleading funnel plot. BMJ. 2006 Sep 16;333(7568):597-600. PMID: 16974018.

30. Sterne JA, Sutton AJ, Ioannidis JP, et al. Recommendations for examining and interpreting funnel plot asymmetry in meta-analyses of randomised controlled trials. BMJ. 2011;343:d4002. PMID: 21784880.

31. Ellis IO, Humphreys S, Michell M, et al. Best Practice No 179. Guidelines for breast needle core biopsy handling and reporting in breast screening assessment. J Clin Pathol. 2004 Sep;57(9):897-902. PMID: 15333647.

32. Compton CC. Reporting on cancer specimens: case summaries and background documentation: A publication of the College of American Pathologists Cancer Committee. 2003.

33. Bossuyt PM, Reitsma JB, Bruns DE, et al. Towards complete and accurate reporting of studies of diagnostic accuracy: The STARD Initiative. Ann Intern Med. 2003 Jan 7;138(1):40-4. PMID: 12513043

Background

Breast Cancer Epidemiology and Clinical Diagnosis

Among women in the United States, breast cancer is the second most common malignancy (after skin cancer), and the second most common cause of cancer death (after lung cancer). Approximately one in eight women in the United States will develop breast cancer during their lifetime.[1] The American Cancer Society estimates that 232,340 new cases of invasive breast cancer and 64,640 new cases of non-invasive breast cancer will be diagnosed in 2013, and 39,620 women will die of breast cancer.

During the earliest stages of breast cancer, there are usually no symptoms. The process of breast cancer diagnosis is initiated by detection of an abnormality through self-examination, physical examination by a clinician, or screening mammography. Data from the Behavioral Risk Factor Surveillance System show that, in 2010, 75.4 percent of U.S. women aged ≥40 years and 79.7 percent of women aged 50 to 74 years reported having a mammogram within the past 2 years. If initial assessment suggests that the abnormality may be breast cancer, the woman may be referred for a biopsy, which is a sampling of cells or tissue from the suspicious lesion. In the United States, the most common indication for breast biopsy is the detection of suspicious abnormalities by screening mammography. Among women screened annually for 10 years, approximately 50 percent will need additional imaging, and 5-7 percent will have biopsies.[2,3] Over a million women have breast biopsies each year in the United States. There are currently three techniques for obtaining samples from suspicious breast lesions: fine-needle aspiration, biopsy with a hollow core needle, or open surgical retrieval of tissue. Fine-needle aspiration samples cells and does not assess tissue architecture, is generally considered less sensitive than core needle and open biopsy methods,[4] and is used less frequently. For these reasons it will not be discussed further in this report. Core-needle biopsy, which retrieves a sample of tissue, and open surgical procedures are therefore the most frequently used biopsy methods.

Samples obtained by any of these methods are evaluated by pathologists and classified into histological categories with the primary goal of determining whether the lesion is benign or malignant. Because core needle biopsy often samples only part of the breast abnormality, there is the risk that a lesion will be classified as benign or as high risk (e.g., atypical ductal hyperplasia, [ADH]) or non-invasive (e.g., ductal carcinoma in situ, DCIS) when invasive cancer is in fact present in unsampled areas. In contrast, open surgical biopsy often samples most or all of the lesion, and it is thought that there is a smaller risk of misdiagnosis. However, while open surgical biopsy methods are considered to be the most accurate, they also appear to carry a higher risk of complications, such as bleeding or infection, compared to core needle biopsy. Therefore, if core needle biopsy is also highly accurate, women and their clinicians may prefer some type of core needle biopsy to open surgical biopsy.

Core needle biopsy may be carried out using a range of techniques. If the breast lesion to be biopsied is not palpable, an imaging method (i.e., stereotactic mammography, ultrasound, or magnetic resonance imaging (MRI)) may be used to locate the lesion. The biopsy may be carried out with needles of varying diameter, and one or more samples of tissue may be taken. Sometimes a vacuum device is used to assist in removing the tissue sample through the needle. It is thought that these and other variations in how core needle biopsy is carried out may affect the accuracy and rate of complications of the biopsy. Imaging methods may also influence the performance of open surgical biopsies because the majority of such biopsies are preceded by an image-guided wire localization procedure. In general, the impact of aspects of biopsy technique on test performance and safety are not clear.

Original Evidence Report and Rationale for the Update

In 2009, the ECRI Evidence-based Practice Center (EPC) conducted a comparative effectiveness review for core needle versus open surgical biopsy.[5,6] The original report provided a detailed description of the technical aspects of alternative biopsy methods and we have not repeated this information here. The original report assessed the diagnostic test performance and adverse events of multiple core needle biopsy techniques and tools, compared to open surgical biopsy, and also evaluated differences between open biopsy and core needle biopsy with regards to patient preference, costs, availability, and other factors. The key conclusions were that core needle biopsies were almost as accurate as open surgical biopsies, had a lower risk of severe complications, and were associated with fewer subsequent surgical procedures. The need for update of the 2009 report was assessed in 2010 by the RAND EPC. Several high-impact general medical and specialty journals were searched, a panel of experts in the field was consulted, and an overall assessment of the need to update the report was produced. The conclusion of the update Surveillance Report was that additional studies and changes in practice render some conclusions of the original report possibly out of date. Specifically, the Surveillance Report noted the following:

- New studies are available regarding—
  - the DCIS underestimation rate of stereotactic vacuum-assisted core needle biopsy
  - test performance of MRI-guided core needle biopsy
  - test performance of freehand automated device core needle technology
- New studies on the test performance of core needle biopsy may allow the exploration of heterogeneity for test performance or harm outcomes

On the basis of the Surveillance Report findings, an updated review of the published literature was considered necessary to synthesize all evidence on currently available methods for core needle and open surgical breast biopsy.

Key Questions

To determine the Key Questions and study selection criteria (population, intervention, comparator, outcome, timing and setting; PICOTS) for this update, we began by considering the criteria used in the original Evidence Report. On the basis of input from clinical experts during the development of our protocol, we made minor revisions to the Key Questions and study eligibility criteria to clarify the focus of the updated review. We specified the following three Key Questions to guide the conduct of the update:

Key Question 1: In women with a palpable or nonpalpable breast abnormality, what is the test performance of different types of core needle breast biopsy compared with open biopsy for diagnosis?

- What factors associated with the patient and her breast abnormality influence the test performance of different types of core needle breast biopsy compared with open biopsy for diagnosis of a breast abnormality?

- What factors associated with the procedure itself influence the test performance of different types of core needle breast biopsy compared with open biopsy for diagnosis of a breast abnormality?
- What clinician and facility factors influence the test performance of core needle breast biopsy compared with open biopsy for diagnosis of a breast abnormality?

Key Question 2: In women with a palpable or nonpalpable breast abnormality, what are the adverse events (harms) associated with different types of core needle breast biopsy compared with open biopsy for diagnosis?

- What factors associated with the patient and her breast abnormality influence the adverse events of core needle breast biopsy compared with the open biopsy technique in the diagnosis of a breast abnormality?
- What factors associated with the procedure itself influence the adverse events of core needle breast biopsy compared with the open biopsy technique in the diagnosis of a breast abnormality?
- What clinician and facility factors influence the adverse events of core needle breast biopsy compared with the open biopsy technique in the diagnosis of a breast abnormality?

Key Question 3: How do open biopsy and various core needle techniques differ in terms of patient preference, availability, costs, availability of qualified pathologist interpretations, and other factors that may influence choice of a particular technique?

Methods

This report updates a previously completed Comparative Effectiveness Review on core needle and open surgical biopsy methods for the diagnosis of breast cancer. To update the report we performed a systematic review of the published scientific literature using established methodologies as outlined in the Agency for Healthcare Research and Quality's (AHRQ) "Methods Guide for Comparative Effectiveness Reviews," which is available at: http://effectivehealth care.ahrq.gov. [7] The main sections in this chapter reflect the elements of the protocol that guided this review. We have followed the reporting requirements of the "Preferred Reporting Items for Systematic Reviews and Meta-analyses" (PRISMA) checklist.[8] All key methodological decisions were made a priori. The protocol was developed with input from external clinical and methodological experts, in consultation with the AHRQ task order officer (TOO), and was posted online to solicit additional public comments. Its PROSPERO registration number is CRD42013005690.

AHRQ Task Order Officer

The AHRQ Task Order Officer (TOO) was responsible for overseeing all aspects of this project. The TOO facilitated a common understanding among all parties involved in the project, resolved ambiguities, and fielded all Evidence-based Practice Center (EPC) queries regarding the scope and processes of the project. The TOO and other staff at AHRQ helped to establish the Key Questions and protocol and reviewed the report for consistency, clarity, and to ensure that it conforms to AHRQ standards.

External Stakeholder Input

A new panel of experts was convened to form the Technical Expert Panel (TEP). The TEP included representatives of professional societies, experts in the diagnosis and treatment of breast cancer (including radiologists and surgeons), and a patient representative. The TEP provided input to help further refine the Key Questions and protocol, identify important issues, and define the parameters for the review of evidence. Discussions among the EPC, TOO, and the TEP occurred during a series of teleconferences and via email.

Key Questions

The final Key Questions are listed at the end of the Background section. The refinement of the Key Questions took into account the patient populations, interventions, comparators, outcomes, and study designs that are clinically relevant for core needle biopsies.

Analytic Framework

We used an analytic framework (Figure 1) that maps the Key Questions within the context of populations, interventions, comparators, and outcomes of interest. The framework was adapted from that used in the original 2009 CER. It depicts the chain of logic that links the test performance of core needle biopsy for the diagnosis of breast abnormalities (Key Question 1) with patient-relevant outcomes (Key Question 3) and adverse events of testing (Key Question 2).

Figure 1. Analytic framework

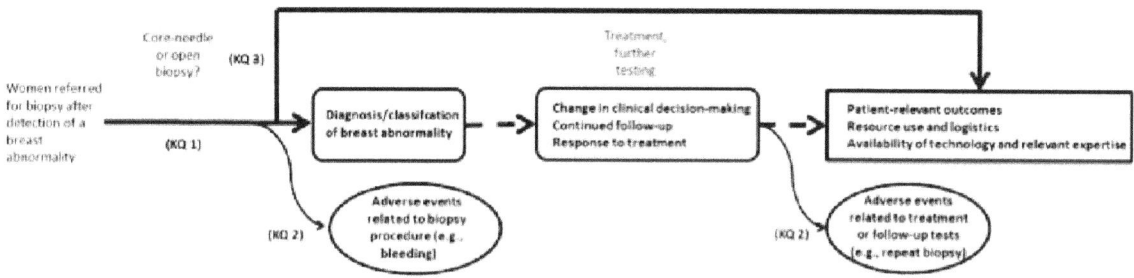

KQ = Key Question.

Scope of the Review

Populations and Conditions of Interest

The population of interest for all Key Questions was women who have been referred for biopsy for the diagnosis of primary breast cancer (including multifocal and bilateral disease) following self-examination, physical examination, or screening mammography. Studies carried out in women who had been previously diagnosed with breast cancer and were being examined for recurrence or to assess the extent of disease (staging) were excluded. The original report excluded studies carried out in women at high risk of breast cancer; however, MRI-guided biopsy is used mainly in this subset of patients. For this reason, following extensive discussions with the TEP, we decided to broaden the scope of the review to include studies carried out in women at high baseline risk of breast cancer (e.g., on the basis of BRCA genetic testing or family history of breast cancer). Of note, studies often do not provide information on the risk of cancer among included patients. Thus we grouped studies into two categories: (1) studies that explicitly reported that more than 15 percent of included patients were at high risk of cancer; (2) studies that either enrolled less than 15 percent of patients at high risk of cancer or did not provide information on baseline risk. Throughout this report, we refer to the latter group as "studies of women at average risk of cancer"; however, we acknowledge that it may include studies enrolling patients at higher-than-average cancer risk but failing to report the relevant information.

Interventions

For all Key Questions, the interventions of interest were core needle and open biopsy done to evaluate whether a breast lesion is malignant. Other uses of biopsy techniques (e.g., use of biopsy to examine the sentinel lymph nodes in women with an established diagnosis of breast cancer) were not considered. Studies were required to have used biopsy instrumentation that is currently commercially available, as studies of discontinued devices are not applicable to current practice.

Comparators (Index and Reference Standard Tests)

For test performance outcomes (Key Question 1) the reference standard was either open surgical biopsy, or followup by clinical examination and/or mammography for at least six months. The diagnostic performance of each core biopsy technique (each index test) was quantified versus the reference standard. Most assessments of diagnostic performance quantify the sensitivity and the specificity of each index test – here each needle core biopsy technique. Sensitivity and specificity are probabilities conditional on true disease status, and are noncomparative in nature. The reference standard is used in their definition, and is not a "comparator test". The comparative diagnostic performance of alternative needle core biopsy techniques was also evaluated. For adverse events and patient-relevant outcomes (outcomes other than diagnostic performance; Key Questions 2 and 3) the comparators of interest were: open surgical biopsy, followup by clinical examination and/or mammography for at least six months, or alternative core needle biopsy methods (e.g., stereotactic mammography versus ultrasound to locate the breast lesion; use versus non-use of vacuum-assistance to extract tissue samples).

Outcomes

For Key Question 1, the outcome of interest was test performance, as assessed by sensitivity (proportion of cancers detected by the reference standard that are also detected by core needle biopsy); specificity (proportion of negative findings according to core needle biopsy that were classified as negative by the reference standard; equal to one minus the false positive rate); underestimation rate for high risk lesions (most often atypical ductal hyperplasia, ADH), defined as the proportion of core needle biopsy findings of high risk lesions that are found to be malignant according to the reference standard); and underestimation rate for ductal carcinoma in situ (DCIS), defined as the proportion of core needle biopsy findings of DCIS that are found to be invasive according to the reference standard.

For Key Question 2 we looked for the following outcomes: rate of inconclusive biopsy findings (e.g. inadequate sampling of lesion); comparisons of repeat biopsy rates between core needle and open surgical biopsy; subsequent false positive and false negative rates on mammography (impact of breast biopsy on future mammographic examinations); dissemination or displacement of cancerous cells along the needle track; and patient-centered outcomes (including bruising, bleeding or hematomas, pain, use of pain medication, infections, fainting or near fainting, time to recover). Because adverse events were not consistently defined across studies, we accepted the definitions used in the individual studies (when available).

For Key Question 3, we considered patient-relevant outcomes (patient preferences for specific procedures, cosmetic results, quality of life, anxiety and other psychological outcomes, time to complete tumor removal [for women with cancer], recurrence rate [for women with cancer, including local, regional, and distant recurrence], cancer-free survival and overall survival); resource use and logistics (costs, resource utilization other than cost [number of additional surgical procedures, procedural time], subsequent surgical procedures, wait time for test results); and availability of technology and relevant expertise (physician experience, availability of equipment, availability of [qualified] pathologists to evaluate biopsy samples).

Timing

We required that the duration of clinical and/or mammography followup was at least six months in studies where open surgical biopsy was not performed.

Setting

Studies in all geographic locations and care settings were evaluated, including general hospitals, academic medical centers, and ambulatory surgical centers, among others.

Study Design and Additional Criteria

We required that studies had been published in peer-reviewed journals as full articles. For all Key Questions, studies were required to have been published in English. Restricting included studies to those published in English, which was also an inclusion criterion in the original review, was deemed unlikely to bias the results of the review and avoids the resource-intensive translation of research articles published in languages other than English.

For Key Question 1 eligible studies were prospective or retrospective cohort studies or randomized controlled trials. Retrospective case studies ("case series"[9]) and other studies sampling patients on the basis of outcomes (e.g. diagnostic case-control studies, or studies selecting cases on the basis of specific histological findings) were excluded. Empirical evidence from meta-epidemiological studies suggests that diagnostic case-control studies may overestimate test performance. Studies were required to report information on the sensitivity, specificity, positive or negative predictive value of tests, or to include data that allow the calculation of one or more of these outcomes. Specifically, studies needed to provide adequate information to reconstruct 2×2 tables of test performance of the index against the reference standard. Table 1 illustrates how index and reference standard results were used to construct such 2×2 tables.

Table 1. Definitions of diagnostic groups based on index and reference standard test results

		Reference Standard Results (open surgery or followup)	
		Malignant (invasive or in situ)	*Benign*
Core Needle Biopsy Results (index test)	*Malignant (invasive or in situ)*	considered TP	considered TP*
	High risk lesion (e.g., ADH)	considered TP	considered FP
	Benign	considered FN	considered TN

*Some study authors specifically stated that diagnoses of malignancy on core needle biopsy were assumed to be correct, whether or not a tumor was observed upon surgical excision. The original version of this review also classified all diagnoses of malignancy on core needle biopsy as true positives.
ADH = atypical ductal hyperplasia; FN = false negative; FP = false positive; TN = true negative; TP = true positive.

Two issues related to the definition of diagnostic test categories merit additional description. First, occasionally core needle biopsy removes the entire target lesion that is being biopsied, rendering subsequent surgical biopsies unable to confirm the findings of the index test procedure. In such cases of core needle diagnoses of malignancy, we considered the core needle results to be true positive. This operational definition was adopted by several of the primary studies we reviewed and the original ECRI report. Second, in our primary analysis (and consistent with the 2009 ECRI report) core needle biopsy identified high risk lesions that on subsequent surgery (or followup) are not found to be associated with malignant disease were considered false positive. To assess the impact of this operational definition on our findings we performed a sensitivity analysis where high risk lesions on index core needle biopsy found to be non-malignant (high risk or benign) on subsequent open biopsy or surgery were excluded from the analyses.

Noncomparative studies of test performance (i.e. studies of a single index test) were required to have enrolled at least 10 participants per arm or per comparison group. This inclusion criterion was intended to reduce the risk of bias from non-representative participants in small studies. Further, smaller studies do not produce precise estimates of test performance and as such are unlikely to substantially affect results. Studies were also required to have followed at least fifty percent of participants to completion. This criterion was intended to reduce the risk of bias from high rates of attrition.

Key Question 2 was addressed by extracting harm-related information for core needle biopsy and open surgical biopsy from studies meeting the criteria for Key Question 1. In addition, we included studies that met all other selection criteria for Key Question 1 except for the use of a reference standard and the reporting of information on test performance outcomes. This allowed us to consider additional sources of evidence that assess adverse events. Finally, for this Key Question, we also reviewed primary research articles, regardless of design (i.e., case reports and case series, case-control studies, cohort studies, randomized trials), that address the dissemination or displacement of cancer cells by the biopsy procedure, a relatively rare harm that is specific to core biopsy.

The original report did not use formal criteria for study selection for Key Question 3. Based on the findings of the original report, we used the same PICOTS criteria described above and considered the following study designs:

- Randomized controlled trials, cohort studies, and cross-sectional studies on patient preferences, cosmetic results of biopsy procedures, physician experience (including studies of the "learning curve" for different biopsy methods and tools).
- Cost studies, including cost-minimization and cost-consequence analyses, were used to obtain information on resource utilization and unit costs. Given the large variability of cost information among different jurisdictions, we only considered studies conducted in the U.S. setting and published after 2004.[10]
- Cost-effectiveness/cost-utility analyses based on primary trials of breast biopsy interventions were used to obtain information on unit costs and resource utilization.[11] Specifically, we considered the components of cost and resource use but did not use cost-effectiveness ratios or other summary measures of cost-effectiveness/utility. As for cost studies, we only considered primary cost-effectiveness/-utility studies conducted in the US setting and published after 2004.[10] We did not use model-based cost-effectiveness results.
- Studies of pathologist qualifications for interpreting core needle biopsy results; including interlaboratory initiatives to standardize diagnostic criteria (e.g., proficiency testing) or minimal competency requirements.
- Surveys of the availability of equipment for obtaining core needle biopsies and of qualified pathologists to examine biopsy samples.

Literature Search and Abstract Screening

We searched MEDLINE®, Embase®, the Cochrane Central Register of Controlled Trials (CENTRAL), the Cochrane Database of Systematic Reviews, the Database of Abstracts of Reviews of Effects (DARE), the Health Technology Assessment Database (HTA), the U.K. National Health Service Economic Evaluation Database (NHS EED), the U.S. National Guideline Clearinghouse (NGC), and the Cumulative Index to Nursing and Allied Health

Literature (CINAHL®); last search on December 16, 2013. Appendix A describes the search strategy we employed which is a revision and expansion of the search strategy used in the original report. Of note, the original report used a search filter for studies of diagnostic tests to increase search specificity; this is a reasonable approach given the large volume of literature on studies on diagnostic biopsy methods for breast cancer. Because this update covered a short time period (from 2009 to 2013) we opted to not use this filter, in order to increase search sensitivity.[12, 13] Our searches covered the time period from six months before the most recent search date in the original report, to ensure adequate overlap.

To identify studies excluded from the original report because they enrolled women at high risk for cancer, the set of abstracts screened for the original report was obtained and rescreened for potentially eligible studies of high risk women. In addition, the list of studies excluded from the original report following full text review was checked to identify studies excluded because they included women at high risk for cancer. We also performed a search for systematic reviews on the topic and used their reference lists of included studies to validate our search strategy and to make sure we identified all relevant studies.

All reviewers screened a common set of 200 abstracts (in 2 pilot rounds, each with 100 abstracts), and discussed discrepancies, in order to standardize screening practices and ensure understanding of screening criteria. The remaining citations were split into nonoverlapping sets, each screened by two reviewers independently. Discrepancies were resolved by consensus involving a third investigator.

We asked the TEP to provide citations of potentially relevant articles. Additional studies were identified through the perusal of reference lists of eligible studies, published clinical practice guidelines, relevant narrative and systematic reviews, Scientific Information Packages from manufacturers, and a search of U.S. Food and Drug Administration databases. All articles identified through these sources were screened for eligibility against the same criteria as for articles identified through literature searches. We sent the final list of included studies to the TEP to ensure that no key publications had been missed.

Study Selection and Eligibility Criteria

Potentially eligible citations were obtained in full text and reviewed for eligibility on the basis of the predefined inclusion criteria. A single reviewer screened each potentially eligible article in full-text to determine eligibility; reviewers were instructed to be inclusive. A second reviewer verified all relevant articles. Disagreements regarding article eligibility were resolved by consensus involving a third reviewer. Appendix B lists all the studies excluded after full-text screening and the reason for exclusion.

Data Abstraction and Management

Data was extracted using electronic forms and entered into the Systematic Review Data Repository (SRDR; http://srdr.ahrq.gov/). The basic elements and design of these forms is similar to those we have used for other reviews of diagnostic tests and includes elements that address population characteristics, sample size, study design, descriptions of the index and reference standard tests of interest, analytic details, and outcome data. Prior to data extraction, forms were customized to capture all elements relevant to the Key Questions. We used separate sections in the extraction forms for Key Questions related to short-term outcomes, including classification of breast abnormalities, intermediate outcomes (such as clear surgical margins), patient-relevant outcomes (such as quality of life), and factors affecting (modifying) test performance. We pilot-tested the forms on several studies extracted by multiple team members to ensure consistency in operational definitions.

A single reviewer extracted data from each eligible study. At least one other team member reviewed and confirmed all data (data verification). Disagreements were resolved by consensus including a third reviewer. We contacted authors (1) to clarify information reported in the papers that is hard to interpret (e.g., inconsistencies between tables and text); and (2) to verify suspected overlap between study populations in publications from the same group of investigators.

Assessment of the Risk of Bias of Individual Studies

We assessed the risk of bias for each individual study using the assessment methods detailed in the AHRQ Methods Guide for Effectiveness and Comparative Effectiveness Review hereafter referred to as the Methods Guide. We used elements from the Quality Assessment for Diagnostic Accuracy Studies instrument (QUADAS version 2), to assess the risk of bias (methodological quality or internal validity) of the diagnostic test studies included in the review (these studies comprise the majority of the available studies).[14-17] The tool assesses four domains of risk of bias related to patient selection, index test, reference standard test, and patient flow and timing. For studies of other designs we used appropriate sets of items to assess risk of bias or methodological "quality": for nonrandomized cohort studies we used items from the Newcastle-Ottawa scale,[18] for randomized controlled trials we used items from the Cochrane Risk of Bias tool,[19] and for studies of resource utilization and costs we used items from the checklist proposed by Drummond et al.[20]

We assessed and reported methodological quality items (as "Yes", "No", or "Unclear/Not Reported") for each eligible study. We then rated each study as being of low, intermediate, or high risk of bias on the basis of adherence to accepted methodological principles. Generally, studies with low risk of bias have the following features: lowest likelihood of confounding due to comparison to a randomized controlled group; a clear description of the population, setting, interventions, and comparison groups; appropriate measurement of outcomes; appropriate statistical and analytic methods and reporting; no reporting inconsistencies; clear reporting of dropouts and a low dropout rate; and no other apparent sources of bias. Studies with moderate risk of bias are susceptible to some bias but not sufficiently to invalidate results. They do not meet all the criteria for low risk of bias owing to some deficiencies, but none are likely to introduce major bias. Studies with moderate risk of bias may not be randomized or may be missing information, making it difficult to assess limitations and potential problems. Studies with high risk of bias are those with indications of bias that may invalidate the reported findings (e.g., observational studies not adjusting for any confounders, studies using historical controls, or studies with very high dropout rates). These studies have serious errors in design, analysis, or reporting and contain discrepancies in reporting or have large amounts of missing information. We discuss the handling of high risk of bias studies in evidence synthesis in the following sections. Studies of different designs were graded within the context of their study design.

Data Synthesis

We summarized included studies qualitatively and presented important features of the study populations, designs, tests used, outcomes, and results in summary tables. Population characteristics of interest included age, race/ethnicity, and palpability of lesion. Design characteristics included methods of population selection and sampling, and followup duration. Test characteristics included imaging-guided versus not imaging-guided, and vacuum-assisted versus not vacuum-assisted methods. We looked for information on test performance, adverse events, patient preferences, and resource utilization including costs.

Statistical analyses were conducted using methods currently recommend for use in Comparative Effectiveness Reviews of diagnostic tests.[21, 22] For all outcomes we assessed heterogeneity graphically (e.g. by inspecting a scatterplot of studies in the receiver operating characteristic, ROC, space) and by examining the posterior distribution of between-study variance parameters.

For Key Question 1 we performed meta-analysis on studies that were deemed sufficiently similar. Based on the technical characteristics of the different tests, and the findings of the original Evidence Report, we developed a mixed effects binomial-bivariate normal regression model that accounted for different imaging methods (e.g. US, stereotactic mammography, MRI), the use of vacuum (yes vs. not), the baseline of risk of cancer of included patients (high versus average risk), and residual (unexplained) heterogeneity.[23-25] This model allowed us to estimate the test performance of alternative diagnostic tests, and perform indirect comparisons among them.[23] Furthermore, it allowed us to model the correlation between sensitivity and specificity and to derive meta-analytic ROC curves.[24, 25] A univariate mixed effects logistic regression (binomial-normal) model was used for the meta-analysis of DCIS and high risk lesion underestimation rates.[26]

We performed meta-regression analyses (e.g. to evaluate the impact of study risk of bias items, or the effect of other study-level characteristics) by extending the model to include additional appropriately coded terms in the regression equations.[27, 28] Such analyses were planned for patient and breast lesion factors (e.g., age, density of breast tissue, microcalcifications, and palpability of the lesions), biopsy procedure factors (e.g., needle size, imaging guidance, vacuum extraction, and number of samples), clinician and facility-related factors (e.g., training of the operator, country were the study was conducted), and risk of bias items. We performed additional sensitivity analyses (e.g., leave-one-out meta-analysis and comparisons of studies added in the update versus studies included in the original report).[29]

For Key Question 2, we found that adverse events were inconsistently reported (across studies) and that the methods for ascertaining their occurrence were often not presented in adequate detail. For this reason we refrained from performing meta-analyses for these outcomes. Instead, we calculated descriptive statistics (medians, 25th and 75th percentiles, minimum and maximum values) across all studies and for specific test types. For Key Question 3, because of the heterogeneity of research designs and outcomes assessed, for all outcomes except the number of surgical procedures, we did not perform meta-analysis but instead chose to summarize the data qualitatively. We performed a meta-analysis comparing core needle and open surgical biopsies with respect to the number of patients who required one versus more than one surgical procedures for treatment, after the establishment of breast cancer diagnosis. This analysis used a standard univariate normal random effects model with a binomial distribution for the within-study likelihood of each biopsy group (core needle vs. open).

All statistical analyses were performed using Bayesian methods; models were fit using Markov Chain Monte Carlo methods and noninformative prior distributions. Theory and empirical comparisons suggest that, when the number of studies is large, this approach produces results similar to those of maximum likelihood methods (which do not require the specification of priors).[30] Results were summarized as medians of posterior distributions with associated 95 percent central credible intervals (CrIs). A CrI denotes a range of values within which the parameter value is expected to fall with 95% probability.

Grading the Strength of Evidence

We followed the Methods Guide[7] to evaluate the strength of the body of evidence for each Key Question with respect to the following domains: risk of bias, consistency, directness, precision, and reporting bias.[7,31] Generally, strength of evidence was downgraded when risk of bias was not low, in the presence of inconsistency, when evidence was indirect or imprecise, or when we suspected that results were affected by selective analysis or reporting.

We determined risk of bias (low, medium, or high) on the basis of the study design and the methodological quality. We assessed consistency on the basis of the direction and magnitude of results across studies. We considered the evidence to be indirect when we had to rely on comparisons of biopsy methods across different studies (i.e., indirect comparisons). We considered studies to be precise if the CrI was narrow enough for a clinically useful conclusion, and imprecise if the CrI was wide enough to include clinically distinct conclusions. The potential for reporting bias ("suspected" vs. "not suspected") was evaluated with respect to publication, selective outcome reporting, and selective analysis reporting. We made qualitative dispositions rather than perform formal statistical tests to evaluate differences in the effect sizes between more precise (larger) and less precise (smaller) studies because such tests cannot distinguish between "true" heterogeneity between smaller and larger studies, other biases, and chance.[32,33] Therefore, instead of relying on statistical tests, we evaluated the reported results across studies qualitatively, on the basis of completeness of reporting, number of enrolled patients, and numbers of observed events. Judgment on the potential for selective outcome reporting bias was based on reporting patterns for each outcome of interest across studies. We acknowledge that both types of reporting bias are difficult to reliably detect on the basis of data available in published research studies. We believe that our searches (across multiple databases), combined with our plan for contacting test manufacturers (for additional data) and the authors of published studies (for data clarification) limited the impact of reporting and publication bias on our results, to the extent possible.

Finally, we rated the body of evidence using four strength of evidence levels: high, moderate, low, and insufficient.[7] These describe our level of confidence that the evidence reflects the true effect for the major comparisons of interest.

Assessing Applicability

We followed the Methods Guide[7] in evaluating the applicability of included studies to patient populations of interest. Applicability to the population of interest was also judged separately on the basis of patient characteristics (e.g., age may affect test performance because the consistency of the breast tissue changes over time), method by which suspicion is established (e.g., mammography vs. other methods may affect test performance through spectrum effects), baseline risk of cancer ("average risk" vs. "high risk" women may affect estimated test performance because of differences in diagnostic algorithms), outcomes (e.g., prevalence of breast cancers diagnosed upon biopsy may also be a marker of spectrum effects), and setting of care (because differences in patient populations, diagnostic algorithms, and available technologies may affect test results).

Peer Review

The initial draft report was pre-reviewed by the TOO and an AHRQ Associate Editor (a senior member of another EPC). Following revisions, the draft report was sent to invited peer reviewers and was simultaneously uploaded to the AHRQ Web site where it was available for public comment for 30 days. All reviewer comments (both invited and from the public) were collated and individually addressed. The revised report and the EPC's responses to invited and public reviewers' comments were again reviewed by the TOO and Associate Editor prior to completion of the report. The authors of the report had final discretion as to how the report was revised based on the reviewer comments, with oversight by the TOO and Associate Editor.

Results

Our literature searches identified 8,637 potentially relevant citations (including 1,127 rescreened from the original ECRI evidence report). After review of the abstracts, the full-length articles of 2,480 of these studies were obtained and examined in full text. Finally, 128 new studies were considered eligible for inclusion in the updated review, for a total of 316 included studies. Figure 2 presents the literature flow and Table 2 summarizes the additions to the original report, separately by Key Question.

Figure 2. Flow chart of included studies

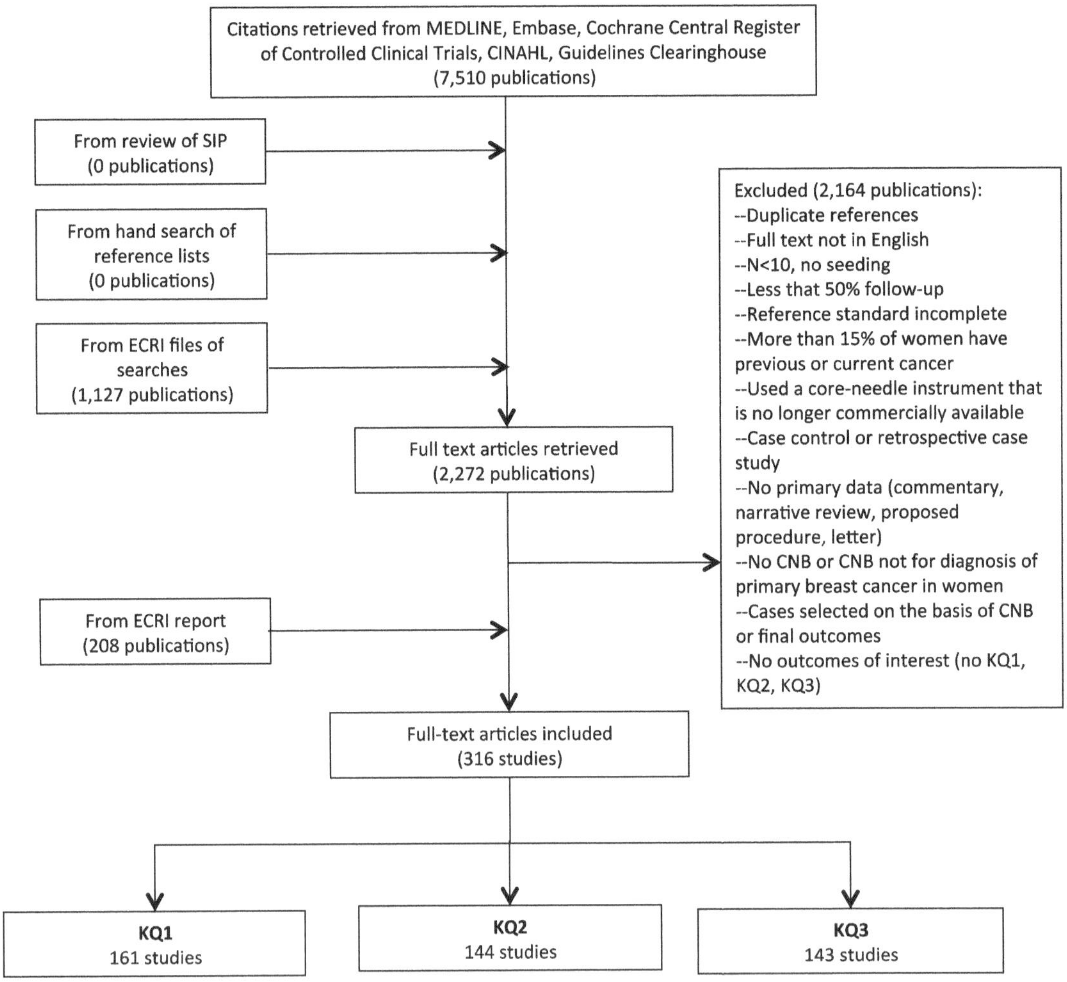

```
Citations retrieved from MEDLINE, Embase, Cochrane Central Register
of Controlled Clinical Trials, CINAHL, Guidelines Clearinghouse
(7,510 publications)

From review of SIP
(0 publications)

From hand search of
reference lists
(0 publications)

From ECRI files of
searches
(1,127 publications)

        ↓
Full text articles retrieved
(2,272 publications)

Excluded (2,164 publications):
--Duplicate references
--Full text not in English
--N<10, no seeding
--Less that 50% follow-up
--Reference standard incomplete
--More than 15% of women have
previous or current cancer
--Used a core-needle instrument that
is no longer commercially available
--Case control or retrospective case
study
--No primary data (commentary,
narrative review, proposed
procedure, letter)
--No CNB or CNB not for diagnosis of
primary breast cancer in women
--Cases selected on the basis of CNB
or final outcomes
--No outcomes of interest (no KQ1,
KQ2, KQ3)

From ECRI report
(208 publications)

        ↓
Full-text articles included
(316 studies)

    ↓           ↓           ↓
   KQ1         KQ2         KQ3
161 studies  144 studies  143 studies
```

CNB = core needle biopsy; KQ = Key Question; N = number of patients; SIP = Scientific Information Packet.

Table 2. Summary of new evidence evaluated in this update*

Key Question	Studies Included in the Original Report	Studies Identified by the Updating Process	Total Number of Studies Synthesized in This Report
Key Question 1: What is the test performance of different types of core needle breast biopsy compared with open biopsy in the diagnosis of breast cancer?	107**	54	161
Key Question 2: What are the adverse events (harms) associated with core needle breast biopsy compared to the open biopsy in the diagnosis of breast cancer?	74	70	144
Key Question 3: How do open biopsy and various core needle techniques differ in terms of patient preference, availability, costs, availability of qualified pathologist interpretations, and other factors that may influence choice of a particular technique?	84	59	143

*Some studies addressed multiple Key Questions
** The original ECRI report included a total of 108 studies; one core needle biopsy study overlapped with one of the studies identified in our update which enrolled a larger patient population; thus the smaller study was excluded from Key Question 1.

Key Question 1: In women with a palpable or nonpalpable breast abnormality, what is the test performance of different types of core needle breast biopsy compared with open biopsy for diagnosis?

Included Studies

Fifty-four new studies identified by this update met the inclusion criteria for Key Question 1. We synthesized these studies with the 106 studies identified by the original evidence report, for a total of 160 studies providing information on test performance outcomes. Studies had been published between 1990 and 2013. Fifty studies were prospectively designed, and 58 were conducted in the United States. Ten studies provided information on more than one group of patients (typically undergoing biopsy with a different biopsy device). In statistical analyses these groups were treated as separate strata, leading to a total of 171 complete 2×2 tables of diagnostic test results, with information on 69,804 breast lesions.

Test Performance for Breast Cancer Diagnosis

Test Performance of Open Surgical Biopsy

Research studies of needle biopsy methods and technical experts generally suggested that open surgical biopsy could be considered a "gold" standard test (i.e. a test without measurement error). One study identified by the original evidence report, provided information on the test performance of open surgical biopsy, using published literature and primary patient data (patient charts) from patients evaluated at a single medical center.[34] Based on a re-review of archived open biopsy material by a second pathologist, patient chart review, study of cases with benign results on biopsy after suspicious mammography results, and expert opinion, the authors concluded that open surgical biopsy may miss one to two percent of breast cancers (i.e. sensitivity of 98% or greater). We found a single clinical study of patients undergoing surgical biopsies who were followed by imaging for 12 months after biopsy. This study reported underestimation in 16.7 percent of ADH lesions (1 of 6 lesions) and 7.1 percent of DCIS lesions (1/14 lesions) diagnosed thorough open biopsy.[35] The small number of lesions in this study precludes reliable conclusions. Because open surgical biopsy samples the entire target lesion or a large part of it, in theory underestimation rates can be reduced to zero.

Test Performance of Core Needle Biopsy Methods

A total of 160 studies contributed information to analyses of test performance of core needle biopsy methods.[35-194] Six studies enrolled women at high risk of cancer development and 154 enrolled women at average risk. The studies reported on a variety of biopsy techniques: 131 study arms reported on the use of a single form of imaging guidance (83 stereotactic; 41 ultrasound; 6 MRI; 1 grid) whereas ten used freehand methods, 29 used multiple methods, including freehand techniques in some cases (and did not report test performance results separately by each method), and one did not report adequate details. Sixty study arms used vacuum-assisted methods to obtain the biopsy sample; 80 used automated methods; 30 used multiple methods; and 1 did not report adequate details. Needle size also varied across studies: 57 used 14G needles, nine used smaller and 46 used larger bores; 48 studies did not report relevant information or used a range of needle sizes. Reference standard tests also differed across studies: 26 used open biopsy on all included patients; 94 used mean or median follow up of between 6 and 24 months for test negative patients, and 40 used mean or median followup of 24 months or more for test negative cases. Details about study design, selection criteria, enrolled populations, biopsy methods and results, are publically available in the SRDR. Consistent with the findings of the original report, the overall risk of bias was considered moderate to high, mainly due to concerns about spectrum bias, retrospective data collection, differential verification, and lack of information regarding the blinding of reference standard test assessors to the index test results. Detailed results from our risk of bias assessment are provided at the end of this section.

The prevalence of malignant disease (invasive or DCIS, at the lesion level) ranged from 1 percent to 94 percent, with a median of 34 percent. The proportion of correct diagnoses ranged from 68 percent to 100 percent, with a median of 96 percent. Table 3 summarizes the results for alternative diagnostic biopsy methods, together with information on the number of lesions evaluated by each test and summary test performance information, for women at average risk of cancer. Table 4 summarizes the same information for women deemed to be at high risk for cancer (e.g. due to genetic factors or strong family history). Figure 3 presents individual study estimates and meta-analytic results in the ROC space for both groups of women. These plots indicate that results were fairly homogeneous across studies for each test and that test sensitivity and specificity were close to 1 (studies cluster at the top left corner of the space). In analyses excluding high risk lesions on core needle biopsy that were also classified as high risk lesions on the reference standard test, the summary sensitivity of the various tests was unaffected; and summary specificity was somewhat increased (Appendix C).

Key findings with respect to test performance (sensitivity, specificity, and positive and negative likelihood ratios[*]) and underestimation rates are summarized narratively below. As mentioned, only six studies reported results on the test performance of various biopsy methods for breast cancer diagnosis in high risk women. Of these studies, only three reported information on underestimation rates (all three for high risk lesions; none for DCIS).

---

[*] To aid in the interpretation of likelihood ratios we remind readers that these statistics can be used to convert pre-test probabilities to post-test probabilities. For example, before testing, assume that a patient has probability of disease $\textit{pre-test } p = 0.1$ and $\textit{pre-test odds} = \dfrac{\textit{pre-test } p}{1 - \textit{pre-test } p} = \dfrac{0.1}{0.9} = 0.11$. If the diagnostic test has a positive likelihood ratio (LR^+) of 15 then the post-test odds are $\textit{post-test odds} = \textit{pre-test odds} \times LR^+ = 0.11 \times 15 = 1.67$. This corresponds to a post-test probability of $\textit{post-test } p = \dfrac{\textit{post-test odds}}{\textit{post-test odds} + 1} = \dfrac{1.67}{1.67 + 1} = 0.625$ (i.e. the post-test probability is approximately 6 times greater than the pre-test value). If the test results had been negative and the test had a negative likelihood ratio (LR^-) of 0.1, the post-tests odds would be $\textit{post-test odds} = \textit{pre-test odds} \times LR^- = 0.11 \times 0.1 = 0.011$, which corresponds to $\textit{post-test } p = \dfrac{0.011}{0.011 + 1} = 0.011$ (i.e. approximately the post-test probability is approximately 10 times lower than the pre-test value). As a rule of thumb, $LR^+ > 10$ and $LR^- < 0.1$ are generally considered clinically meaningful.

Table 3. Summary estimates of test performance for alternative core needle biopsy methods – women at average risk of cancer

Biopsy Method or Device	N Studies [N biopsies] for Sensitivity & Specificity	Sensitivity	Specificity	N Studies [N biopsies] for DCIS Underestimation	DCIS Underestimation Probability	N Studies [N biopsies] for High Risk Lesion Underestimation	High Risk Lesion Underestimation Probability
Freehand, automated	10 [786]	0.91 (0.80 to 0.96)	0.98 (0.95 to 1.00)	0 [0]	NA	1 [6]	0.88 (0.32 to 1.00)
US-guided, automated	27 [16287]	0.99 (0.98 to 0.99)	0.97 (0.95 to 0.98)	14 [307]	0.38 (0.26 to 0.51)	21 [601]	0.25 (0.16 to 0.36)
US-guided, vacuum-assisted	12 [1543]	0.97 (0.92 to 0.99)	0.98 (0.96 to 0.99)	5 [48]	0.09 (0.02 to 0.26)	9 [20]	0.11 (0.02 to 0.33)
Stereotactically guided, automated	37 [9535]	0.97 (0.95 to 0.98)	0.97 (0.96 to 0.98)	18 [664]	0.26 (0.19 to 0.36)	29 [357]	0.47 (0.37 to 0.58)
Stereotactically guided, vacuum-assisted	43 [14667]	0.99 (0.98 to 0.99)	0.92 (0.89 to 0.94)	34 [1899]	0.11 (0.08 to 0.14)	40 [1002]	0.18 (0.13 to 0.24)
MRI-guided, automated	2 [89]	0.90 (0.57 to 0.99)	0.99 (0.91 to 1.00)	0 [0]	NA	1 [1]	0.49 (0.02 to 0.97)
MRI-guided, vacuum-assisted	1 [10]	1.00 (0.98 to 1.00)	0.91 (0.54 to 0.99)	1 [1]	0.00 (0.00 to 0.38)	0 [0]	NA
Multiple methods/other	33 [26028]	0.99 (0.98 to 0.99)	0.96 (0.93 to 0.97)	18 [628]	0.22 (0.15 to 0.30)	25 [866]	0.32 (0.23 to 0.41)

All numbers are medians with 95% CrIs, unless otherwise stated.
CrI = credible interval; DCIS = ductal carcinoma in situ; MRI = magnetic resonance imaging; N = number; NA = not applicable; US = ultrasound.

Table 4. Summary estimates of test performance for alternative core needle biopsy methods – women at high risk of cancer

Biopsy Method or Device	N Studies (N biopsies) for Sensitivity and Specificity	Sensitivity (95% CrI)	Specificity (95% CrI)
Stereotactically guided, automated	1 [416]	0.97 (0.82 to 1.00)	0.97 (0.91 to 0.99)
Stereotactically guided, vacuum-assisted	2 [311]	0.99 (0.93 to 1.00)	0.93 (0.79 to 0.98)
MRI-guided, automated	2 [56]	0.90 (0.58 to 0.98)	0.99 (0.92 to 1.00)
MRI-guided, vacuum-assisted	1 [76]	1.00 (0.98 to 1.00)	0.92 (0.61 to 0.99)

No studies provided information on the test performance of freehand or US-guided biopsy methods, or the use of multiple methods in populations of women at high risk of cancer.
Results are based on bivariate model with risk group as a covariate.
CrI = credible interval; DCIS = ductal carcinoma in situ; MRI = magnetic resonance imaging; N = number; US = ultrasound.

Figure 3. Scatterplot of results in the receiver operating characteristic space and summary receiver operating characteristic curves of alternative core needle biopsy methods for the diagnosis of breast cancer

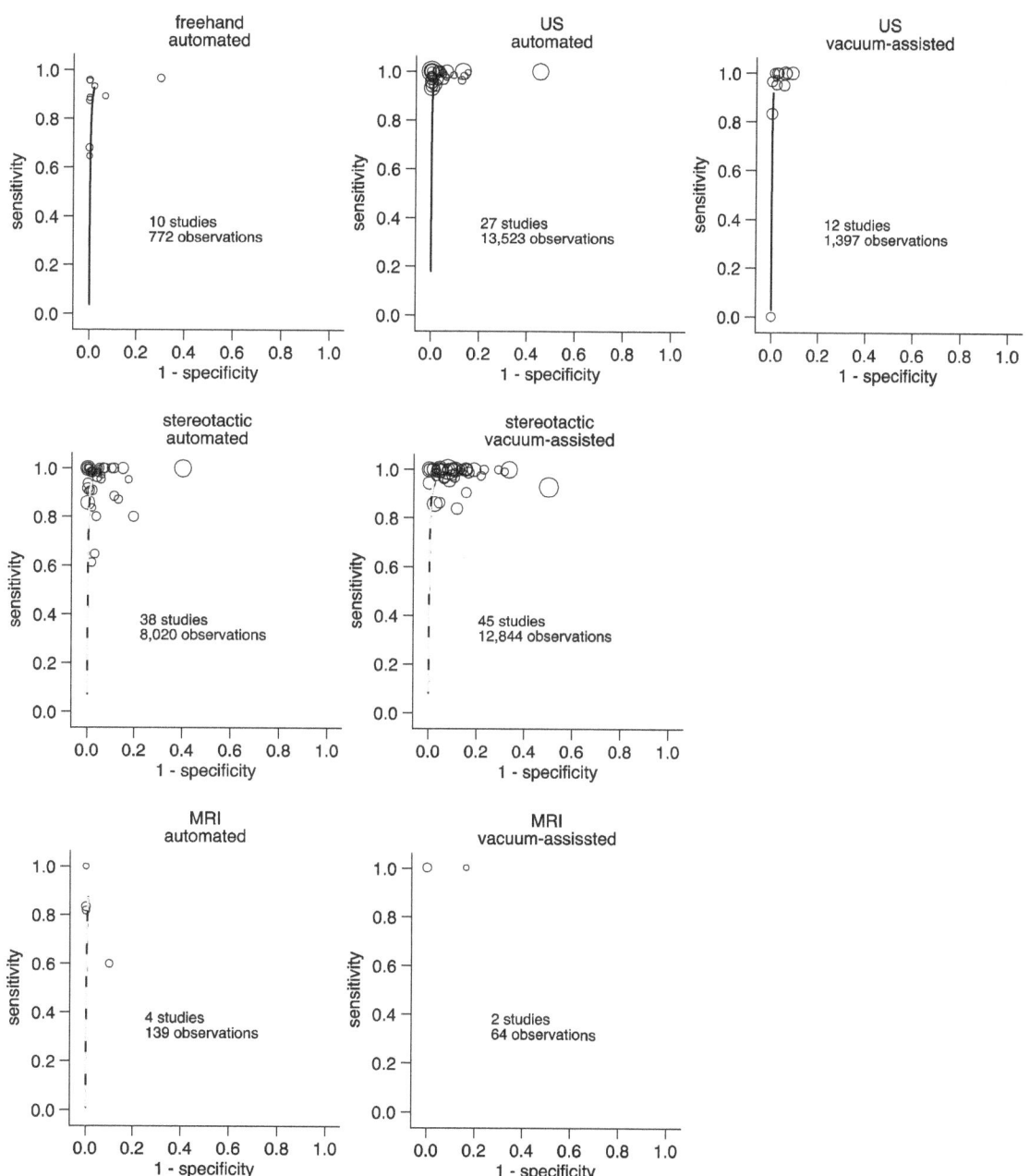

Solid black lines represent results for average risk women; dashed gray lines represent results for high risk women (when studies were available). The numbers of observations and studies include cohorts of women both at average and high risk of cancer. The number of observations reflects the total number of data points in the analysis; some studies contributed patient-level and others lesion-level results. MRI = magnetic resonance imaging; US = ultrasound.

Freehand Core Needle Biopsies

Women at average risk of cancer: Ten cohorts reported data on the accuracy of nonguided (i.e., freehand) core needle biopsies performed with automated biopsy devices. The summary sensitivity was 0.91 (95% CrI, 0.80 to 0.96) and the summary specificity was 0.98 (95% CrI, 0.95 to 1.00), corresponding to a positive likelihood ratio of 58.4 (95% CrI, 19.0 to 226.9) and a negative likelihood ratio of 0.09 (95% CrI, 0.04 to 0.20). Only one study provided information on the high risk lesion underestimation rate (five cancers misclassified as high risk lesions among a total of six such lesions on core needle biopsy). No studies provided information on the DCIS underestimation rate.

Women at high risk of cancer: No studies provided information on the test performance (sensitivity, specificity, or underestimation rates) of freehand core needle biopsy techniques in women at high risk of breast cancer.

Ultrasound Guided Automated Device Core Needle Biopsies

Women at average risk of cancer: Twenty-seven cohorts of 16,287 biopsies used ultrasound guidance and an automated biopsy device. The summary sensitivity was 0.99 (95% CrI, 0.98 to 0.99) and the summary specificity was 0.97 (95% CrI, 0.95 to 0.98), corresponding to a positive likelihood ratio of 33.5 (95% CrI, 20.7 to 56.9) and a negative likelihood ratio of 0.01 (95% CrI, 0.01 to 0.02). Fourteen studies provided information on the DCIS underestimation; the summary rate was 0.38 (95% CrI, 0.26 to 0.51). Twenty-one studies provided information on high risk lesion underestimation; the summary rate was 0.25 (95% CrI, 0.16 to 0.36).

Women at high risk of cancer: No studies provided information on the test performance (sensitivity, specificity, or underestimation rates) of ultrasound-guided automated core needle biopsy techniques in women at high risk of breast cancer.

Ultrasound Guided Vacuum-Assisted Core Needle Biopsies

Women at average risk of cancer: Twelve cohorts of 1,543 biopsies used ultrasound guidance and a vacuum-assisted device to perform breast biopsies. The summary sensitivity was 0.97 (95% CrI, 0.92 to 0.99) and the summary specificity was 0.98 (95% CrI, 0.96 to 0.99), corresponding to a positive likelihood ratio of 57.7 (95% CrI, 25.8 to 138.7) and a negative likelihood ratio of 0.03 (95% CrI, 0.01 to 0.08). Five studies provided information on DCIS underestimation: the summary rate was 0.09 (95% CrI, 0.02 to 0.26). Nine studies provided information on high risk lesion underestimation: the summary rate was 0.11 (95% CrI, 0.02 to 0.33).

Women at high risk of cancer: No studies provided information on the test performance (sensitivity, specificity, or underestimation rates) of ultrasound-guided automated core needle biopsy techniques in women at high risk of breast cancer.

Stereotactically Guided Automated Device Core Needle Biopsies

Women at average risk of cancer: Thirty-seven cohorts of 9,535 biopsies used stereotactic guidance and an automated biopsy device. The summary sensitivity was 0.97 (95% CrI, 0.95 to 0.98) and the summary specificity was 0.97 (95% CrI, 0.96 to 0.98), corresponding to a positive likelihood ratio of 33.6 (95% CrI, 22.6 to 50.9) and a negative likelihood ratio of 0.03 (95% CrI, 0.02 to 0.05). Eighteen studies provided information on DCIS underestimation; the summary rate was 0.26 (95% CrI, 0.19 to 0.36). Twenty-nine cohorts provided information on high risk lesion underestimation; the summary rate was 0.47 (95% CrI, 0.37 to 0.58).

Women at high risk of cancer: One study reported information on the test performance of stereotactically guided automated core needle biopsy methods. Using model-based results, sensitivity was 0.97 (0.82 to 1.00) and specificity was 0.97 (0.91 to 0.99). No studies provided information on the underestimation rate of stereotactically guided automated core needle biopsy methods in women at high risk of breast cancer.

Stereotactically Guided Vacuum-Assisted Core Needle Biopsies

Women at average risk of cancer: Forty-three cohorts of 14,667 biopsies used stereotactic guidance and a vacuum-assisted device to perform core needle biopsies. The summary sensitivity was 0.99 (95% CrI, 0.98 to 0.99) and the summary specificity was 0.92 (95% CrI, 0.89 to 0.94), corresponding to a positive likelihood ratio of 12.8 (95% CrI, 9.4 to 17.9) and a negative likelihood ratio of 0.01 (95% CrI, 0.01 to 0.02). Thirty-four studies provided information on DCIS underestimation; the summary rate was 0.11 (95% CrI, 0.08 to 0.14). Forty studies provided information on high risk lesion underestimation; the summary underestimation rate was 0.18 (95% CrI, 0.13 to 0.24).

Women at high risk of cancer: Two studies provided information on the test performance of stereotactically guided vacuum assisted core needle biopsies. The summary sensitivity was 0.99 (95% CrI 0.93 to 1.00) and summary specificity was 0.93 (0.79 to 0.98). One of the two studies also reported that two cancer cases were underestimated by the biopsy diagnosis, among a total of 17 high risk lesions (for an underestimation rate of 12%).

MRI-Guided Automated Core Needle Biopsies

Women at average risk of cancer: Two cohorts reported data on the accuracy of MRI-guided biopsies performed with automated biopsy devices. The summary sensitivity was 0.90 (95% CrI, 0.58 to 0.99) and the summary specificity was 0.99 (95% CrI, 0.92 to 1.00), corresponding to a positive likelihood ratio of 62.3 (95% CrI, 9.4 to 726.3) and a negative likelihood ratio of 0.10 (95% CrI, 0.01 to 0.44). None of the studies provided information on the DCIS underestimation rate. One study provided information on the high risk lesion underestimation rate (one biopsy-detected high risk lesion was found to be malignant).

Women at high risk of cancer: Two cohorts provided information on the test performance of MRI-guided automated core needle biopsies among women at high risk for cancer. The summary sensitivity was 0.90 (95% CrI 0.57 to 0.99) and summary specificity was 0.99 (0.91 to 1.00). One of the two studies also reported that no cancers were diagnosed in the two women considered to have high risk lesions on core needle biopsy (i.e. no underestimation was observed in the study).

MRI-Guided Vacuum-Assisted Core Needle Biopsies

Women at average risk of cancer: One cohort reported data on the accuracy of MRI-guided biopsies performed with automated biopsy devices. All malignant lesions (n=3) were identified on pathologic examination of biopsy samples (model-based sensitivity 1.00, 95% CrI, 0.98 to 1.00); none of the nonmalignant lesions (n=7) were false positives (model-based specificity 0.91, CrI, 0.54 to 0.99). No cancer was diagnosed in the one woman considered to have DCIS on core needle biopsy (i.e. no DCIS underestimation was observed in the study). The study did not provide information on the high risk lesion underestimation rate.

Women at high risk of cancer: One cohort provided information on the test performance of MRI-guided vacuum-assisted core needle biopsies among women at high risk for cancer. The model-based sensitivity was 1.00 (95% CrI 0.98 to 1.00) and summary specificity was 0.92 (0.61 to 0.99). The study also reported that no cancers developed in the seven women considered to have high risk lesions on core needle biopsy (i.e. no underestimation was observed in the study).

Populations Biopsied with Multiple Core Needle Methods (or Other Methods)

Women at average risk of cancer: An additional 33 cohorts reported results from populations of women undergoing core needle biopsy with diverse methods. The majority of these studies (31 of 33) did not stratify their results by biopsy method (with respect to imaging guidance or use of vacuum); this group also included one study using grid guidance, and one study that did not report information on the use of vacuum assistance. In this heterogeneous group of studies, the summary sensitivity was 0.99 (95% CrI, 0.98 to 0.99) and the summary specificity was 0.96 (95% CrI, 0.93 to 0.97), corresponding to a positive likelihood ratio of 22.2 (95% CrI, 15.1 to 32.9) and a negative likelihood ratio of 0.01 (95% CrI, 0.01 to 0.02). Eighteen studies provided information on the DCIS underestimation; the summary DCIS underestimation rate was 0.22 (95% CrI, 0.15 to 0.30). Twenty-five studies provided information on high risk lesion underestimation; the summary underestimation rate was 0.32 (95% CrI, 0.23 to 0.41).

Women at high risk of cancer: No studies of high risk women were included in this subgroup.

Contextualizing the Results of Test Performance Meta-Analyses

To contextualize the results of the test performance meta-analyses presented in the preceding sections we evaluated the impact of testing in a hypothetical cohort of 1,000 women, under alternative scenarios for disease prevalence. Because delayed diagnosis on the basis of biopsy results is the most important (adverse) outcome related to testing we highlight here results based on false negative biopsies (and their complement, true positive biopsies) in Figure A. In populations with low cancer prevalence, the number of cases where treatment may be delayed on the basis of biopsy results (i.e., false negative biopsies) is expected to be small (e.g., for all ultrasound or stereotactically guided biopsy methods less than five out of 1,000 women, if prevalence is 10 percent or less). As prevalence increases the number of false negative results increases for all biopsy methods, but more rapidly for MRI-guided automated and freehand methods, which had the lowest sensitivity. However, results for MRI-guided automated methods were based on only six studies. Figure 4 also presents numerical results for a prevalence of 25 percent, which is approximately the prevalence of breast cancer among women referred for breast biopsy in the United States. All stereotactically and U.S.-guided methods, and MRI-guided vacuum assisted methods are expected to have fewer than ten false negative results (for every 1000 women undergoing biopsy), even when prevalence is as high as 0.30.

To illustrate the dependence of the number of true positive results among patients who are test positive by breast biopsy on the prevalence of disease, we calculated positive predictive values over a range of prevalences for different biopsy methods (Figure 5). These results suggest that even in low breast cancer prevalence settings (of 5 to 10 percent), 70 to 80 percent of women who test positive will truly have breast cancer for all tests except stereotactically and MRI-guided, vacuum-assisted biopsy methods. These two methods are associated with somewhat lower positive predictive values (approximately 50 to 60 percent) in low-prevalence settings, reflecting their lower specificity (compared to other tests). However, as the prevalence increases, the positive predictive value approaches 1 for all tests.

The above comparisons (test outcomes in a hypothetical cohort of known prevalence and positive predictive value calculations) can serve as aids for contextualizing the test performance meta-analysis results presented above. However, they do not reflect the uncertainty around the meta-analytic summary estimates. The following section presents the results of formal (indirect) comparisons among alternative core needle biopsy methods.

Figure 4. Outcomes of testing in a hypothetical cohort of 1,000 women

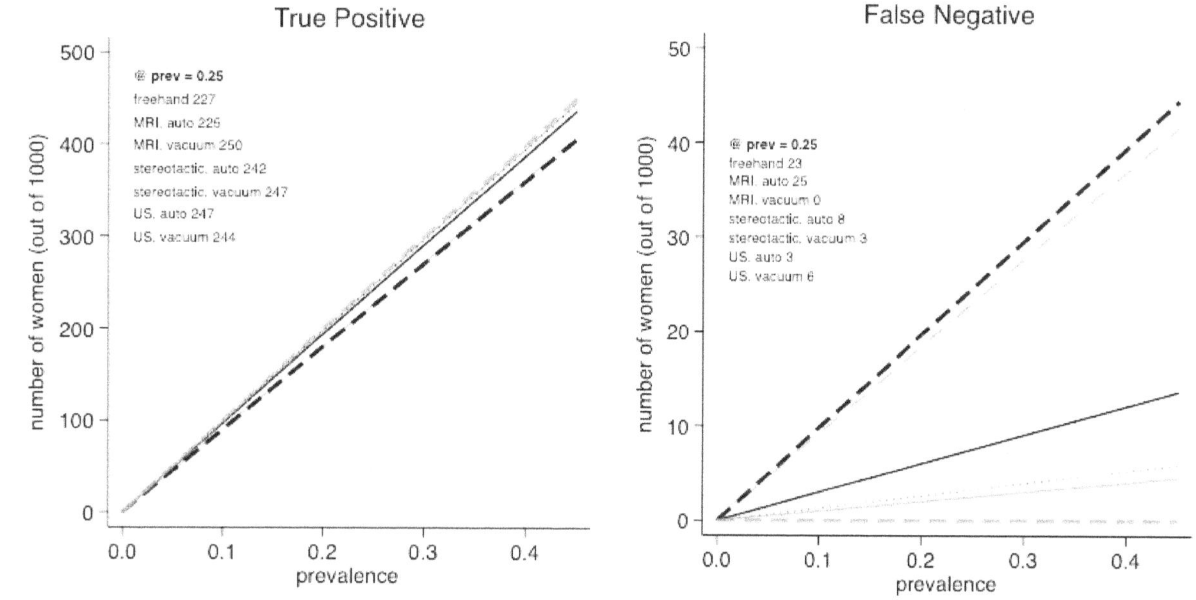

True Positive

@ prev = 0.25
freehand 227
MRI, auto 229
MRI, vacuum 250
stereotactic, auto 242
stereotactic, vacuum 247
US, auto 247
US, vacuum 244

False Negative

@ prev = 0.25
freehand 23
MRI, auto 25
MRI, vacuum 0
stereotactic, auto 8
stereotactic, vacuum 3
US, auto 3
US, vacuum 6

Lines correspond to different test modalities: grey dashed-dotted = freehand; black solid = stereotactically guided, automated; grey solid = stereotactically guided, vacuum-assisted; black dotted = US-guided, automated; grey dotted = U.S.-guided, vacuum-assisted; black dashed = MRI-guided, automated; grey dashed = MRI-guided, vacuum assisted.

Figure 5. Positive predictive value of alternative biopsy methods

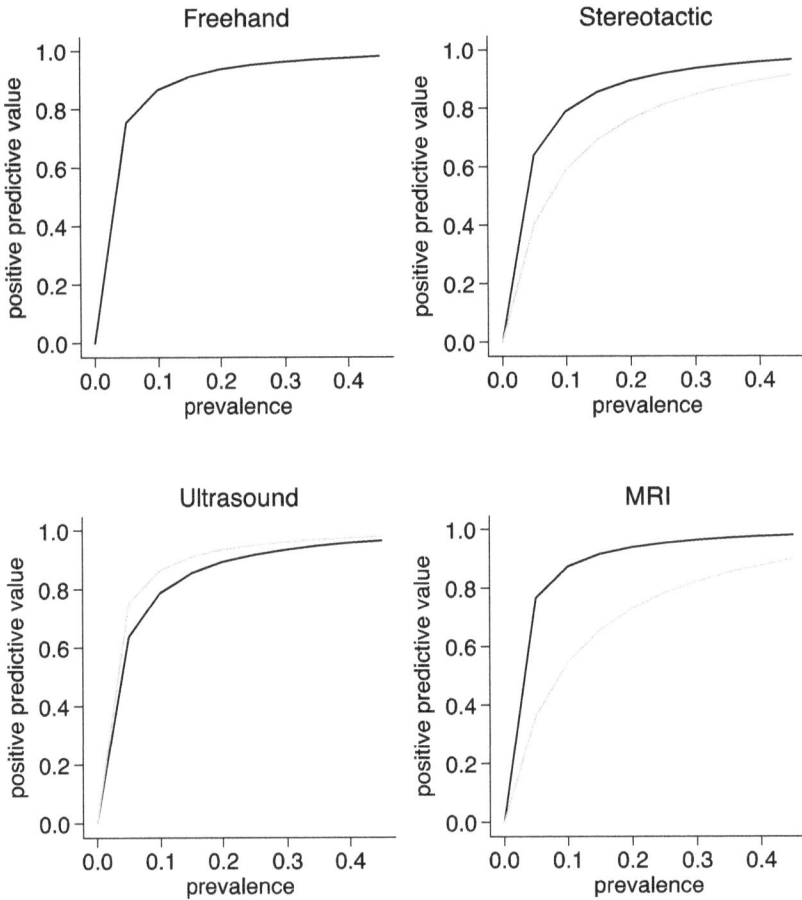

MRI = magnetic resonance imaging. Black lines are used for automated and gray lines for vacuum-assisted core needle biopsy methods.

Comparative Test Performance

To compare test performance across different biopsy methods we used indirect (meta-regression-based) comparisons. Table 5 presents comparisons between pairs of biopsy methods using the same imaging guidance for sensitivity and specificity. We only examined comparisons between biopsy methods using the same imaging modality because lesion characteristics (e.g., palpability, ability to visualize a lesions) strongly influence the choice of imaging modality. In general, differences among tests were relatively small: for example, differences in sensitivity or specificity never exceeded 0.1 (i.e., 10 percent absolute difference). Stereotactically guided automated biopsy had a specificity that was higher by 0.05 compared to vacuum-assisted biopsy methods, and a sensitivity that was 0.02 lower. Comparisons among MRI-guided biopsy methods were imprecise, reflecting the small number of available studies.

Table 5. Differences in sensitivity between pairs of biopsy methods (meta-regression based indirect comparisons)

Biopsy Methods Compared	Difference in Sensitivity	Difference in Specificity
US-guided, automated vs. vacuum-assisted	0.01 (-0.01, 0.06)	-0.01 (-0.03, 0.01)
Stereotactically guided, automated vs. vacuum-assisted	**-0.02 (-0.04, -0.01)**	**0.05 (0.02, 0.08)**
MRI-guided, automated vs. vacuum assisted	**-0.10 (-0.43, -0.01)**	0.07 (-0.03, 0.43)

All results are shown as medians of differences (95% CrI). Positive values denote that the method on the first-listed biopsy method has higher performance that the comparator (second listed method). CrIs that do not include the null value (0) are highlighted in bold. CrI = credible interval; MRI = magnetic resonance imaging.

Factors That Affect Test Performance

We considered evidence on the impact of patient or study level factors on test performance from two complementary sources: (1) within-study evidence (i.e. comparisons of test performance over levels of a factor within the patient population enrolled in a study) and (2) evidence from meta-regression analyses (that combine information across studies). Ideally, all studies would consistently report comparisons of test performance across well-defined subgroups (e.g., by patient, or lesion characteristics). Such within-study comparisons are more informative than comparisons across studies: factors related to study setting are common for all patients within the same study and other patient differences can be addressed (at least to some extent) by appropriate analytic methods (e.g., regression adjustment). In the absence of such information, one has to rely on indirect (across-study) comparisons that are generally less convincing because they cannot account for all differences across included populations. Overall, on the basis of both sources of information (within-study analyses and meta-regression analyses), we found that evidence was insufficient to support any specific factor as a modifier of test performance. Detailed results are presented below.

Within-Study Evidence

Twenty studies (14 identified by the original review and 6 included in the current update) of 11,280 patients provided information on factors that affect test performance. Specifically, 16 studies provided information on patient and lesion-related factors, 10 on procedural factors, and 3 on clinician and facility factors (some studies provided information on multiple factors). The majority of studies (140 of 160) did not allow investigation of the impact of any factors on test performance. The 20 included studies were reported inconsistently and often lacked details necessary for formal statistical assessment of the impact of various factors on test performance. These findings raise concerns regarding selective analysis and outcome reporting with respect to modifiers of test performance. Table 6 summarizes the findings of individual studies.

Table 6. Studies evaluating factors that may affect test performance (20 studies, reporting on multiple factors each)

Author, Year [PMID]	Biopsy Method	Factors Evaluated	Key Findings
Patient and lesion factors			
Cusick et al., 1990 [2183373]	Freehand	Lesion size	Smaller lesions (<2 cm in diameter) were more likely to be misdiagnosed.
Barreto et al. 1991 [2044776]	Freehand	Lesion size; Lesion location; Patient age	Tumor size did not affect the accuracy of the procedure. All lesions in the study were > 2 cm in diameter. Lesions in the right breast were more likely to be misdiagnosed. Patient age was not related to accuracy.
Makkun et al. 2011 [no PMID]	Ultrasound-guided automated device	Lesion type	The accuracy of biopsy in palpable lesions was 100%, while the accuracy of biopsy in nonpalpable lesions was 79.16%
Povoski et al. 2011 [21835024]	Ultrasound-guided automated device	Size of lesion; BI-RADS classification;	There was no difference between the median size of the lesion in cases of false negative biopsies and the median size in all cases biopsied. Among women undergoing interval followup after biopsy, the rate of false negatives was 0% for lesions initially classified as BI-RADS 3, 0.6% for lesions classified BI-RADS 4, and 2.8% for lesions classified BI-RADS 5.
Wiratkapun et al. 2012 [22252182]	Ultrasound-guided automated device	Patient age; breast density; lesion type; BI-RADS classification; lesion location	There was no statistically significant relationship between underestimation and patient age, breast density, lesion size, lesion visibility on mammography, lesion type (pure mass vs. mass with calcification), lesion BI-RADS classification (4 vs. 5). Lesions in the lower outer quadrant of the breast were more often underestimated. There was a tendency for younger women with larger mass lesions located at the lower quadrants of the breast and with BI-RADS 5 lesions not seen on mammography to have underestimated lesions.
Dahlstrom et al. 1996 [8735717]	Stereotactically guided automated device	Lesion type	There was no difference in the number of cores needed for diagnosis of microcalcifications, densities, or stellate lesions.
Koskela et al. 2005 [16020555]	Stereotactically guided automated device	Lesion type	There were zero false-negatives out of 97 procedures performed on masses on mammography, but 4 false-negatives out of 108 procedures performed on lesions with microcalcifications.
Walker et al. 1997 [no PMID]	Stereotactically guided automated device	Lesion type	The sensitivity of core needle biopsy was much lower for microcalcifications than for any other type of lesion.
Lomoschitz et al. 2004 [15273332]	Stereotactically guided, vacuum-assisted	Lesion type	Biopsies were equally accurate for lesions with microcalcifications and lesions detected as masses on mammography.
Pfarl et al, 2002 [12438044]	Stereotactically guided, vacuum-assisted	Lesion type	Biopsies were equally accurate for lesions with microcalcifications and lesions detected as masses on mammography.

Table 6. Studies evaluating factors that may affect test performance (20 studies, reporting on multiple factors each) (continued)

Author, Year [PMID]	Biopsy Method	Factors Evaluated	Key Findings
Reiner et al. 2009 [19565246]	Stereotactically guided, vacuum-assisted	Lesion type	The agreement rate between core needle biopsy and surgery was higher in nonpapillary lesions than in papillary lesions, but this difference was not statistically significant. 5 of 6 cases of underestimation occurred in papillary lesions, and the one false negative occurred in a nonpapillary lesion.
Venkataraman et al. 2012 [22127375]	Stereotactically guided, vacuum-assisted	Patient age; lesion size	There was no correlation between patient age and upgrade. However, there was a positive correlation between size of the lesion and upgrade.
Abdsaleh et al. 2003 [12630998]	Multiple methods	Patient breast density	Technical failures were more likely to occur in women with very dense breast tissue.
Ciatto et al. 2007 [16823506]	Multiple methods	Lesion type	False negative results were 2.7% for palpable lesions, 2.2% for nonpalpable lesions, 2.3% for masses on mammography, 1.4% for distortions on mammography, and 2.5% for microcalcifications.
Cipolla et al. 2006 [16473738]	Multiple methods	Lesion type	Correspondence between core needle biopsy and surgical biopsy results was 100% for palpable lesions but only 88% for nonpalpable lesions.
Fajardo et al. 2004 [15035520]	Multiple methods	Lesion type	Sensitivity was 97.4% for biopsies of masses detected on mammography and 90.7% for biopsies of nonpalpable lesions and lesions with microcalcifications.
Procedural factors			
de Lucena et al. 2007 [17663457]	Ultrasound-guided automated device	Number of cores	Taking >2 cores did not improve accuracy. Taking >2 cores did not reduce the rate of false negatives. The 6 tumors (out of 101) that were falsely diagnosed as benign by core needle biopsy would not have been correctly diagnosed even if up to six cores were taken.
Fishman et al. 2003 [12601206]	Ultrasound-guided automated device	Number of cores	Taking >2 cores improved the accuracy of the biopsy, with 4 cores being the optimal number. 1 case of DCIS would have been missed if fewer than 4 cores had been taken; the other 13 tumors identified in the study would have been correctly diagnosed if only 2 cores had been taken.
Kirshenbaum et al. 2003 [484822]	Ultrasound-guided automated device	Number of cores	1 core was diagnostic in 82.6% of cases, 2 cores in 90.5% of cases, 3 cores in 97.9% of cases, 4 cores in 98.9% of cases, and 5 cores in 100% of cases. 100% of malignant lesions were diagnosed after the fourth core.
Wiratkapun et al. 2012 [22252182]	Ultrasound-guided automated device	Number of cores	There was no statistically significant relationship between underestimation and number of biopsy cores.
Dahlstrom et al. 1996 [8735717]	Stereotactically guided automated device	Number of cores	One core was diagnostic in 71% of cases, two cores in 84% of cases, three cores in 90% of cases, four cores in 91% of cases, and five cores in 93% of cases.

Table 6. Studies evaluating factors that may affect test performance (20 studies, reporting on multiple factors each) (continued)

Author, Year [PMID]	Biopsy Method	Factors Evaluated	Key Findings
Koskela et al. 2005 [16020555]	Stereotactically guided automated device	Number of cores	Comment that more than three cores must be taken from lesions before an accurate diagnosis can be made.
Lomoschitz et al. 2004 [15273332]	Stereotactically guided, vacuum-assisted	Number of cores	12 cores were necessary for accurate diagnosis, but taking >12 cores did not improve accuracy.
Venkataraman et al. 2012 [22127375]	Stereotactically guided, vacuum-assisted	Number of cores	There was no correlation between number of cores and upgrade.
Abdsaleh et al. 2003 [12630998]	Multiple methods	Number of cores; breast density	Taking 2 cores instead of one increased the accuracy of the procedure. Technical failures were more likely to occur in women with very dense breast tissue.
Helbich et al. 1997 [9169689]	Multiple methods	Patient position	Patients were randomly assigned to undergo stereotactic biopsies in either seated or prone position. The accuracy data were not reported separately for each group, but the authors commented that patient position did not affect the biopsy procedure.

Clinician and facility factors

Barreto et al. 1991 [2044776]	Freehand	Operator experience	Operator inexperience appeared to be related to misdiagnosis.
Pfarl et al, 2002 [12438044]	Stereotactically guided, vacuum-assisted	Operator experience	For 6 of the seven false-negatives, the biopsy had been performed by an operator who had previously performed fewer than 15 stereotactic-guided biopsies.
Ciatto et al. 2007 [16823506]	Multiple methods	Operator experience	Sensitivity of core needle biopsies improved as the operators (radiologists) gained experience, from 88% in the first year of the study to 96% in the eighth year of the study.

BI-RADS = Breast Imaging-Reporting and Data System; PMID = PubMed identification number.

Meta-Regression Analyses

Meta-regression analyses were possible for the following factors: needle gauge, choice of reference standard, the proportion of lesions that were palpable, country where the study was performed, whether multiple centers contributed patients to a study, study design, and risk of bias. All models accounted for the biopsy method used (i.e., imaging guidance method and type of device) and the population's risk of cancer (average vs. high). Table 7 summarizes the findings of the meta-regression analyses. The credible intervals for all examined factors included the null value (indicating the lack of difference in sensitivity or specificity), with the exception of increased sensitivity in studies conducted in the United States (vs. any other country); and higher specificity in studies using followup of 6 to 24 months (as compared to studies using surgical pathology results for all patients) and studies with a prospective design (as compared to studies with a retrospective design). These results must be interpreted with caution, because they rely on indirect comparisons across studies. Furthermore, because these results represent odds ratios for test performance outcomes that are close to 1 (e.g., sensitivity and specificity for all tests were above 0.9), readers should keep in mind that small differences among subgroups of studies can result in (very) large odds ratio values. For example, if the summary sensitivities in two subgroups are 0.99 and 0.98, the odds ratio for sensitivity is approximately 2 ≈ (0.99/0.01)/(0.98/0.02).

Table 7. Meta-regression analysis for test performance outcomes

Modifier Category	Potential Modifier	Comparison	Relative Odds for Sensitivity (95% CrI)	Relative Odds for Specificity (95% CrI)
Biopsy procedure factors	Needle gauge	14G vs <14G	0.55 (0.12, 2.26)	1.59 (0.57, 5.41)
		≥15G vs. <14	0.35 (0.07, 1.66)	0.46 (0.12, 1.74)
		Unclear/NR vs. <14G	0.92 (0.28, 2.71)	**2.69 (1.12, 6.63)**
	Reference standard	≥2 yrs vs. open biopsy	1.84 (0.74, 4.35)	1.42 (0.75, 2.54)
		6mo to 2 yrs vs. open biopsy	1.59 (0.75, 3.49)	**1.84 (1.05, 3.35)**
Lesion factors	Lesion palpability*	>80% palpable lesions vs. ≤80%	1.04 (0.36, 2.88)	0.96 (0.37, 2.00)
		palpability NR vs. ≤80%	0.94 (0.36, 2.39)	0.93 (0.40, 1.88)
Clinician and facility factors	Country where the study was performed	United States vs. other countries	**1.79 (1.02, 3.15)**	0.96 (0.63, 1.49)
	Multicenter study	≥1 centers vs. single center	1.34 (0.49, 3.65)	1.11 (0.56, 2.29)
	Study design	Prospective vs. retrospective	1.36 (0.70, 2.73)	**2.11 (1.33, 3.37)**
		Unclear/NR vs. retrospective	0.95 (0.50, 1.88)	**2.07 (1.29, 3.30)**
Study risk of bias		Intermediate vs. high	0.56 (0.19, 1.52)	1.27 (0.61, 2.32)
		Low vs. high	0.56 (0.17, 1.67)	1.66 (0.78, 3.35)

*Excluding studies of freehand biopsy (because all lesions in such studies were palpable).
Relative odds for sensitivity compare the odds of a positive test result among patients with cancer over the levels of the modifier. Relative odds for specificity compare the odds of a negative test among patients without cancer over the levels of the modifier. Both metrics are obtained from the bivariate meta-analysis model and are exponentiated coefficients from logistic regression; thus, they can be interpreted as odds ratios. Results were adjusted for biopsy technique and baseline risk of breast cancer (high vs. average). CrI = credible interval; NR = not reported; yrs = years.

Risk of Bias Assessment for Studies Addressing Key Question 1

Overall, on the basis of 14 items related to risk of bias, we deemed 12 studies to be at low risk of bias, 111 to be at moderate risk of bias, and 37 to be at high risk of bias. Given our relatively strict selection criteria related to study design and completeness of followup, it is not surprising that the majority of studies reported enrolling consecutive or randomly selected patients (66 percent), were successful in enrolling 85 percent of all eligible patients (63 percent), and reported complete data on at least 85 percent of all enrolled patients (71 percent). However, only 41 percent of studies were judged to be free of spectrum bias, 68 percent were conducted retrospectively (or did not report relevant information), and 84 percent did not apply a "gold" standard reference test on all patients. In most studies (86 percent) the index test was interpreted by readers blinded to the reference standard test results. However, the vast majority of studies (99 percent) either did not provide information on whether index test results were available to interpreters of the reference standard or reported that blinding was not used. Finally, information on the incorporation of clinical information in the interpretation of the index and reference standard tests was judged inadequate in the majority of studies (99 percent for both items).

Key Question 2: In women with a palpable or nonpalpable breast abnormality, what are the adverse events (harms) associated with core needle breast biopsy compared to the open biopsy technique in the diagnosis of breast cancer?

This section summarizes findings from a total of 144 studies (70 new studies and 74 from the original evidence report) reporting information on at least one of the outcomes relevant to Key Question 2.[35, 39, 41, 42, 45-47, 49, 53, 58, 62, 63, 67, 73, 75, 78, 80, 82-84, 87, 91-93, 96, 98, 102-104, 107, 108, 110, 113, 117, 121, 123, 125-131, 135-137, 141, 143, 148-151, 153, 155, 157, 161-163, 165, 167, 168, 170, 173-176, 178, 181, 182, 184, 186-188, 190, 192-261]

Overall, studies were considered to be of low to moderate risk of bias. Of note, 76 of the 160 core needle biopsy studies included in Key Question 1 did not provide any information on adverse events, and thus do not allow us to determine whether any adverse events were observed (and not reported). As such, they are uninformative for this Key Question. Further, selective outcome reporting was considered likely for all adverse events examined, because of the large proportion of studies with unclear or missing data.

Adverse Events of Open Biopsy

Very few of the included studies reported information about complications associated with open surgical biopsy. The original evidence report reported findings from a study published in 1993 and a narrative review published in 2007. The study found that 10.2 percent of a series of 425 wire-localized open biopsy procedures were complicated by vasovagal reactions.[235] The narrative review reported that 2 to 10 percent of breast surgeries are complicated by hematoma formation, and that 3.8 percent are complicated by infections.[250] The original evidence report also identified two studies on core needle biopsy with information on adverse events of open biopsy. One study reported that 6.3 percent of open surgical biopsies were complicated by infections.[192] A second study reported that 2.1 percent of open biopsy procedures were complicated by the development of an abscess, but none of the 234 ultrasound-guided vacuum-assisted core needle procedures had abscess development.[125] Finally, we found one study reporting that four of 100 surgical biopsies required repeat biopsy compared to two of 100 vacuum-assisted core needle biopsies[35] and one study reporting low levels of pain with open biopsy when local lidocaine was used.[259]

Adverse Events of Core Needle Biopsy

We identified 141 studies reporting information on at least one of the adverse events of interest following core needle biopsy (69 new studies and 72 from the original evidence report). Of these studies, 26 reported information related to the dissemination or displacement of cancerous cells during the biopsy procedure, and 112 allowed for the calculation of event rates for hematomas, bleeding, vasovagal reactions, and infections. Table 8 summarizes information for the incidence of these adverse events. Overall, their incidence was low: in more than 50 percent of studies reporting information, the percentage of patients experiencing each of the aforementioned outcomes was less than 2 percent; in 75 percent of studies the event rate was less than 1 percent for infections, less than 5 percent for bleeding and vasovagal reactions, and less than 9 percent for hematoma formation. Results for these outcomes, stratified by biopsy technique, are discussed below. Information on less commonly reported adverse events (including seeding) is summarized narratively in the following sections.

Table 8. Adverse events associated with core needle biopsy for breast cancer diagnosis

Outcome	Number of Studies*	Number of Procedures	Median % of Procedures Where an Event Was Observed (25th – 75th percentile)	Minimum-Maximum Percentage of Procedures Where an Event Was Observed
Hematoma	58	32,584	1.44 (0.25-8.57)	0.00-100.00
Bleeding	46	21,545	1.21 (0.33-3.97)	0.00-100.00
Bleeding requiring treatment	47	22,600	0.00 (0.00-0.14)	0.00-6.45
Infection	40	25,688	0.00 (0.00-0.33)	0.00-2.91
Vasovagal reaction	39	14,482	1.27 (0.37-3.88)	0.00-10.90

*Number of studies providing information on the outcome
max = maximum; min = minimum; perc. = percentile.

Hematomas and Bleeding

Fifty-eight studies including 32,584 core needle biopsy procedures reported information on hematoma formation. In 50 percent of these studies the event rate for hematomas was less than 1.44 percent, and in 75 percent the event rate was less than 8.57 percent. The highest rates of hematoma formation were observed in studies of vacuum-assisted procedures. For example, in 75 percent of studies of ultrasound-guided vacuum-assisted procedures, the event rate for hematomas was 23.24 percent or greater, while no hematomas were reported in three studies of ultrasound-guided biopsies without vacuum assistance. The median hematoma event rate for studies of stereotactic-guided vacuum-assisted biopsies was 1.59 percent, whereas the maximum event rate in studies of stereotactic-guided biopsies without vacuum-assistance was 1.25 percent. Due to incomplete (and potentially selective) reporting, these percentages should be interpreted with caution; however, vacuum-assisted procedures do appear to have a higher rate of hematoma formation than other core needle biopsy methods. Eight cohorts (reported in a total of 5 studies) of ultrasound-guided vacuum-assisted biopsy identified for this update reported that in 1,487 procedures only one hematoma required surgical intervention.[219] The event rates in these studies was similar to the event rate for hematomas requiring treatment calculated across 24 studies included in the original evidence report. No other newly identified studies reported information on the number of hematomas requiring treatment.

Forty-six studies of 21,545 core needle biopsy procedures reported information on bleeding. In 50 percent of these studies the event rate for bleeding was less than 1.21 percent, and in 75 percent the event rate was less than 3.97 percent. In 25 percent of studies of stereotactic-guided vacuum-assisted procedures the event rate for bleeding was 3.75 percent or greater, while the maximum event rate reported in studies of stereotactic-guided biopsies without vacuum assistance was 1.55 percent. The highest event rate in studies of ultrasound-guided vacuum-assisted biopsy was just under 8 percent, while the single study of ultrasound-guided biopsy without vacuum assistance that contained information on bleeding reported an event rate of 5.26 percent. With the same caveats as for hematoma formation, vacuum-assisted procedures appeared to be associated with bleeding more often than nonvacuum-assisted procedures. Overall, bleeding was a rare complication. In addition to the studies reporting bleeding, we identified one study in which 19 percent of 1177 patients undergoing ultrasound guided vacuum-assisted biopsy had skin ecchymosis without hematoma.[219] One study of stereotactic-guided vacuum-assisted biopsy identified in our updated searches reported that of 485 women biopsied, one patient was observed in the hospital for one day due to persistent bleeding. A second study of stereotactic-guided vacuum-assisted biopsy identified in our updated searches reported that of 64 women undergoing stereotactic-guided vacuum-assisted biopsy, one patient required surgery to stop bleeding.[170] The event rates in these two studies are consistent with the 0.34 percent of vacuum-assisted procedures reported in the previous report to be complicated by bleeding that required treatment. No other newly identified studies reported information on bleeding events that required treatment. Overall, 47 studies provided information on bleeding events that required additional treatment; more than half of the studies reported than no bleeding events requiring treatment were observed and the rate was lower than 0.14 percent in 75 percent of the studies.

Nine studies of various core needle techniques that were included in the original report specified that bruising occurred after core needle biopsy procedures. Three of the nine reported that bruising was a common event, two reported that approximately 50 percent of patients had bruising, and four studies reported that 45 out of 976 patients (4.6%) had severe bruising. We identified two additional studies that reported information on bruising. One study of stereotactic-guided biopsy without vacuum assistance noted that 1.2 percent of 200 patients reported tenderness, swelling or bruising at the biopsy site following the biopsy.[67] The second study reported that 2 of 101 patients undergoing stereotactic vacuum-assisted biopsy experienced mild bruising that resolved without treatment.[207]

Table 9 summarizes information on hematomas and bleeding (total and cases requiring treatment), stratified by biopsy technique.

Table 9. Core needle biopsy procedures and rates of hematoma formation and bleeding

Outcome	Biopsy Technique	N Studies	Number of Procedures	Median % of Procedures Where an Event Was Observed (25th to 75th percentile)	Minimum-Maximum Percentage of Procedures Where an Event Was Observed
Hematoma formation	all devices	58	32,584	1.44 (0.25-8.57)	0.00-100.00
	freehand, automated	2	1,487	0.00-0.00	
	US, automated	3	937	0.00-3.24	
	US, vacuum-assisted	8	3,291	13.20 (3.76-23.24)	0.99-36.27
	stereotactic, automated	5	1,706	0.97 (0.77-1.00)	0.00-1.25
	stereotactic, vacuum-assisted	22	12,345	1.59 (0.69-8.57)	0.00-100.00
	MRI, automated	2	116	NA	1.33-4.88
	MRI, vacuum-assisted	1	58	NA	43.10
	other	15	12,644	1.07 (0.00-7.20)	0.00-79.12
Bleeding	all devices	46	21,545	1.21 (0.33-3.97)	0.00-100.00
	freehand, automated	3	1,732	NA	0.14-3.97
	US, automated	1	190	NA	NA
	US, vacuum-assisted	6	2,251	2.52 (1.14-4.95)	0.70-7.84
	stereotactic, automated	5	1,144	0.48 (0.00-1.29)	0.00-1.55
	stereotactic, vacuum-assisted	19	13,584	0.78 (0.30-3.75)	0.14-26.94
	MRI, automated	0	0	NA	NA
	MRI, vacuum-assisted	1	10	0.00	0.00
	other	11	2,634	2.10 (0.44-4.24)	0.00-100.00
Bleeding requiring treatment	all devices	47	22,600	0.00 (0.00-0.14)	0.00-6.45
	freehand, automated	3	1,732	NA	0.00-0.00
	US, automated	2	1,152	NA	0.00-0.00
	US, vacuum-assisted	7	2,321	0.00 (0.00-1.14)	0.00-4.95
	stereotactic, automated	3	496	NA	0.00-0.00
	stereotactic, vacuum-assisted	18	13,452	0.00 (0.00-0.20)	0.00-3.03
	MRI, automated	0	0	NA	NA
	MRI, vacuum-assisted	1	10	0.00	NA
	other	13	3,437	0.00 (0.00-0.00)	0.00-6.45

We only report the minimum and maximum percentage of events when three or fewer studies were available for a biopsy technique. When a single study reported information we simply list the percentage of procedures associated with complications. MRI = magnetic resonance imaging; NA = not applicable; US = ultrasound.

Infections

Across 40 studies, including 25,688 core needle procedures, the median percentage of infectious complications was 0.00 percent. One study, identified by the original evidence report, reported that a patient developed an abscess that required surgical treatment in a series of 268 stereotactically guided vacuum-assisted procedures.[168] One study identified by this update reported that 2 of 118 patients undergoing stereotactic vacuum-assisted biopsy developed infections that required antibiotics.[248] Table 10 summarizes information on infections, stratified by biopsy technique.

Table 10. Core needle biopsy procedures and rates of infectious complications

Biopsy Technique	N Studies	Number of Procedures	Median % of Procedures Where an Event Was Observed (25th – 75th percentile)	Minimum-Maximum Percentage of Procedures Where an Event Was Observed
All devices	40	25,688	0.00 (0.00-0.33)	0.00-2.91
Freehand, automated	3	1,637	NA	0.00-2.00
US, automated	4	1,675	0.05 (0.00-0.92)	0.00-1.74
US, vacuum-assisted	4	1,962	0.00 (0.00-0.99)	0.00-1.98
Stereotactic, automated	10	2,321	0.00 (0.00-0.63)	0.00-2.91
Stereotactic, vacuum-assisted	9	4,803	0.00 (0.00-0.20)	0.00-0.89
MRI, automated	0	0	NA	NA
MRI, vacuum-assisted	0	0	NA	NA
Other techniques	10	13,290	0.10 (0.00-0.26)	0.00-2.20

We only report the minimum and maximum percentage of events when three or fewer studies were available for a biopsy technique. MRI = magnetic resonance imaging; NA = not applicable; US = ultrasound.

Pain and Use of Pain Medications

The original report identified three vacuum-assisted biopsy procedures reported to have been terminated after patients complained of severe pain, and we identified one study of 4086 stereotactic-guided vacuum-assisted procedures in which four biopsies were suspended due to pain.[233] No studies reported procedure termination due to patient complaints of pain in any other types of biopsy procedures. Twenty-five studies of a wide variety of biopsy methods reported information about patient pain during the procedure (pain was assessed heterogeneously and for that reason we did not calculate overall event rates).

Eleven studies reported information on the use of pain medications. One of these studies reported that 100 percent of patients were sent home with narcotics after an open biopsy procedure, and only three patients required narcotics after a core needle procedure.[102] Twenty patients were reported to have required acetaminophen after a core needle procedure.[125] Note that being sent home with a medication may not necessarily mean the patients required or used the medication.

Vasovagal Reactions

Thirty-nine studies with 14,482 procedures reported information about the occurrence of vasovagal reactions (fainting or near-fainting) during core needle biopsy. The median event rate in these studies was 1.27 percent, although one study reported an event rate of nearly 11 percent. More than 40 percent of the vasovagal reactions occurred in patients who were reported to have been positioned sitting upright for the biopsy procedure (many of the studies did not report patient position so the other 60 percent of vasovagal reactions could have occurred in patients positioned in a variety of positions, or could have occurred primarily in seated patients).

Table 11 summarizes information on vasovagal reactions, stratified by biopsy technique.

Table 11. Core needle biopsy procedures and rates of vasovagal reactions

Biopsy Technique	N Studies	Number of Procedures	Median % of Procedures Where an Event Was Observed (25th – 75th percentile)	Minimum-Maximum Percentage of Procedures Where an Event Was Observed
All devices	39	14,482	1.27 (0.37-3.88)	0.00-10.90
Freehand, automated	1	1,431	NA	0.00-0.00
US, automated	2	235	NA	0.53-8.89
US, vacuum-assisted	3	2,532	NA	0.43-1.43
Stereotactic, automated	12	1,978	1.44 (0.51-3.47)	0.00-8.33
Stereotactic, vacuum-assisted	13	5,843	1.90 (0.34-5.41)	0.00-10.90
MRI, automated	0	0	NA	NA
MRI, vacuum-assisted	1	10	NA	0.00
Other techniques	7	2,453	1.78 (0.99-2.20)	0.00-3.47

We only report the minimum and maximum percentage of events when three or fewer studies were available for a biopsy technique. When a single study reported information we simply list the percentage of procedures associated with complications. MRI = magnetic resonance imaging; NA = not applicable; US = ultrasound.

Impact of Biopsy Procedure on Usual Activities and Time to Recovery

Three studies provided information on the impact of biopsy procedures on usual activities. The first study reported that of 34 women undergoing ultrasound-guided vacuum-assisted breast biopsy, 16 (47%) women stated that the procedure did not interfere with usual activity, 14 (41%) stated that there was minor interference, and four (12%) felt that there was mild interference.[125] The second study reported four cases in which the patient felt constrained in her daily life due to the procedure.[216] The third study reported vacuum-assisted biopsy results in less psychological/physical stress when compared to surgical procedures.[35]

A single study provided information regarding time to recovery, measured by asking patients how long it had taken for them to return to their normal activities after the biopsy procedure.[80] This study reported that the average time of recovery was 3.5 days for open biopsy procedures and 1.5 days for stereotactically guided automated gun core needle biopsy procedures.

Impact of Biopsy Procedure on Subsequent Mammographic Procedures

Five studies reported information about the impact of core needle biopsies on subsequent mammographic examinations. Three studies reported on stereotactic-guided vacuum-assisted core needle procedures. These studies enrolled 3,748 patients, of whom 3,345 (89.2%) were reported to have no mammographically visible scarring after the biopsy procedure. Only seven of the patients were reported to have scars that were potentially diagnostically confusing on subsequent mammographic procedures. In the fourth study, 91 patients underwent stereotactic- or ultrasound-guided vacuum-assisted core needle biopsy. The researchers reported that at 6-month followup there was no evidence of scarring, architectural distortion, alterations of the skin, fat necrosis, or other changes that are frequently observed after surgical breast biopsy.[216] In the fifth study, patients underwent mammography at 6 or 12 months, and the authors reported that mammograms showed structural distortions at the biopsy site in the 100 women who underwent surgical biopsy, and no sequelae in the 100 women who received vacuum-assisted core needle biopsy.[35]

Miscellaneous Reported Adverse Events

The original report identified eight studies with information on pneumothorax, seizures, vomiting, or acute inflammation, and we identified one additional study reporting vomiting and one additional study reporting inflammation. Four studies of 2,600 patients reported that four cases of pneumothorax, none of which required treatment, had occurred. None of these four studies used the same core needle biopsy method. Two studies reported that one patient per study (out of 3,487 patients in total) had suffered a seizure during a stereotactic-guided vacuum-assisted procedure. One study of 268 patients undergoing stereotactic-guided vacuum-assisted biopsies reported that three patients developed acute inflammation at the biopsy site after the procedure. One study of 485 women undergoing stereotactic-guided vacuum-assisted biopsies reported that two patients developed signs of inflammation judged to be mastitis. Two studies reported that a patient vomited during the procedure; one of these studies was of 185 stereotactic-guided vacuum-assisted procedures and the second was of 236 vacuum-assisted procedures using either stereotactic or ultrasound guidance. We did not identify any new studies reporting any other significant adverse events associated with core biopsy procedures.

Dissemination and Displacement of Cancerous Cells During the Biopsy Procedure

To address the potential dissemination or displacement of cancerous cells by breast biopsy we did not use the study-design evaluation criteria for Key Questions 1 and 2; instead, we considered any clinical study that addressed the topic (including case reports and case series). Full details of the included studies are available in SRDR.

We reviewed 14 studies that used histopathology to demonstrate dissemination or displacement of cells by core needle biopsy procedures (four new studies and 10 studies included in the original report). Nine studies had a cohort design, and five were case series or case reports.

The percentage of needle tracks previously reported to contain displaced cancerous cells ranged from 0 to 65 percent. We identified a cohort study that reported that the percentage of ultrasound-guided biopsies with cancerous cells in the needle wash material ranged from 33 percent to 69 percent.[244] The original report observed that the risk of finding displaced cancerous cells was increased by greater duration of the biopsy procedure,[230] multiple needle passes,[243] and a short interval between core needle biopsy and surgical excision,[205] while the risk was decreased by diagnosis of invasive lobular carcinoma[243] and the use of vacuum-assisted core needle biopsy.[205] The incidence of positive cytological findings in needle wash material was also greater with multiple needle passes and automated device (versus vacuum-assisted) biopsy.[244]

Although the clinical significance of these displaced cancerous cells is debated,[205] we found four case reports of patients developing tumors at the site of prior core needle biopsies, which supplement the six case reports previously identified for this review.[199, 201, 218, 224, 246] Four of these ten women were reported to have not received radiation therapy for the primary tumor; for the other six women it was not reported whether they had received radiation therapy.

The previous evidence report found four studies with 1,879 women that explored the risk of tumor recurrence following biopsy.[202, 208, 220, 221] Three of these four studies reported that women who did not have a preoperative needle biopsy had a higher rate of tumor recurrence than women who did receive a preoperative needle biopsy;[202, 208, 221] the fourth study reported the opposite. We identified an additional cohort study, published in 2011, that reported no development of tumors along the needle track among more than a thousand women receiving a core needle biopsy diagnosis of cancer in early 2008 through 2009.[253] The majority of the women in the original four studies were treated with breast-conserving surgery and radiation therapy; the newly identified fifth study did not report whether women received radiation therapy.

The original evidence report found three studies with 3,103 women that investigated the risk of seeding the lymph nodes with cancerous cells after biopsy procedures.[210, 232, 234] Two of the three studies reported that the method of biopsy did not affect the rate of positive sentinel lymph nodes; the third study reported that the rate of metastases to the sentinel lymph node was higher in women who underwent some form of preoperative biopsy. We found two new studies examining the topic of epithelial cell displacement into lymph nodes after biopsy. One study described 15 cases of epithelial cell displaced into the lymph node subcapsular sinus in a series of axillary lymph node dissections taken approximately 2 weeks after either core needle or open breast biopsy.[200] The authors stated that this was probably the result of mechanical transport of cells during biopsy and that the clinical implications are likely not significant. The second study examined epithelial displacement into lymphovascular spaces in the breast core needle biopsy specimens of seven women who were diagnosed with pure DCIS after core needle biopsy and surgical excision.[222] These women did not have recurrences or metastases after 24 to 84 months followup. The authors suggest that because this epithelial displacement is seen in the initial core biopsy sample, the presence of tumor cell clusters in lymphovascular spaces may not reflect lymphovascular invasion.[197]

The original evidence report identified a case series report of 25 cases of false-positive sentinel lymph nodes, in which the false-positives appeared to be caused by displacement of benign epithelial cells during a biopsy procedure.[197] Twelve of the false-positive cases had undergone core needle biopsy prior to the sentinel lymph procedure, 12 had undergone wire-localization open biopsy, and one had undergone a fine-needle aspiration procedure. Findings of false-positive sentinel lymph nodes are clinically important because the findings are likely to lead to adverse events from unnecessary treatment. Because 22 of the 25 cases had intraductal papilloma at the biopsy site, the authors of the case series report suggested using caution when interpreting sentinel lymph node histopathology in cases where intraductal papilloma was noted during the initial biopsy procedure.

Factors That Modify the Association of Biopsy Procedures With Adverse Events

Due to the small number of studies providing information on any of the factors of interest and the poor reporting of adverse events across studies, we believe that the evidence is insufficient to establish any specific factor (other than patient positioning for vasovagal events and the use of vacuum for bleeding, as discussed in preceding sections) as a determinant of the rate of adverse events among women undergoing biopsy for breast cancer diagnosis. Information extracted from individual studies is summarized in Table 12.

Table 12. Studies evaluating factors that may affect the incidence of adverse events

Author, Year [PMID]	Biopsy Technique	Factors Evaluated	Key Findings
Patient and lesion factors			
Lin et al., 2000 [not indexed]	Ultrasound guided vacuum-assisted	Breast density	Among 8 women with hematomas and pre-biopsy mammograms, 75% had breasts classified as dense. No patients with breasts classified as fatty developed hematomas.
Wang et al., 2012 [21300503]	Ultrasound guided vacuum-assisted	Lesion size	No statistically significant difference was observed in mean lesion size for cases with and without hematoma.
Zografos et al. 2008 [18814132]	Stereotactic-guided vacuum-assisted	BI-RADS classification, patient age	There was no statistically significant association between hematoma formation and BI-RADS classification or patient age.
Frank et al., 2007 [17661855]	Stereotactic-guided automated gun	Patient age	Pain was not associated with patient age (p=0.11).
Chetlen et al., 2013 [23789678]	Multiple methods	Medications received at the time of biopsy	Non–clinically significant hematomas developed in 22 of 102 (21.6%) procedures performed on patients taking antithrombotic medications vs. 67 of 515 procedures (13.0%) performed on patients not on antithrombotic therapy. The probability of development of a non–clinically significant hematoma was 21.6% in association with antithrombotic therapy and 13.0% without anti-thrombotic therapy (p = 0.025). This finding was confirmed in multivariable logistic regression analysis. The mean log volume of hematoma in patients taking antithrombotics did not differ significantly from that in patients not taking antithrombotics (p = 0.126). In analyses adjusted for needle size, the association of antithrombotic treatment with log volume remained nonstatistically significant (p = 0.07).
Procedural factors			
McMahon et al. 1992 [1422715]	Freehand	Needle gauge	18G core needle procedure were associated with significantly less pain than 14G core needle procedures, but there was no significant difference in pain between 14G and 16G procedures.
Wong and Hisham 2003 [484085]	Freehand	Needle gauge	No difference in the amount of pain experienced by patients undergoing a 14G core needle procedure vs. a 16G core needle procedure.
Zagouri et al., 2011 [21709018]	Stereotactic-guided vacuum-assisted	Number of cores	In women who underwent additional sampling (96 cores vs. the standard 24-36), the rate of clinically significant hematomas doubled from 3.5% to 7.5%.
Frank et al., 2007 [17661855]	Stereotactic-guided automated gun	Number of cores, duration of procedure	Pain was associated with the number of biopsy cores (p=0.032) and the duration of the procedure (p=0.046).

Table 12. Studies evaluating factors that may affect the incidence of adverse events (continued)

Author, Year [PMID]	Biopsy Technique	Factors Evaluated	Key Findings
Schaefer et al., 2012 [22381441]	Multiple methods	Needle gauge; biopsy device	There were significantly higher rates of bleeding (p<0.001) and hematoma (p=0.029) in the Mammotome 8G than in the Mammotome 11G group. There were no significant differences in bleeding rates (p=0.799) or hematoma rates (p=0.596) between the ATEC 12G and the ATEC 9G group. There were no significant differences in bleeding or hematoma rates in the Mammotome 8G group and the ATEC 9G group, but there was less bleeding (p=0.015) and fewer hematomas (p=0.001) in the Mammotome 11G group than in the ATEC 12G group.
Seror et al., 2012 [21310570]	Multiple methods	Needle gauge/probe	There was no difference in pain with different probe sizes (12 mm, 15 mm, and 20 mm).
Szynglarewicz et al., 2011 [21367573]	Multiple methods	Vacuum-assistance; biopsy device	Biopsy with an automated device was significantly more painful than biopsy with a vacuum-assisted hand-held device (p<0.01).
Chetlen et al., 2013 [23789678]	Multiple methods	Needle gauge; number of cores	The proportion of hematoma formation after biopsy with 9G needles was 29.5% vs. 3.6% after biopsy with 12G or 14G needles (the difference was statistically significant and remained significant in multivariable logistic regression analysis). The mean log volume of hematoma comparing larger versus smaller gauge needles was not statistically significantly different (p = 0.08). In analyses adjusted for antithrombotic treatment, the association of needle size with log volume became statistically significant (p = 0.048). The paper stated that the mean and median numbers of tissue samples obtained from patients who developed and those who did not develop a hematoma were not statistically significantly different. However the reported p-values were both statistically significant (p < 0.001). The authors noted that the number of tissue samples was strongly correlated with needle gauge.
Clinician and facility factors			
Kirshenbaum et al., 2003 [12876040]	Multiple methods	Operator experience	The majority of vasovagal reactions occurred when inexperienced operators performed the biopsy procedures.

PMID = PubMed identification number.

Key Question 3: How do open biopsy and various core needle techniques differ in terms of patient preference, availability, costs, availability of qualified pathologist interpretations, and other factors that may influence choice of a particular technique?

We identified 59 new studies[35, 41, 43, 49, 62, 78, 86, 96, 118, 121, 134, 137, 138, 142, 163, 170, 174, 198, 206, 211, 213, 217, 226, 229, 236, 239, 255, 259, 262-292] that addressed various aspects of KQ3. Together with the 84 studies[39, 42, 46, 47, 50, 54, 58, 73, 75, 91, 104, 107, 115-117, 125, 127, 141, 143, 149, 167, 181, 182, 184, 188, 230, 249, 293-349] included in the original evidence report, this section synthesizes evidence from 143 studies. Generally, our findings confirmed those of the original evidence report. In the following subsections, we first discuss aspects of diagnostic biopsy important to patients, followed by economic factors that may influence the choice of a particular technique, and then proceed to summarize information on other factors, including the availability of equipment, procedure duration time, time to complete tumor removal, wait time for test results, and recurrence rates. Because of the nature of this Key Question and the heterogeneity of the sources of information used to address each outcome of interest, we did not attempt to grade the strength of evidence for most outcomes considered for this Key Question (this is consistent with the original evidence report).

Anxiety and Distress

We identified 12 studies[35, 121, 198, 211, 226, 266, 268, 276, 281, 282, 286, 288] that looked at levels of anxiety and distress related to biopsy procedures. This outcome was not specifically examined in the original report, and we base our conclusions on the studies retrieved for this update. Overall, patients reported increased levels of anxiety and distress immediately before or during the procedure, and these levels were reduced after the procedure. One study reported mean anxiety levels just before the procedure to be well above normal on State Trait Anxiety Inventory (STAI) (mean 48; normal=35.9), Impact of Event Scale (mean 26; normal < 8.5), Center for Epidemiological Studies-Depression Scale (mean 16; normal 8), and Perceived Stress Scale (mean 19; normal=12.6).[268] This was corroborated by a second study that reported participants prebiopsy STAI-S and STAI-T T scores were two standard deviations higher than the mean T score (T-score mean 50, SD 10).[281] Yet another study reported that one procedure out of 602 could not be completed because of patient anxiety.[121] One study found greater anxiety in surgical biopsy patients than in those receiving core needle vacuum-assisted biopsies.

Four studies,[226, 266, 282, 288] three of which were randomized controlled trials, looked at a range of options to ameliorate stress during core needle biopsy procedures, with relaxation, medication, empathy, and hypnosis all showing reductions in stress either just before or during the procedure. One randomized controlled trial reported on stress levels in three groups of patients (those receiving usual care, relaxation, or medication to reduce anxiety). All three groups had preprocedural state anxiety levels that were significantly higher than normal and reported significant reductions in anxiety 24 hours after the procedure. Patients in the medication group reported significantly less anxiety during the procedure, when compared with the usual care and relaxation groups.[266] They also reported that there was no statistically significant difference in anxiety levels during the procedure for those who underwent stereotactically guided versus ultrasound-guided procedures.[266] A second randomized controlled trial looked at the use of empathy and hypnosis in relieving anxiety. The authors found that standard care patients experienced an increase in anxiety during the procedure, patients who were given empathy experienced no change in anxiety during the procedure, and patients receiving hypnosis experienced a decrease in anxiety during the procedure. A final randomized controlled trial reported that the main effect of an education intervention on anxiety was that those in the control group tended to have lower postconsultation anxiety than those in the education group.

Procedure Preference

We found two studies[198, 286] that specifically addressed procedure preference in addition to the 20[39, 46, 58, 73, 91, 125, 181, 182, 299, 303, 304, 306, 309, 311, 312, 317, 321, 322, 331, 347] in the original evidence report. Both of the new studies reported a positive experience with core needle biopsy, relative to surgical biopsy. One study reported that women who had previously experienced only core needle or surgical biopsy were willing to wait a median of 3.2 weeks longer to avoid surgical than to avoid core needle biopsy; while women who had experienced both were willing to wait 2.4 weeks longer to avoid surgical than to avoid core needle biopsy.[286] This supports the findings of the original report: the majority of studies reported core needle biopsies to be preferable to open biopsies. However, a single study reported the reverse: a survey of 59 patients (20 open biopsy, 20 fine needle aspiration, and 19 core needle biopsy) from Detroit, Michigan in 1997 and 1998 found that 90 percent were satisfied with their open surgical biopsy compared to only 80 percent satisfied with a vacuum-assisted core needle biopsy, though the authors reported that this difference was not statistically significant at the p=0.05 level.[299] The original evidence report also noted that the majority of the studies reported such information as that the patients tolerated the procedure well or would recommend it to others in the future. One study reported that 99 percent of image-guided core needle biopsy patients rated their overall experience as positive and 97 percent said they would recommend the center to a family member or friend if they needed a biopsy.[198] Another study reported that patients preferred the decubitus position to the prone position.[182] Two studies reported that vacuum-assisted procedures were more comfortable than other types of core needle biopsies.[317] Two other studies reported that patients lost less time to core needle procedures than to open procedures.[309]

Surgical Procedures Avoided

We identified 12 new studies[35, 49, 86, 96, 118, 137, 170, 263, 269, 274, 289, 290] providing information on the number of surgical procedures avoided by the use of core needle biopsy methods for breast cancer diagnosis. Including the 30 studies[42, 47, 50, 58, 115-117, 143, 167, 293-295, 297, 304, 305, 308, 319, 320, 324, 325, 327, 329, 332, 335, 340, 342, 344-346, 349] considered in the original report, a total of 42 studies provide information on this outcome. In general, studies found that core needle biopsy obviated the need for surgery for a substantial proportion of women, ranging from 29 to 87 percent. Of the 42 studies, ten reported comparisons against open surgical biopsy with respect to the number of patients requiring only one surgical procedure (vs. more than one). Meta-analysis of these studies suggested that the odds of requiring only one surgical procedure were almost 15 times higher among women receiving core needle biopsy; odds ratio = 14.8 (95% CrI, 7.2 to 50.2). This result should be interpreted with caution because of the possibility of confounding by indication. Women may have been selected for a specific diagnostic approach on the basis of clinical or other factors, which may also be associated with the need for additional surgical interventions.

Cosmetic Results

We identified three new studies that addressed cosmetic results[62, 239, 255] with core needle or open biopsy. Two reported that core needle biopsy produced minimal scars that were acceptable to the patients, and the third reported that vacuum-assisted core needle biopsy produced "better cosmetic effects compared to open excision."[255] The original evidence report identified 10 other studies[46, 104, 125, 143, 181, 299, 306, 322, 331, 347] that included information on cosmetic results for vacuum-assisted core needle biopsy and reported that patients were generally satisfied with the cosmetic results. Only one of the 10 studies included in the original report compared a group of patients undergoing core needle biopsy to a group of patients undergoing open biopsy.[299] This study reported a greater satisfaction with appearance of the breast 2 years after surgery in core needle patients (95 percent very satisfied) than in open biopsy patients (25 percent very satisfied).[299]

Resource Utilization and Costs

We found two additional studies on the relative costs of core needle biopsy.[134, 290] The results below reflect a total of ten studies, including eight studies identified in the original report.[107, 188, 310, 313, 330, 333, 339, 341] The original report concluded that the costs of surgical biopsy are considerably greater than those of core needle biopsy. In this update we identified one study (2008) reporting average charges for core needle biopsy at $10,500 and excision biopsy at $11,500.[290] The authors based their costs on the calculation of mean patient charges for initial diagnostic procedure and subsequent necessary surgeries, which were compared for patients undergoing biopsy for BI-RADS-5 lesions between 1998 and 2002. The authors recommend core needle biopsy as the initial diagnostic approach for highly suspicious lesions, based upon improved pathologic margins and fewer surgical procedures rather than significant costs savings.

Another study compared per-procedure costs of core needle biopsy and fine needle biopsy. Based on reimbursements for facility fees, but excluding professional fees, the costs were $477.92 versus $166.34, respectively.[134]

The original evidence report reported on the relative costs of open surgical biopsy and various core needle biopsy techniques in six studies. The studies reviewed factors that included purchase price of devices, personnel time and costs, the costs of processing and analyzing samples, patient volume, whether the device is used as a complementary procedure, and what mammography results determine the use of a core needle biopsy technique. The original report also noted that MRI-guidance is the most expensive method of performing core needle biopsies.[350] We did not find any new studies comparing the costs or cost-effectiveness of different core needle or imaging techniques.

We did not identify any new studies for resource utilization. The two studies discussed in the original evidence report[188, 330] stated that vacuum-assisted procedures and procedures that required dedicated prone tables required more physician and room time.

Physician Experience

We identified seven new studies,[265, 271, 277-279, 283, 285] which, together with the 10 studies included in the original report,[127, 141, 188, 303, 314, 315, 323, 326, 336, 338] support the conclusions that greater experience with particular devices improves accuracy, shortens procedure duration times, and leads to a decrease in the number of open biopsies. One study reported a trend that indicated that in a training program, the fellows were able to establish an accurate diagnosis with fewer core biopsy samples in their later cases (i.e. as the training progressed and they gained experience).[265] A second study introduced a training program for breast lesion excision system biopsy, for which they reported that fellows who had previous experience in vacuum-assisted biopsy could perform the new procedure after four procedures (median), while those without previous exposure showed proficiency after nine procedures (median). This was compared to the

12 procedures required for a new user to become proficient with vacuum-assisted biopsy.[278] A survey of 79 fellows who had graduated from approved breast fellowships between 2005 and 2009 reported that many physicians feel poorly prepared to do ultrasound-guided (41 poorly prepared; 16 moderately prepared; 22 well prepared) or stereotactic (57 poorly prepared; 7 moderately prepared; 15 well prepared) core needle biopsies.[285] A report of data from the National Accreditation Program for Breast Centers showed that the two most common deficiencies for breast centers were in standards for ultrasound-guided biopsy (24 of 238 centers failed) and for stereotactic core needle biopsy (17 of 238 centers failed).[279] Two new studies reported on the effects of training programs. The first reported that residents performed 83 percent of vacuum-assisted biopsies and 86 percent of core needle biopsies successfully after a training program and that their comfort level increased at least one level.[271] The other showed that surgeon-directed, multi-year, quality improvement workshops across 12 hospitals improved preoperative core biopsy rates.[277]

Availability of a Qualified Pathologist

We did not identify any new studies for this outcome. The two studies included in the original report showed conflicting results, with one reporting that whether the specimen was read by a local or central pathologist had little effect as agreement rates were very high,[300] and the second reporting that the pathologist's lack of experience with the TruCut device explains its poor performance.[311]

Availability of Equipment/Utilization

The original report identified three studies reporting on the impact of equipment availability and utilization,[301, 344, 348] to which we added four[217, 284, 288, 289] more for a total of seven. The original report concluded that wait times are longer for open procedures and dedicated prone biopsy tables. We found a randomized controlled trial that reported that patients who waited 4 days or more for a core needle biopsy procedure were less satisfied than patients who waited 3 days or less (p=0.007).[288] We did not find any new studies reporting the overall wait times for core needle biopsies or comparing wait times for core needle vs. open biopsy procedures. Other studies looked at utilization rates of core needle biopsies over time. One study reported that the nonoperative diagnosis rates in core needle biopsy had increased from 49 percent in 1995/96 to 87 percent in 2000/01 to 94 percent in 2005/06.[289] A second study reported that with a stable total patient population and constant number of open and needle-localized procedures, stereotactic breast biopsies had increased from 56 in 1995 to 68 in 1996, 118 in 1997, and 172 in 1998.[217] They further reported that diagnostic yield had increased in the stereotactic era.[217] A third study reported a similar increase in core needle biopsy utilization between January 1992 and March 1998, with a corresponding decrease in open biopsies.[284]

Procedure Duration Time

We identified an additional 17 studies[41, 43, 78, 121, 137, 138, 163, 174, 206, 211, 213, 226, 236, 259, 270, 275, 287] that reported results for procedure duration across various types of biopsy. When these studies are added to the 40 studies[39, 42, 46, 47, 50, 54, 58, 73, 75, 91, 141, 143, 149, 181, 182, 184, 188, 230, 249, 296, 298, 302, 303,

[307, 309, 316-318, 323, 326, 328, 330, 331, 333, 334, 337, 338, 343, 347, 349] identified in the original evidence report, reported procedure times range between 3 and 128 minutes. This large range is probably the result of different definitions for procedure time. For example, one study reported times for "total procedure" (from signing of informed consent to end of preparation for next patient) as 26.7 minutes for ultrasound guided core biopsy and 47.5 minutes for stereotactic core biopsy; "room time" (from signing of informed consent to end of procedure) as 23.1 minutes for ultrasound guided core biopsy and 36.5 minutes for stereotactic core biopsy; and "physician time" (time radiologist located lesion to time enough samples had been obtained) as 12.3 minutes for ultrasound guided core biopsy and 18.6 minutes for stereotactic core biopsy.[287]

Mean procedure times for ultrasound-guided core needle biopsies ranged from 3 to 60 minutes, based on 11 original[39, 50, 91, 143, 188, 303, 309, 316, 330, 337, 343] and five new studies,[206, 213, 226, 270, 287] while stereotactically guided core needle procedures tended to take longer, with mean procedure times ranging from 10 to 100 minutes (15 original[42, 46, 54, 58, 75, 91, 141, 175, 181, 182, 296, 316, 317, 330, 349] plus five new studies [137, 174, 211, 236, 287]). Twelve studies (four new[41, 43, 78, 163] and eight from the original report[149, 249, 323, 326, 328, 333, 334, 338] studies) gave mean times for MRI-guided procedures, ranging from 8 to 70 minutes.

Vacuum-assisted core biopsies had reported mean or median durations of 3 to 70 minutes, based on 28 studies (19 original[39, 42, 46, 58, 143, 181, 230, 249, 298, 302, 303, 323, 326, 328, 330, 331, 333, 334, 347] and 9 new[41, 43, 121, 137, 138, 206, 213, 236, 287]). Two studies gave mean times for open procedures, ranging from 40 to 45 minutes depending on tumor size.[259, 298]

Time to Complete Tumor Removal

We identified nine studies[142, 229, 262, 264, 267, 272, 273, 280, 290] that reported results for time in days from biopsy to surgery for tumor removal. There were no studies addressing this specific outcome in the original report. Overall times from biopsy to tumor removal ranged from 5 to 153 days. One study directly compared wait times for core needle and surgical biopsies, reporting an average time from initial procedure to final surgical procedure for core needle biopsy as 27 days and excisional biopsy as 22 days.[290] The rest of the studies gave results for core needle biopsy only, with means ranging from 14 to 62 days and medians ranging from 9 to 83 days. One study reported that the implementation of a Rapid Diagnosis and Support Program reduced the time from biopsy to surgery from 51.54 to 33.36 days.[262] A second study reported that excisional biopsy is a factor in the increase in delays between first physician encounter and surgery from 1992 to 2005.[264]

Wait Time for Test Results

We found seven studies that discussed wait times for core needle biopsy results.[142, 198, 262, 272, 273, 291, 292] There were two studies included in the original report, for a total of nine studies addressing this outcome. Overall, core needle wait times ranged from 1 to 114 days, with most reported as between 1 and 1.3 days. The two studies in the original report that compared wait times after core needle and open biopsies showed that wait times for core needle biopsy results are shorter by an average of 7 to 10 days. One study reported that using a microwave processor (a nonstandard processing method that is not in widespread use) to reduce wait times for test results reduced the average wait for results ($P<0.001$).[142] Another study reported that the implementation of a Rapid Diagnosis and Support Program reduced wait times from 3.92 to 3.35 days.[262] One study looked specifically at the reasons for diagnostic delays that exceeded 90 days and found that many diagnostic delays were the result of false negative results that were caused by sampling errors.[291] Two studies assessed patient satisfaction with wait times. One found that most participants (88 percent) thought the wait for test results (usually the day after the biopsy by phone) was reasonable.[198] The other reported an improvement in patient satisfaction scores sense of timeliness of provision of diagnostic test results from 4.5 (of 5) before the implementation of the Rapid Diagnosis and Support Program to 4.75 after its implementation.[262]

Recurrence Rates

We found one study that discussed recurrence rates among core needle biopsy patients.[213] In this study, 143 lesions in 86 patients were completely excised using an ultrasound-guided Mammotome system. Excision was considered complete when a fluid-filled cavity or air bubbles were demonstrated by ultrasound. Of these 143 lesions, only one lesion recurred within six months. A second biopsy showed breast adenosis, the same diagnosis as the original biopsy.

Discussion

Key Findings and Assessment of the Strength of Evidence

In this update of the 2009 Comparative Effectiveness Review on breast biopsy methods we synthesized evidence from a total of 316 studies (128 new studies and 188 from the original report). We found few studies providing information on the test performance of open surgical biopsy. In contrast, the evidence base on core needle biopsy methods now includes a large number of studies reporting on almost 70,000 breast lesions. This allowed us to assess the comparative performance of tests (when using the same type of imaging guidance), in addition to updating the 2009 report's evaluation of the performance of individual biopsy methods. Tables E-G summarize our assessment of the strength of evidence. Following the original evidence report, and in view of the paucity of evidence on open surgical biopsy, we refrained from rating the strength of evidence for this technique for all Key Questions. For Key Questions 1 and 2, we assessed the strength of evidence by integrating our (subjective) judgments on the risk of bias of included studies, the consistency of their findings, the directness of the available data, and the precision of quantitative results. For Key Question 3 we only rated the strength of evidence for the outcome of additional surgical procedures required after biopsy. We did not rate the strength of evidence for other Key Question 3 outcomes because of the diversity of designs employed and outcomes addressed (see the Methods section for our approach to rating the strength of evidence). Interested readers should consult Appendix D for the detailed assessment of the strength of evidence.

Test Performance and Comparative Test Performance

Among women at average risk of cancer, core needle biopsy using ultrasound or stereotactic guidance had average sensitivities ranging from 0.97 to 0.99 and average specificities ranging from 0.92 to 0.98. Freehand biopsy methods appeared to have lower average sensitivity (0.91) compared to other methods, but similar specificity (0.98). Stereotactically guided automated techniques were associated with lower sensitivity and higher specificity compared to stereotactically guided vacuum-assisted methods. Although these results were fairly precise, they were derived from indirect comparisons across studies of moderate to high risk of bias. MRI-guided biopsies were evaluated in only six studies with small sample sizes, leading to substantial uncertainty around estimates of test performance. Table 13 summarizes our assessment of the strength of evidence for alternative biopsy methods in women at average risk of cancer and for comparisons among biopsy methods using the same imaging guidance modality. Of note, we rated the strength of evidence on both *absolute* and *comparative* test performance, whereas the original report considered *absolute* test performance only.

We did not find a difference in test performance between women at low and high risk of breast cancer. Because the number of studies of women at high risk of cancer was small, comparisons of test performance between low and high risk women had substantial uncertainty and results were not sufficient to support definitive conclusions. Evidence on modifiers of test performance was also sparse for all biopsy methods, raising concerns about selective outcome and analysis reporting.

Table 13. Strength of evidence about comparative test performance in women at average risk of breast cancer

Outcome	Comparison or Biopsy Method	Overall Rating	Key Findings and Comments
Test performance of individual biopsy methods	Freehand	Low	– Sensitivity: 0.91 (0.80 to 0.96) – Specificity: 0.98 (0.95 to 1.00)
	Ultrasound, automated	Moderate	– Sensitivity: 0.99 (0.98 to 0.99) – Specificity: 0.97 (0.95 to 0.98)
	Ultrasound, vacuum-assisted	Moderate	– Sensitivity: 0.97 (0.92 to 0.99) – Specificity: 0.98 (0.96 to 0.99)
	Stereotactically guided, automated	Moderate	– Sensitivity: 0.97 (0.95 to 0.98) – Specificity: 0.97 (0.96 to 0.98)
	Stereotactically guided, vacuum-assisted	Moderate	– Sensitivity: 0.99 (0.98 to 0.99) – Specificity: 0.92 (0.89 to 0.94)
	MRI-guided, automated	Insufficient	– Sensitivity: 0.90 (0.57 to 0.99) – Specificity: 0.99 (0.91 to 1.00)
	MRI-guided, vacuum-assisted	Insufficient	– Sensitivity: 1.00 (0.98 to 1.00) – Specificity: 0.91 (0.54 to 0.99)
Comparison of test performance among alternative biopsy methods	Ultrasound-guided, automated vs. vacuum-assisted	Low	– Difference in sensitivity: 0.01 (-0.01 to 0.06) [no difference] – Difference in specificity: -0.01 (-0.03 to 0.01) [no difference]
	Stereotactically guided, automated vs. vacuum-assisted	Low	– Difference in sensitivity: -0.02 (-0.04 to -0.01) [vacuum-assisted is better] – Difference in specificity: 0.05 (0.02 to 0.08) [automated is better]
	MRI-guided, automated vs. vacuum-assisted	Insufficient	– Difference in sensitivity: -0.10 (-0.43 to -0.01) [vacuum-assisted is better] – Difference in specificity: 0.07 (-0.03 to 0.43) [no difference]
Modifiers of test performance for women at average and high risk of breast cancer	All biopsy methods	Insufficient	– Few studies provided within-sample information for each modifier of interest; meta-regression results rely on cross-study comparisons so consistency of effects cannot be assessed – Within-study (direct) evidence was sparse; between study evidence relied on indirect comparisons across studies – In meta-regression analyses CrIs were wide; extreme odds ratio values were often observed because sensitivity and specificity for all tests were very close to 1 (see Results)

CrIs = credible interval; MRI = magnetic resonance imaging.

Underestimation Rates

Underestimation rates varied among alternative biopsy methods and were often imprecisely estimated because of the relatively small number of lesions contributing data for these analyses. In general, underestimation was less common with stereotactically guided vacuum-assisted biopsy methods, as compared to stereotactically or ultrasound-guided automated methods. Our assessment of the strength of evidence for this outcome is summarized in Table 14.

Table 14. Strength of evidence for underestimation rates in women at average risk of cancer

Outcome	Comparison or Biopsy Method	Overall Rating	Key Findings and Comments
DCIS underestimation	Ultrasound-guided, automated	Low	– Average underestimation probability: 0.38 (0.26 to 0.51) [14 studies]
	Ultrasound-guided, vacuum-assisted	Low	– Average underestimation probability: 0.09 (0.02 to 0.26) [5 studies]
	Stereotactically guided, automated	Low	– Average underestimation probability: 0.26 (0.19 to 0.36) [18 studies]
	Stereotactically guided, vacuum-assisted	Low	– Average underestimation probability: 0.11 (0.08 to 0.14) [34 studies]
	Other biopsy methods	Insufficient	No available studies or few studies with small numbers of lesions.
High risk lesion underestimation rate	Ultrasound-guided, automated	Low	– Average underestimation probability: 0.25 (0.16 to 0.36) [21 studies]
	Ultrasound-guided, vacuum-assisted	Low	– Average underestimation probability: 0.11 (0.02 to 0.33) [9 studies]
	Stereotactically guided, automated	Low	– Average underestimation probability: 0.47 (0.37 to 0.58) [29 studies]
	Stereotactically guided, vacuum-assisted	Low	– Average underestimation probability: 0.18 (0.13 to 0.24) [40 studies]
	Other biopsy methods	Insufficient	No available studies or few studies with small numbers of lesions

DCIS = ductal carcinoma in situ.

Adverse Events and Additional Surgeries After Biopsy

In general, adverse events were reported inconsistently, raising concerns about selective outcome and analysis reporting. Few studies provided information on the harms of open surgical biopsy. Core needle biopsy was only infrequently associated with serious adverse events or adverse events requiring additional treatment. Comparisons between open and core needle biopsy are based on indirect comparisons and expert opinion, with limited empirical evidence. Open biopsy appeared to be associated with an increased incidence of adverse events (including serious adverse events) compared to core needle biopsy. Our assessment of the strength of evidence for adverse events is summarized in Table 15.

Among core needle biopsy methods, vacuum-assisted methods appeared to be associated with increased bleeding and hematoma formation. Sitting upright during the biopsy procedure was associated with more vasovagal reactions. Information about the dissemination or displacement of cancer cells during the biopsy procedure was provided by a small number of studies with various designs. Cancer cell seeding along the needle tract was a rare outcome. Studies reported that women were generally satisfied with the cosmetic results of core needle procedures.

Women diagnosed with breast cancer by core needle biopsy were able to have their cancer treated with a single surgical procedure, more often than women diagnosed by open surgical biopsy. Although the magnitude of this association was large (the ratio of the odds was almost 15), women and their physicians are likely to choose biopsy methods on the basis of factors (e.g., lesion location, or characteristics of the lesion on imaging) that may also be associated with the need for additional surgeries. Thus, confounding by indication is likely, and we rated the strength of evidence for this association as moderate. A difference in the rate of additional surgeries among women diagnosed with alternative biopsy methods is likely, but we have less confidence that it is an effect of the biopsy methods *per se* or that the magnitude of the difference is known.

Table 15. Strength of evidence assessment for adverse events of biopsy

Outcomes	Test or Comparison	Overall Rating	Key Findings
Bleeding (any severity)	Alternative core needle biopsy methods	Low	– Median %: 1.21 (25th perc. = 0.33; 75th perc.= 3.97) – Selective outcome and analysis reporting likely – Few studies reported bleeding requiring treatment; the event rate was low (<0.40 perc.) in those studies
Bleeding events that require treatment	Alternative core needle biopsy methods	Low	– Median %: 0 (25th perc. = 0; 75th perc.= 0.14) – Selective outcome and analysis reporting likely – Few studies reported bleeding requiring treatment; the event rate was low
Hematoma formation	Alternative core needle biopsy methods	Low	– Median %: 1.44 (25th perc. = 0.25; 75th perc.= 8.57) – Selective outcome and analysis reporting likely
Infectious complications	Alternative core needle biopsy methods	Low	– Median %: 0 (25th perc. = 0; 75th perc.= 0.33) – Selective outcome and analysis reporting likely
Vasovagal reactions:	Alternative core needle biopsy methods	Low	– Median %: 1.27 (25th perc. = 0.37; 75th perc.= 3.88) – Potential for selective outcome and analysis reporting
Pain and severe pain	Alternative core needle biopsy methods	Low	25 studies of a wide variety of biopsy methods reported information about patient pain during the procedure (pain was assessed heterogeneously across studies).
Other adverse events	Alternative core needle biopsy methods	Insufficient	– Most events were reported by a single study precluding assessment of consistency – Individual studies did not provide adequate information for precise estimation of the event rate) – Only informal indirect comparisons among biopsy methods were possible – Selective outcome and analysis reporting likely
Modifiers of adverse events – vasovagal reactions	Sitting upright during the biopsy procedure	Low	– Vasovagal reactions were more common among patients sitting during the biopsy procedure – Results were reported in few studies (11 studies; 8 from the original evidence report and 3 from this update) – Selective outcome and analysis reporting likely
Modifiers of adverse events – bleeding	Vacuum-assisted versus nonvacuum assisted biopsy methods	Low	– Vacuum-assisted procedures were generally associated with increased rates of bleeding and hematoma formation – Bleeding events were generally uncommon – Comparisons among biopsy methods were based on informal indirect comparisons (across studies) – Selective outcome and analysis reporting likely
All other modifiers of adverse events	Comparisons among alternative core needle biopsy methods	Insufficient	– Most factors assessed by a single study limiting our ability to assess consistency – Selective outcome and analysis reporting likely – Within-study comparisons provided direct evidence

perc. = percentile.

Limitations of the Evidence Base

We believe that the evidence regarding the performance of core needle biopsy for diagnosis of breast lesions is limited in the following ways:

- Published evidence on the test performance and adverse events of open surgical biopsy was sparse.
- Available studies, particularly for Key Questions 1 and 2, were at moderate to high risk of bias and the publications we reviewed did not follow the Standards for Reporting of Diagnostic Accuracy (STARD) guidelines.[351] Information on patient selection criteria, patient or lesion characteristics (e.g., granular reporting of pathology results), was often missing or inconsistently reported. Information on adverse events and patient-relevant outcomes was often incomplete, potentially selectively reported. Studies did not use standardized definitions and ascertainment methods for adverse events. Pathology results

were not reported with adequate granularity in the majority of cases.
- Studies typically used lesions (or biopsy procedures) as the unit of analysis, instead of patients. This way, patients with multiple lesions contributed multiple observations to the analyses. Lesions belonging to the same patient are likely to have similar characteristics (i.e. they are correlated). Unfortunately, studies reported results in a way that did not allow for the correlation to be accounted for in our statistical models. As such, our analyses (and those of the original report) assume independence among lesions. If the correlation among lesions in the same patient is high (positive and close to one) individual study and meta-analytic results will underestimate uncertainty and may also be biased (the direction of bias is unpredictable). However, unless each patient contributes large numbers of lesions that are highly correlated, the underestimation of uncertainty will not be large. Further, bias is unlikely unless patients contributing large numbers of lesions also have lesions that are substantially harder (or easier) to diagnose compared to those of other patients. Without additional data on the test performance on individual lesions within patients it is not possible to ascertain the impact of this factors on our results.
- Studies provided limited information to assess the impact of various patient-, lesion-, procedure-, or system- related factors on the outcomes of breast biopsy. For example, the impact of patient age, breast density, lesion type, training and experience of the operators, and error rates of pathologists who read the samples, on test performance, adverse events, or clinical outcomes could not be assessed.
- We found very few studies on MRI-guided biopsy for women at average or high risk of cancer. Because MRI-guided biopsy is likely reserved for diagnostically challenging cases (e.g., when lesions cannot be visualized by other modalities) and may be available in specialized care settings indirect (i.e. across studies) comparisons between MRI-guided and other biopsy procedures may be confounded by factors unrelated to the diagnostic value of the tests compared.
- There is limited information on the comparative effectiveness of alternative biopsy methods on patient-relevant outcomes, resource use and logistics, and availability of technology and expertise for different core needle biopsy techniques.

Strengths and Limitations of This Review

We conducted an up-to-date review of the benefits and risks of breast biopsy methods for breast cancer diagnosis, with respect to test performance, underestimation rates, adverse events, and patient-relevant outcomes. Previous reviews on this topic have focused on special patient populations (e.g., patients with nonpalpable lesions), selected outcomes (e.g. DCIS underestimation[352] or seeding[353]), or biopsy methods (e.g., ultrasound-guided biopsy[354]). Nonetheless, our work has several limitations, which – to a large extent – reflect the limitations of the underlying evidence base. Studies were deemed to be of moderate to high risk of bias because of characteristics related to their design and conduct, limiting our ability to draw strong conclusions. Information for several outcomes of interest was not reported from all available studies (e.g., underestimation rates, adverse events) raising concerns about selective outcome and analysis reporting. Information on study- or population level characteristics that could be modifiers of test performance, adverse events, or clinical outcomes, was inadequate. Thus, our ability to explore between-study heterogeneity was limited. Further, because we relied on published information and did not have access to individual patient data, we were unable to evaluate the impact of patient- or lesion-level factors on outcomes of interest.

The reference standard in the reviewed studies was a combination of clinical followup and pathologic confirmation (following open biopsy or excisional surgery). We assumed that these diagnostic methods have negligible measurement error (i.e., that they represent a "gold" standard). It is unlikely that this assumption is exactly true (e.g., some degree of diagnostic error is possible for pathologic examination, and clinical followup may provide less than perfectly accurate information). However, we believe that the error rate of the reference standard is low enough that its influence on our estimates is unlikely to be substantial.

Applicability of Review Findings

The existing evidence base on core needle biopsy of breast lesions in women at average risk of cancer appears to be applicable to clinical practice in the United States. Studies enrolled patients with an average age similar to that of women undergoing breast biopsy in the United States, and for indications that represent the most prevalent indications in U.S. clinical practice (i.e. mammographic findings of suspicious lesions). While fewer than half of the studies in this review were conducted in the United States, almost all were carried out in either the United States or in industrialized European or Asian countries where core-biopsy methods are likely sufficiently similar to those used in the United States. However, the applicability of our findings to women at high risk of breast cancer may be limited because we found few studies explicitly reporting on groups of patients at high baseline risk of breast cancer on the basis of factors such as genetic testing, or family history of disease. Of note, this may be an instance of incomplete reporting rather than a true characterization of the baseline risk of included populations (i.e. some high risk populations may have been misclassified as "average risk").

Evidence Gaps and Ongoing Research

Table 16 summarizes the evidence gaps with regards to the Key Questions of diagnostic test performance and adverse events. A search on ClinicalTrials.gov for randomized trials comparing alternative biopsy methods did not identify trials examining biopsy techniques for breast cancer diagnosis (last search: Dec 5, 2013; 141 records retrieved).

Table 16. Evidence gaps for biopsy methods for the diagnosis of breast cancer

Key Question	Category	Evidence Gap
Comparative effectiveness of core needle biopsy and open surgical biopsy	General	Limited information on the diagnostic test performance of open surgical biopsy was available. However, expert opinion and research studies consider open biopsies to have very low measurement error (but not exactly zero).
	Population	Limited information for women specified to be at high baseline risk of breast cancer.
	Interventions & Comparators	Limited information on MRI-guided biopsy methods (all patient populations). For other biopsy methods a large body of evidence was available; however studies were at moderate to high risk of bias and poorly reported.
	Outcomes	Information on underestimation rates was relatively limited. Pathology results were not reported using consistent or sufficiently granular classification schemes.
	Modifiers of test performance	Optimal core needle biopsy method for specific subgroups of patients, lesion characteristics.

Table 16. Evidence gaps for biopsy methods for the diagnosis of breast cancer (continued)

Key Question	Category	Evidence Gap
Adverse events of core needle biopsy and open surgical biopsy	General	Information for adverse events of interest was incompletely and (potentially) selectively reported.
	Interventions & Comparators	Evidence comparing the adverse events of open and alternative core needle biopsy methods was limited.
	Outcomes	Limited information was available for key adverse events of interest. Reporting in existing studies was inconsistent and potentially selective. Outcome ascertainment was not standardized.
	Modifiers of adverse events	Information on factors that affect the incidence of adverse events is sparse. Unclear what subgroups of patients and lesions may be most likely to experience adverse events.
Patient-relevant and resource-related outcomes	General	Comparative effectiveness information among alternative biopsy techniques (both open and core needle) was very sparse and indirect. Comparisons between methods are susceptible to confounding and selection bias.
	Population	Evidence is limited both for women at average and high risk of breast cancer.
	Outcomes	The balance of benefits and risks associated with alternative breast biopsy with respect to clinical outcomes, quality of life, and resource use has not been comprehensively assessed.

MRI = magnetic resonance imaging.

Future Research Needs

- Studies of test performance are needed to evaluate MRI-guided biopsy methods. Ideally, these studies will be large (powered to achieve adequate precision), prospectively designed, multicenter investigations enrolling patients representative of those seen in clinical practice. Patient selection criteria and the characteristics of included populations should be reported in detail. Studies should use standardized histological classification systems for pathological classification the specialty and experience of those performing the biopsy procedure should be reported. The reference standard for test negative cases should be regular monitoring for an adequate period of time (e.g., 2 years).
- Although a large number of studies were available for other core needle biopsy methods we believe that additional well-designed and fully reported prospective cohort studies are needed, primarily for addressing questions about the impact of patient-, lesion-, procedure-, or system-level factors on test performance, adverse events, and patient-relevant outcomes. Given that a large number of core needle biopsies are performed annually in diverse settings, such studies could be conducted at relatively low cost.
- Large-scale databases of prospectively-collected observational data on breast biopsy procedures and outcomes could be used to evaluate the effectiveness of alternative biopsy methods with respect to short and long term outcomes, and potential modifying factors. Such studies would need to collect detailed information on baseline factors that may be associated with both the choice of biopsy method and the outcomes of interest (e.g., lesion size, palpability, imaging characteristics, etc.), to adjust for potential confounding factors. Comparisons across methods should be performed only among patients that would be candidates for assessment with all methods being compared.
- In all future studies, baseline risk of cancer development should be characterized using consistent and widely accepted criteria to allow appropriate subgroup analyses.

- We believe that a randomized comparison of alternative biopsy methods is unlikely to be fruitful because existing studies indicate that biopsy procedures have sensitivities and specificities that are fairly similar and close to 1. Under these conditions randomized trials comparing alternative biopsy methods would need to enroll very large numbers of participants to allow reliable comparisons between tests.
- Additional information is also needed to define what patient and lesion factors may correspond with accuracy or adverse events of specific techniques. Future research needs to be better reported for progress to be made on these questions.

Conclusions

A large body of evidence indicates that ultrasound and stereotactically guided core needle biopsy procedures have sensitivity and specificity close to that of open biopsy procedures, and are associated with fewer adverse events. The strength of the evidence on the test performance of these methods is deemed moderate because studies are at medium to high risk of bias, but provide precise results and exhibit low heterogeneity. Freehand procedures have lower sensitivity than imaging-guided methods. The strength of conclusions about the comparative test performance of automated and vacuum-assisted devices (when using the same imaging guidance) is deemed low, because of concerns about the risk of bias of included studies and the reliance on indirect comparisons. There were insufficient data to draw conclusions for MRI-guided biopsy or women at high baseline risk of cancer. Harms were reported inconsistently, raising concerns about selective outcome and analysis reporting. There is low strength of evidence that vacuum-assisted procedures appear to have a higher risk of bleeding than automated methods. There is moderate strength of evidence that women diagnosed with breast cancer by core needle biopsy are more likely to have their cancer treated with a single surgical procedure, compared with women diagnosed by open surgical biopsy.

Abbreviations

ADH	Atypical ductal hyperplasia
AHRQ	Agency for healthcare Research and Quality
CrI	Credible interval
DCIS	Ductal carcinoma in situ
EPC	Evidence-based Practice Center
FN	False negative
FP	False positive
MRI	Magnetic resonance imaging
PICOTS	Populations-Interventions-Comparators-Outcomes-Timing-Setting
PRISMA	Preferred Reporting Items for Systematic Reviews and Meta-Analyses
QUADAS	Quality Assessment of Diagnostic Accuracy Studies
ROC	Received operating characteristic
SRDR	Systematic Review Data Repository
STARD	Standards for Reporting of Diagnostic Accuracy
TEP	Technical expert panel
TOO	Task Order Officer
TN	True negative
TP	True positive
US	Ultrasound

References

1. American Cancer Society. Breast Cancer Facts & Figures 2013-2014. Atlanta, GA: American Cancer Society; 2013. www.cancer.org/acs/groups/content/@research/documents/document/acspc-040951.pdf. Accessed March 26, 2014.

2. Hubbard RA, Kerlikowske K, Flowers CI, et al. Cumulative probability of false-positive recall or biopsy recommendation after 10 years of screening mammography: a cohort study. Ann Intern Med. 2011 Oct 18;155(8):481-92. PMID: 22007042.

3. Elmore JG, Barton MB, Moceri VM, et al. Ten-year risk of false positive screening mammograms and clinical breast examinations. N Engl J Med. 1998 Apr 16;338(16):1089-96. PMID: 9545356.

4. Yu YH, Wei W, Liu JL. Diagnostic value of fine-needle aspiration biopsy for breast mass: a systematic review and meta-analysis. BMC Cancer. 2012;12:41. PMID: 22277164.

5. Bruening W, Schoelles K, Treadwell J, et al. Comparative Effectiveness of Core-Needle and Open Surgical Biopsy for the Diagnosis of Breast Lesions. Comparative Effectiveness Review No. 19 (Prepared by the ECRI Institute Evidence-based Practice Center under Contract No. 290-02-0019). AHRQ Publication No. 10-EHC007-EF. Rockville, MD: Agency for Healthcare Research and Quality; December 2009. www.ncbi.nlm.nih.gov/books/NBK45220/pdf/TOC/pdf. Accessed April 25, 2013.

6. Bruening W, Fontanarosa J, Tipton K, et al. Systematic review: comparative effectiveness of core-needle and open surgical biopsy to diagnose breast lesions. Ann Intern Med. 2010 Feb 16;152(4):238-46. PMID: 20008742.

7. Agency for Healthcare Research and Quality. Methods Guide for Effectiveness and Comparative Effectiveness Reviews. Rockville, MD: Agency for Healthcare Research and Quality; April 2012. www.effectivehealthcare.ahrq.gov/ehc/products/60/318/MethodsGuide_Prepublication-Draft_20120523.pdf. Accessed April 25, 2013.

8. Moher D, Liberati A, Tetzlaff J, et al. Preferred reporting items for systematic reviews and meta-analyses: the PRISMA statement. Int J Surg. 2010;8(5):336-41. PMID: 20171303.

9. Dekkers OM, Egger M, Altman DG, et al. Distinguishing case series from cohort studies. Ann Intern Med. 2012 Jan 3;156(1 Pt 1):37-40. PMID: 22213493.

10. Drummond M, Barbieri M, Cook J, et al. Transferability of economic evaluations across jurisdictions: ISPOR Good Research Practices Task Force report. Value Health. 2009 Jun;12(4):409-18. PMID: 19900249.

11. Ramsey S, Willke R, Briggs A, et al. Good research practices for cost-effectiveness analysis alongside clinical trials: the ISPOR RCT-CEA Task Force report. Value Health. 2005 Sep-Oct;8(5):521-33. PMID: 16176491.

12. Leeflang MM, Scholten RJ, Rutjes AW, et al. Use of methodological search filters to identify diagnostic accuracy studies can lead to the omission of relevant studies. J Clin Epidemiol. 2006 Mar;59(3):234-40. PMID: 16488353.

13. Whiting P, Westwood M, Burke M, et al. Systematic reviews of test accuracy should search a range of databases to identify primary studies. J Clin Epidemiol. 2008 Apr;61(4):357-64. PMID: 18313560.

14. Whiting PF, Rutjes AW, Westwood ME, et al. QUADAS-2: a revised tool for the quality assessment of diagnostic accuracy studies. Ann Intern Med. 2011 Oct 18;155(8):529-36. PMID: 22007046.

15. Whiting P, Rutjes AW, Reitsma JB, et al. The development of QUADAS: a tool for the quality assessment of studies of diagnostic accuracy included in systematic reviews. BMC Med Res Methodol. 2003 Nov 10;3:25. PMID: 14606960.

16. Whiting P, Rutjes AW, Dinnes J, et al. Development and validation of methods for assessing the quality of diagnostic accuracy studies. Health Technol Assess. 2004 Jun;8(25):iii, 1-234. PMID: 15193208.

17. Whiting PF, Weswood ME, Rutjes AW, et al. Evaluation of QUADAS, a tool for the quality assessment of diagnostic accuracy studies. BMC Med Res Methodol. 2006 Mar 6;6:9. PMID: 16519814.

18. Wells G, Shea B, O'Connell D, et al. The Newcastle-Ottawa Scale (NOS) for assessing the quality of nonrandomised studies in meta-analyses. www.ohri.ca/programs/clinical_epidemiology/oxford.asp. Accessed 29 April 2013.

19. Higgins JP, Altman DG, Gotzsche PC, et al; Cochrane Bias Methods Group/Cochrane Statistical Methods Group. The Cochrane Collaboration's tool for assessing risk of bias in randomised trials. BMJ. 2011 Oct 18;343:d5928. PMID: 22008217.

20. Drummond MF, Jefferson TO. Guidelines for authors and peer reviewers of economic submissions to the BMJ. The BMJ Economic Evaluation Working Party. BMJ. 1996 Aug 3;313(7052):275-83. PMID: 8704542.

21. Trikalinos TA, Balion CM. Chapter 9: options for summarizing medical test performance in the absence of a "gold standard." J Gen Intern Med. 2012 Jun;27 Suppl 1:S67-75. PMID: 22648677.

22. Trikalinos TA, Balion CM, Coleman CI, et al. Chapter 8: meta-analysis of test performance when there is a "gold standard." J Gen Intern Med. 2012 Jun;27 Suppl 1:S56-66. PMID: 22648676.

23. Hamza TH, van Houwelingen HC, Stijnen T. The binomial distribution of meta-analysis was preferred to model within-study variability. J Clin Epidemiol. 2008 Jan;61(1):41-51. PMID: 18083461.

24. Rutter CM, Gatsonis CA. A hierarchical regression approach to meta-analysis of diagnostic test accuracy evaluations. Stat Med. 2001 Oct 15;20(19):2865-84. PMID: 11568945.

25. Arends LR, Hamza TH, van Houwelingen JC, et al. Bivariate random effects meta-analysis of ROC curves. Med Decis Making. 2008 Sep-Oct;28(5):621-38. PMID: 18591542.

26. Stijnen T, Hamza TH, Ozdemir P. Random effects meta-analysis of event outcome in the framework of the generalized linear mixed model with applications in sparse data. Stat Med. 2010 Dec 20;29(29):3046-67. PMID: 20827667.

27. Hamza TH, van Houwelingen HC, Heijenbrok-Kal MH, et al. Associating explanatory variables with summary receiver operating characteristic curves in diagnostic meta-analysis. J Clin Epidemiol. 2009 Dec;62(12):1284-91. PMID: 19398297.

28. van Houwelingen HC, Arends LR, Stijnen T. Advanced methods in meta-analysis: multivariate approach and meta-regression. Stat Med. 2002 Feb 28;21(4):589-624. PMID: 11836738.

29. Olkin I. Diagnostic statistical procedures in medical meta-analyses. Stat Med. 1999 Sep 15-30;18(17-18):2331-41. PMID: 10474143.

30. Dahabreh IJ, Trikalinos TA, Lau J, et al. An Empirical Assessment of Bivariate Methods for Meta-Analysis of Test Accuracy. Rockville (MD); 2012.

31. Singh S, Chang SM, Matchar DB, et al. Grading a body of evidence on diagnostic tests. In: Chang SMM, D. B. Smetana, G. W. Umscheid, C. A., ed Methods Guide for Medical Test Reviews. AHRQ Publication No. 12-EHC017. Rockville, MD: Agency for Healthcare Research and Quality; June 2012:chapter 7. www.ncbi.nlm.nih.gov/books/NBK98241/ Accessed April 25, 2013.

32. Lau J, Ioannidis JP, Terrin N, et al. The case of the misleading funnel plot. BMJ. 2006 Sep 16;333(7568):597-600. PMID: 16974018.

33. Sterne JA, Sutton AJ, Ioannidis JP, et al. Recommendations for examining and interpreting funnel plot asymmetry in meta-analyses of randomised controlled trials. BMJ. 2011;343:d4002. PMID: 21784880.

34. Antley CM, Mooney EE, Layfield LJ. A comparison of of accuracy rates between open biopsy, cutting-needle biopsy, and fine-needle aspiration biopsy of the breast: a 3-year experience. The Breast Journal. 1998;4(1):3-8.

35. Pistolese CA, Ciarrapico A, Perretta T, et al. Cost-effectiveness of two breast biopsy procedures: surgical biopsy versus vacuum-assisted biopsy. Radiol Med. 2012 Jun;117(4):539-57. PMID: 22020428.

36. Abdsaleh S, Azavedo E, Lindgren PG. Semiautomatic core biopsy. A modified biopsy technique in breast diseases. Acta Radiol. 2003 Jan;44(1):47-51. PMID: 12630998.

37. Ahmed ME, Ahmad I, Akhtar S. Ultrasound guided fine needle aspiration cytology versus core biopsy in the preoperative assessment of non-palpable breast lesions. J Ayub Med Coll Abbottabad. 2010 Apr-Jun;22(2):138-42. PMID: 21702288.

38. Akita A, Tanimoto A, Jinno H, et al. The clinical value of bilateral breast MR imaging: is it worth performing on patients showing suspicious microcalcifications on mammography? Eur Radiol. 2009 Sep;19(9):2089-96. PMID: 19350244.

39. Alonso-Bartolome P, Vega-Bolivar A, Torres-Tabanera M, et al. Sonographically guided 11-G directional vacuum-assisted breast biopsy as an alternative to surgical excision: utility and cost study in probably benign lesions. Acta Radiol. 2004 Jul;45(4):390-6. PMID: 15323390.

40. Ambrogetti D, Bianchi S, Ciatto S. Accuracy of percutaneous core biopsy of isolated breast microcalcifications identified by mammography. Experience with a vacuum-assisted large-core biopsy device. Radiol Med. 2003 Oct;106(4):313-9. PMID: 14612823.

41. An YY, Kim SH, Kang BJ, et al. Usefulness of magnetic resonance imaging-guided vacuum-assisted breast biopsy in Korean women: a pilot study. World J Surg Oncol. 2013 Aug 16;11(1):200. PMID: 23948057.

42. Apesteguia L, Mellado M, Saenz J, et al. Vacuum-assisted breast biopsy on digital stereotaxic table of nonpalpable lesions non-recognisable by ultrasonography. Eur Radiol. 2002 Mar;12(3):638-45. PMID: 11870480.

43. Arazi-Kleinman T, Skair-Levy M, Slonimsky E, et al. JOURNAL CLUB: Is screening MRI indicated for women with a personal history of breast cancer? Analysis based on biopsy results. AJR Am J Roentgenol. 2013 Oct;201(4):919-27. PMID: 24059385.

44. Barreto V, Hamed H, Griffiths AB, et al. Automatic needle biopsy in the diagnosis of early breast cancer. Eur J Surg Oncol. 1991 Jun;17(3):237-9. PMID: 2044776.

45. Bauer RL, Sung J, Eckhert KH, Jr., et al. Comparison of histologic diagnosis between stereotactic core needle biopsy and open surgical biopsy. Ann Surg Oncol. 1997 Jun;4(4):316-20. PMID: 9181231.

46. Beck RM, Gotz L, Heywang-Kobrunner SH. Stereotaxic vacuum core breast biopsy--experience of 560 patients. Swiss Surg. 2000;6(3):108-10. PMID: 10894010.

47. Becker L, Taves D, McCurdy L, et al. Stereotactic core biopsy of breast microcalcifications: comparison of film versus digital mammography, both using an add-on unit. AJR Am J Roentgenol. 2001 Dec;177(6):1451-7. PMID: 11717106.

48. Bernardi D, Borsato G, Pellegrini M, et al. On the diagnostic accuracy of stereotactic vacuum-assisted biopsy of nonpalpable breast abnormalities. Results in a consecutive series of 769 procedures performed at the Trento Department of Breast Diagnosis. Tumori. 2012 Jan-Feb;98(1):113-8. PMID: 22495711.

49. Boarki K, Labib M. The role of US guided handheld vacuum assisted breast core biopsy (VACB) in the surgical management of breast nodules: preliminary report of KCCC experience. Gulf J Oncolog. 2008 Jul(4):39-44. PMID: 20084774.

50. Bolivar AV, Alonso-Bartolome P, Garcia EO, et al. Ultrasound-guided core needle biopsy of non-palpable breast lesions: a prospective analysis in 204 cases. Acta Radiol. 2005 Nov;46(7):690-5. PMID: 16372687.

51. Brancato B, Crocetti E, Bianchi S, et al. Accuracy of needle biopsy of breast lesions visible on ultrasound: audit of fine needle versus core needle biopsy in 3233 consecutive samplings with ascertained outcomes. Breast. 2012 Aug;21(4):449-54. PMID: 22088803.

52. Brenner RJ, Bassett LW, Fajardo LL, et al. Stereotactic core-needle breast biopsy: a multi-institutional prospective trial. Radiology. 2001 Mar;218(3):866-72. PMID: 11230668.

53. Britton PD, Flower CD, Freeman AH, et al. Changing to core biopsy in an NHS breast screening unit. Clin Radiol. 1997 Oct;52(10):764-7. PMID: 9366536.

54. Burbank F. Stereotactic breast biopsy of atypical ductal hyperplasia and ductal carcinoma in situ lesions: improved accuracy with directional, vacuum-assisted biopsy. Radiology. 1997 Mar;202(3):843-7. PMID: 9051043.

55. Cangiarella J, Waisman J, Symmans WF, et al. Mammotome core biopsy for mammary microcalcification: analysis of 160 biopsies from 142 women with surgical and radiologic followup. Cancer. 2001 Jan 1;91(1):173-7. PMID: 11148574.

56. Caruso ML, Gabrieli G, Marzullo G, et al. Core Biopsy as Alternative to Fine-Needle Aspiration Biopsy in Diagnosis of Breast Tumors. Oncologist. 1998;3(1):45-9. PMID: 10388083.

57. Chang JM, Won JK, Lee KB, et al. Comparison of shear-wave and strain ultrasound elastography in the differentiation of benign and malignant breast lesions. AJR Am J Roentgenol. 2013 Aug;201(2):W347-56. PMID: 23883252.

58. Chapellier C, Balu-Maestro C, Amoretti N, et al. Vacuum-assisted breast biopsies. Experience at the Antoine Lacassagne Cancer Center (Nice, France). Clin Imaging. 2006 Mar-Apr;30(2):99-107. PMID: 16500540.

59. Cho N, Moon WK, Park JS, et al. Nonpalpable breast masses: evaluation by US elastography. Korean J Radiol. 2008 Mar-Apr;9(2):111-8. PMID: 18385557.

60. Ciatto S, Houssami N, Ambrogetti D, et al. Accuracy and underestimation of malignancy of breast core needle biopsy: the Florence experience of over 4000 consecutive biopsies. Breast Cancer Res Treat. 2007 Mar;101(3):291-7. PMID: 16823506.

61. Cipolla C, Fricano S, Vieni S, et al. Validity of needle core biopsy in the histological characterisation of mammary lesions. Breast. 2006 Feb;15(1):76-80. PMID: 16473738.

62. Cornelis A, Verjans M, Van den Bosch T, et al. Efficacy and safety of direct and frontal macrobiopsies in breast cancer. Eur J Cancer Prev. 2009 Aug;18(4):280-4. PMID: 19352188.

63. Cross MJ, Evans WP, Peters GN, et al. Stereotactic breast biopsy as an alternative to open excisional biopsy. Ann Surg Oncol. 1995 May;2(3):195-200. PMID: 7641014.

64. Crowe Jr JP, Patrick RJ, Rybicki LA, et al. Does ultrasound core breast biopsy predict histologic finding on excisional biopsy? The American Journal of Surgery. 2003;186:397-99.

65. Crystal P, Koretz M, Shcharynsky S, et al. Accuracy of sonographically guided 14-gauge core-needle biopsy: results of 715 consecutive breast biopsies with at least two-year follow-up of benign lesions. J Clin Ultrasound. 2005 Feb;33(2):47-52. PMID: 15674836.

66. Cusick JD, Dotan J, Jaecks RD, et al. The role of Tru-Cut needle biopsy in the diagnosis of carcinoma of the breast. Surg Gynecol Obstet. 1990 May;170(5):407-10. PMID: 2183373.

67. Dahlstrom JE, Jain S, Sutton T, et al. Diagnostic accuracy of stereotactic core biopsy in a mammographic breast cancer screening programme. Histopathology. 1996 May;28(5):421-7. PMID: 8735717.

68. Dahlstrom JE, Jain S. Histological correlation of mammographically detected microcalcifications in stereotactic core biopsies. Pathology (Phila). 2001 Nov;33(4):444-8. PMID: 11827410.

69. de Lucena CE, Dos Santos Junior JL, de Lima Resende CA, et al. Ultrasound-guided core needle biopsy of breast masses: How many cores are necessary to diagnose cancer? J Clin Ultrasound. 2007 Sep;35(7):363-6. PMID: 17663457.

70. Delle Chiaie L, Terinde R. Three-dimensional ultrasound-validated large-core needle biopsy: is it a reliable method for the histological assessment of breast lesions? Ultrasound Obstet Gynecol. 2004 Apr;23(4):393-7. PMID: 15065192.

71. Dhillon MS, Bradley SA, England DW. Mammotome biopsy: impact on preoperative diagnosis rate. Clin Radiol. 2006 Mar;61(3):276-81. PMID: 16488210.

72. Dillon MF, Hill AD, Quinn CM, et al. The accuracy of ultrasound, stereotactic, and clinical core biopsies in the diagnosis of breast cancer, with an analysis of false-negative cases. Ann Surg. 2005 Nov;242(5):701-7. PMID: 16244544.

73. Doyle AJ, Collins JP, Forkert CD. Decubitus stereotactic core biopsy of the breast: technique and experience. AJR Am J Roentgenol. 1999 Mar;172(3):688-90. PMID: 10063861.

74. Doyle AJ, Murray KA, Nelson EW, et al. Selective use of image-guided large-core needle biopsy of the breast: accuracy and cost-effectiveness. AJR Am J Roentgenol. 1995 Aug;165(2):281-4. PMID: 7618540.

75. Elvecrog EL, Lechner MC, Nelson MT. Nonpalpable breast lesions: correlation of stereotaxic large-core needle biopsy and surgical biopsy results. Radiology. 1993 Aug;188(2):453-5. PMID: 8327696.

76. Faizi KS, Hameed T, Azim K, et al. Diagnostic accuracy of Trucut biopsy in the detection of breast lumps. Pakistan Journal of Medical and Health Sciences. 2012;6(4):979-82.

77. Fajardo LL, Pisano ED, Caudry DJ, et al. Stereotactic and sonographic large-core biopsy of nonpalpable breast lesions: results of the Radiologic Diagnostic Oncology Group V study. Acad Radiol. 2004 Mar;11(3):293-308. PMID: 15035520.

78. Fischbach F, Eggemann H, Bunke J, et al. MR-guided freehand biopsy of breast lesions in a 1.0-T open MR imager with a near-real-time interactive platform: preliminary experience. Radiology. 2012 Nov;265(2):359-70. PMID: 22923721.

79. Fishman JE, Milikowski C, Ramsinghani R, et al. US-guided core-needle biopsy of the breast: how many specimens are necessary? Radiology. 2003 Mar;226(3):779-82. PMID: 12601206.

80. Frazee RC, Roberts JW, Symmonds RE, et al. Open versus stereotactic breast biopsy. Am J Surg. 1996 Nov;172(5):491-3; discussion 4-5. PMID: 8942551.

81. Fuhrman G, Cederbom G, Champagne J, et al. Stereotactic core needle breast biopsy is an accurate diagnostic technique to assess nonpalpable mammographic abnormalities. J La State Med Soc. 1996 Apr;148(4):167-70. PMID: 8935619.

82. Fuhrman GM, Cederbom GJ, Bolton JS, et al. Image-guided core-needle breast biopsy is an accurate technique to evaluate patients with nonpalpable imaging abnormalities. Ann Surg. 1998 Jun;227(6):932-9. PMID: 9637557.

83. Georgian-Smith D, D'Orsi C, Morris E, et al. Stereotactic biopsy of the breast using an upright unit, a vacuum-suction needle, and a lateral arm-support system. AJR Am J Roentgenol. 2002 Apr;178(4):1017-24. PMID: 11906893.

84. Gisvold JJ, Goellner JR, Grant CS, et al. Breast biopsy: a comparative study of stereotaxically guided core and excisional techniques. AJR Am J Roentgenol. 1994 Apr;162(4):815-20. PMID: 8140997.

85. Gruber R, Jaromi S, Rudas M, et al. Histologic work-up of non-palpable breast lesions classified as probably benign at initial mammography and/or ultrasound (BI-RADS category 3). Eur J Radiol. 2013 Mar;82(3):398-403. PMID: 22429299.

86. Gruber R, Walter E, Helbich TH. Impact of stereotactic 11-g vacuum-assisted breast biopsy on cost of diagnosis in Austria. Eur J Radiol. 2011 Jan;77(1):131-6. PMID: 19853395.

87. Hahn SY, Shin JH, Han BK, et al. Sonographically-guided vacuum-assisted biopsy with digital mammography-guided skin marking of suspicious breast microcalcifications: comparison of outcomes with stereotactic biopsy in Asian women. Acta Radiol. 2011 Feb 1;52(1):29-34. PMID: 21498322.

88. Hamed H, De Freitas R, Rasbridge S, et al. A prospective randomized study of two gauges of biopty-cut needle in diagnosis of early breast cancer. Breast. 1995;4(2):135-6.

89. Han BK, Choe YH, Ko YH, et al. Stereotactic core-needle biopsy of non-mass calcifications: outcome and accuracy at long-term follow-up. Korean J Radiol. 2003 Oct-Dec;4(4):217-23. PMID: 14726638.

90. Head JF, Haynes AE, Elliott MC, et al. Stereotaxic localization and core needle biopsy of nonpalpable breast lesions: two-year follow-up of a prospective study. Am Surg. 1996 Dec;62(12):1018-23. PMID: 8955240.

91. Helbich TH, Mayr W, Schick S, et al. Coaxial technique: approach to breast core biopsies. Radiology. 1997 Jun;203(3):684-90. PMID: 9169689.

92. Heywang-Kobrunner SH, Heinig A, Hellerhoff K, et al. Use of ultrasound-guided percutaneous vacuum-assisted breast biopsy for selected difficult indications. Breast J. 2009 Jul-Aug;15(4):348-56. PMID: 19500104.

93. Heywang-Kobrunner SH, Schaumloffel U, Viehweg P, et al. Minimally invasive stereotaxic vacuum core breast biopsy. Eur Radiol. 1998;8(3):377-85. PMID: 9510569.

94. Houserkova D, Prasad SN, Svach I, et al. The value of dynamic contrast enhanced breast MRI in mammographically detected BI-RADS 5 microcalcifications. Biomed Pap Med Fac Univ Palacky Olomouc Czech Repub. 2008 Jun;152(1):107-15. PMID: 18795084.

95. Huang PC, Cheung YC, Lo YF, et al. A comparison of spring-loaded and vacuum-assisted techniques for stereotactic breast biopsy of impalpable microcalcification lesions: experience at Chang Gung Memorial Hospital at Linkou. Chang Gung Med J. 2011 Jan-Feb;34(1):75-83. PMID: 21392477.

96. Huang YC, Ho CY. Stereotactic 11-guage Vacuum-assisted Breast Biopsy: Experience of 420 Cases with Microcalcification on Mammography of Non-palpable Lesions. J Radiol Sci. 2011 December;36(4):195-202.

97. Ioffe OB, Berg WA, Silverberg SG, et al. Mammographic-histopathologic correlation of large-core needle biopsies of the breast. Mod Pathol. 1998 Aug;11(8):721-7. PMID: 9720499.

98. Jackman RJ, Lamm RL. Stereotactic histologic biopsy in breasts with implants. Radiology. 2002 Jan;222(1):157-64. PMID: 11756720.

99. Jackman RJ, Marzoni FA, Jr., Rosenberg J. False-negative diagnoses at stereotactic vacuum-assisted needle breast biopsy: long-term follow-up of 1,280 lesions and review of the literature. AJR Am J Roentgenol. 2009 Feb;192(2):341-51. PMID: 19155393.

100. Jackman RJ, Nowels KW, Rodriguez-Soto J, et al. Stereotactic, automated, large-core needle biopsy of nonpalpable breast lesions: false-negative and histologic underestimation rates after long-term follow-up. Radiology. 1999 Mar;210(3):799-805. PMID: 10207484.

101. Jales RM, Sarian LO, Peralta CF, et al. Complex breast masses: assessment of malignant potential based on cyst diameter. J Ultrasound Med. 2012 Apr;31(4):581-7. PMID: 22441915.

102. Johnson AT, Henry-Tillman RS, Smith LF, et al. Percutaneous excisional breast biopsy. Am J Surg. 2002 Dec;184(6):550-4; discussion 4. PMID: 12488164.

103. Kettritz U, Morack G, Decker T. Stereotactic vacuum-assisted breast biopsies in 500 women with microcalcifications: radiological and pathological correlations. Eur J Radiol. 2005 Aug;55(2):270-6. PMID: 16036159.

104. Kettritz U, Rotter K, Schreer I, et al. Stereotactic vacuum-assisted breast biopsy in 2874 patients: a multicenter study. Cancer. 2004 Jan 15;100(2):245-51. PMID: 14716757.

105. Khattar SC, Torp-Pedersen S, Horn T, et al. Ultrasound-guided biopsy of palpable breast masses. Eur J Ultrasound. 1997;6(1):1-7.

106. Kim HS, Kim MJ, Kim EK, et al. US-guided vacuum-assisted biopsy of microcalcifications in breast lesions and long-term follow-up results. Korean J Radiol. 2008 Nov-Dec;9(6):503-9. PMID: 19039266.

107. Kirshenbaum KJ, Voruganti T, Overbeeke C, et al. Stereotactic core needle biopsy of nonpalpable breast lesions using a conventional mammography unit with an add-on device. AJR Am J Roentgenol. 2003 Aug;181(2):527-31. PMID: 12876040.

108. Kirshenbaum K, Keppke A, Hou K, et al. Reassessing specimen number and diagnostic yield of ultrasound guided breast core biopsy. Breast J. 2012 Sep;18(5):464-9. PMID: 22775971.

109. Kirwan SE, Denton ER, Nash RM, et al. Multiple 14G stereotactic core biopsies in the diagnosis of mammographically detected stellate lesions of the breast. Clin Radiol. 2000 Oct;55(10):763-6. PMID: 11052877.

110. Koskela AK, Sudah M, Berg MH, et al. Add-on device for stereotactic core-needle breast biopsy: how many biopsy specimens are needed for a reliable diagnosis? Radiology. 2005 Sep;236(3):801-9. PMID: 16020555.

111. Lai JT, Burrowes P, MacGregor JH. Diagnostic accuracy of a stereotaxically guided vacuum-assisted large-core breast biopsy program in Canada. Can Assoc Radiol J. 2001 Aug;52(4):223-7. PMID: 11512293.

112. Latosinsky S, Cornell D, Bear HD, et al. Evaluation of stereotactic core needle biopsy (SCNB) of the breast at a single institution. Breast Cancer Res Treat. 2000 Apr;60(3):277-83. PMID: 10930116.

113. Levin MF, Papoff WJ, Doan L, et al. Stereotaxic percutaneous core biopsy versus surgical biopsy of nonpalpable breast lesions using a standard mammographic table with an add-on device. Can Assoc Radiol J. 2001 Feb;52(1):29-32. PMID: 11247262.

114. Liberman L, Dershaw DD, Glassman JR, et al. Analysis of cancers not diagnosed at stereotactic core breast biopsy. Radiology. 1997 Apr;203(1):151-7. PMID: 9122384.

115. Liberman L, Ernberg LA, Heerdt A, et al. Palpable breast masses: is there a role for percutaneous imaging-guided core biopsy? AJR Am J Roentgenol. 2000 Sep;175(3):779-87. PMID: 10954467.

116. Liberman L, Feng TL, Dershaw DD, et al. US-guided core breast biopsy: use and cost-effectiveness. Radiology. 1998 Sep;208(3):717-23. PMID: 9722851.

117. Liberman L, Kaplan JB, Morris EA, et al. To excise or to sample the mammographic target: what is the goal of stereotactic 11-gauge vacuum-assisted breast biopsy? AJR Am J Roentgenol. 2002 Sep;179(3):679-83. PMID: 12185043.

118. Liberman L, Sama MP. Cost-effectiveness of stereotactic 11-gauge directional vacuum-assisted breast biopsy. AJR Am J Roentgenol. 2000 Jul;175(1):53-8. PMID: 10882245.

119. Lin WC, Hsu GC, Yu CP, et al. Value of sonographically guided needle sampling of cystic versus solid components in the diagnosis of complex cystic breast masses. Acta Radiol. 2009 Jul;50(6):595-601. PMID: 19452336.

120. Lomoschitz FM, Helbich TH, Rudas M, et al. Stereotactic 11-gauge vacuum-assisted breast biopsy: influence of number of specimens on diagnostic accuracy. Radiology. 2004 Sep;232(3):897-903. PMID: 15273332.

121. Luparia A, Durando M, Campanino P, et al. Efficacy and cost-effectiveness of stereotactic vacuum-assisted core biopsy of nonpalpable breast lesions: analysis of 602 biopsies performed over 5 years. Radiol Med. 2011 Apr;116(3):477-88. PMID: 21225359.

122. Mainiero MB, Philpotts LE, Lee CH, et al. Stereotaxic core needle biopsy of breast microcalcifications: correlation of target accuracy and diagnosis with lesion size. Radiology. 1996 Mar;198(3):665-9. PMID: 8628852.

123. Makkun S, Prueksadee J, Chayakulkheeree J, et al. The accuracy of ultrasound guided 14-gauge core needle breast biopsy: Correlation with surgical excision or long term follow-up. Asian Pacific Journal of Tropical Disease. 2011:222-6.

124. Makoske T, Preletz R, Riley L, et al. Long-term outcomes of stereotactic breast biopsies. Am Surg. 2000 Dec;66(12):1104-8; discussion 8-9. PMID: 11149580.

125. March DE, Coughlin BF, Barham RB, et al. Breast masses: removal of all US evidence during biopsy by using a handheld vacuum-assisted device--initial experience. Radiology. 2003 May;227(2):549-55. PMID: 12676972.

126. Margolin FR, Leung JW, Jacobs RP, et al. Percutaneous imaging-guided core breast biopsy: 5 years' experience in a community hospital. AJR Am J Roentgenol. 2001 Sep;177(3):559-64. PMID: 11517047.

127. McMahon AJ, Lutfy AM, Matthew A, et al. Needle core biopsy of the breast with a spring-loaded device. Br J Surg. 1992 Oct;79(10):1042-5. PMID: 1422715.

128. Meloni GB, Becchere MP, Soro D, et al. Percutaneous vacuum-assisted core breast biopsy with upright stereotactic equipment. Indications, limitations and results. Acta Radiol. 2002 Nov;43(6):575-8. PMID: 12485254.

129. Meyer JE, Christian RL, Lester SC, et al. Evaluation of nonpalpable solid breast masses with stereotaxic large-needle core biopsy using a dedicated unit. AJR Am J Roentgenol. 1996 Jul;167(1):179-82. PMID: 8659367.

130. Meyer JE, Smith DN, Lester SC, et al. Large-core needle biopsy of nonpalpable breast lesions. JAMA. 1999 May 5;281(17):1638-41. PMID: 10235159.

131. Mikhail RA, Nathan RC, Weiss M, et al. Stereotactic core needle biopsy of mammographic breast lesions as a viable alternative to surgical biopsy. Ann Surg Oncol. 1994 Sep;1(5):363-7. PMID: 7850536.

132. Morris EA, Liberman L, Trevisan SG, et al. Histologic heterogeneity of masses at percutaneous breast biopsy. Breast J. 2002 Jul-Aug;8(4):187-91. PMID: 12100109.

133. Mueller-Holzner E, Frede T, Daniaux M, et al. Ultrasound-guided core needle biopsy of the breast: does frozen section give an accurate diagnosis? Breast Cancer Res Treat. 2007 Dec;106(3):399-406. PMID: 17318378.

134. Nagar S, Iacco A, Riggs T, et al. An analysis of fine needle aspiration versus core needle biopsy in clinically palpable breast lesions: a report on the predictive values and a cost comparison. Am J Surg. 2012 Aug;204(2):193-8. PMID: 22464444.

135. Nguyen M, McCombs MM, Ghandehari S, et al. An update on core needle biopsy for radiologically detected breast lesions. Cancer. 1996 Dec 1;78(11):2340-5. PMID: 8941004.

136. Ohsumi S, Takashima S, Aogi K, et al. Breast biopsy for mammographically detected non-palpable lesions using a vacuum-assisted biopsy device (Mammotome) and an upright-type stereotactic mammography unit. Jpn J Clin Oncol. 2001 Nov;31(11):527-31. PMID: 11773259.

137. Ohsumi S, Taira N, Takabatake D, et al. Breast biopsy for mammographically detected nonpalpable lesions using a vacuum-assisted biopsy device (Mammotome) and upright-type stereotactic mammography unit without a digital imaging system: experience of 500 biopsies. Breast Cancer. 2012 Apr 5PMID: 22477266.

138. Order BM, Schaefer PJ, Peters G, et al. Evaluation of two different vacuum-assisted breast biopsy systems: Mammotome(R) system 11G/8G vs. ATEC(R) system 12G/9G. Acta Radiol. 2013 Mar 1;54(2):137-43. PMID: 23319718.

139. Parker SH, Burbank F, Jackman RJ, et al. Percutaneous large-core breast biopsy: a multi-institutional study. Radiology. 1994 Nov;193(2):359-64. PMID: 7972743.

140. Parker SH, Jobe WE, Dennis MA, et al. US-guided automated large-core breast biopsy. Radiology. 1993 May;187(2):507-11. PMID: 8475299.

141. Parker SH, Lovin JD, Jobe WE, et al. Stereotactic breast biopsy with a biopsy gun. Radiology. 1990 Sep;176(3):741-7. PMID: 2167501.

142. Parkin E, Hindocha S, Subar D, et al. An initial experience with rapid microwave processing in the one-stop breast clinic. World J Surg. 2010 Dec;34(12):3036-41. PMID: 20703464.

143. Perez-Fuentes JA, Longobardi IR, Acosta VF, et al. Sonographically guided directional vacuum-assisted breast biopsy: preliminary experience in Venezuela. AJR Am J Roentgenol. 2001 Dec;177(6):1459-63. PMID: 11717107.

144. Peters N, Hoorntje L, Mali W, et al. Diagnostic performance of stereotactic large core needle biopsy for nonpalpable breast lesions in routine clinical practice. Int J Cancer. 2008 Jan 15;122(2):468-71. PMID: 17935136.

145. Peters NHGM, Meeuwis C, Bakker CJG, et al. Feasibility of MRI-guided large-core-needle biopsy of suspiscious breast lesions at 3T. Eur Radiol. 2009;19:1639-44.

146. Pettine S, Place R, Babu S, et al. Stereotactic breast biopsy is accurate, minimally invasive, and cost effective. Am J Surg. 1996 May;171(5):474-6. PMID: 8651388.

147. Pfarl G, Helbich TH, Riedl CC, et al. Stereotactic 11-gauge vacuum-assisted breast biopsy: a validation study. AJR Am J Roentgenol. 2002 Dec;179(6):1503-7. PMID: 12438044.

148. Pfleiderer SO, Brunzlow H, Schulz-Wendtland R, et al. Two-year follow-up of stereotactically guided 9-G breast biopsy: a multicenter evaluation of a self-contained vacuum-assisted device. Clin Imaging. 2009 Sep-Oct;33(5):343-7. PMID: 19712812.

149. Pfleiderer SO, Reichenbach JR, Azhari T, et al. A manipulator system for 14-gauge large core breast biopsies inside a high-field whole-body MR scanner. J Magn Reson Imaging. 2003 Apr;17(4):493-8. PMID: 12655591.

150. Philpotts LE, Hooley RJ, Lee CH. Comparison of automated versus vacuum-assisted biopsy methods for sonographically guided core biopsy of the breast. AJR Am J Roentgenol. 2003 Feb;180(2):347-51. PMID: 12540431.

151. Pistolese CA, Ciarrapico AM, Della Gatta F, et al. Cost-effectiveness analysis of two vacuum-assisted breast biopsy systems: Mammotome and Vacora. Radiol Med. 2009 Aug;114(5):743-56. PMID: 19484585.

152. Pitre B, Baron PL, Baron LF, et al. Stereotactic core biopsy of the breast: results of one-year follow-up of 101 patients. Am Surg. 1997 Dec;63(12):1124-7. PMID: 9393264.

153. Povoski SP, Jimenez RE, Wang WP. Ultrasound-guided diagnostic breast biopsy methodology: retrospective comparison of the 8-gauge vacuum-assisted biopsy approach versus the spring-loaded 14-gauge core biopsy approach. World J Surg Oncol. 2011;9:87. PMID: 21835024.

154. Puglisi F, Pertoldi B, Ramello M, et al. Diagnostic accuracy of perforated compression grid approach for mammographically guided core needle biopsy of breast lesions. Cancer Lett. 1999 Nov 15;146(2):181-8. PMID: 10656624.

155. Reiner CS, Helbich TH, Rudas M, et al. Can galactography-guided stereotactic, 11-gauge, vacuum-assisted breast biopsy of intraductal lesions serve as an alternative to surgical biopsy? Eur Radiol. 2009 Dec;19(12):2878-85. PMID: 19565246.

156. Rosenblatt R, Fineberg SA, Sparano JA, et al. Stereotactic core needle biopsy of multiple sites in the breast: efficacy and effect on patient care. Radiology. 1996 Oct;201(1):67-70. PMID: 8816522.

157. Sauer G, Deissler H, Strunz K, et al. Ultrasound-guided large-core needle biopsies of breast lesions: analysis of 962 cases to determine the number of samples for reliable tumour classification. Br J Cancer. 2005 Jan 31;92(2):231-5. PMID: 15611793.

158. Schueller G, Jaromi S, Ponhold L, et al. US-guided 14-gauge core-needle breast biopsy: results of a validation study in 1352 cases. Radiology. 2008 Aug;248(2):406-13. PMID: 18641246.

159. Schulz-Wendtland R, Kramer S, Lang N, et al. Ultrasonic guided microbiopsy in mammary diagnosis: indications, technique and results. Anticancer Res. 1998 May-Jun;18(3C):2145-6. PMID: 9703772.

160. Scopa CD, Koukouras D, Spiliotis J, et al. Comparison of fine needle aspiration and Tru-Cut biopsy of palpable mammary lesions. Cancer Detect Prev. 1996;20(6):620-4. PMID: 8939348.

161. Sim LS, Kei PL. Upright stereotactic vacuum-assisted needle biopsy of suspicious breast microcalcifications. J Med Imaging Radiat Oncol. 2008 Aug;52(4):358-64. PMID: 18811759.

162. Smith DN, Rosenfield Darling ML, Meyer JE, et al. The utility of ultrasonographically guided large-core needle biopsy: results from 500 consecutive breast biopsies. J Ultrasound Med. 2001 Jan;20(1):43-9. PMID: 11149527.

163. Smith LF, Henry-Tillman R, Mancino AT, et al. Magnetic resonance imaging-guided core needle biopsy and needle localized excision of occult breast lesions. Am J Surg. 2001 Oct;182(4):414-8. PMID: 11720683.

164. Smyth AT, Cederbom GJ. Core biopsy of breast lesions. J La State Med Soc. 1994 Nov;146(11):499-501. PMID: 7806950.

165. Soo MS, Ghate S, Delong D. Stereotactic biopsy of noncalcified breast lesions: utility of vacuum-assisted technique compared to multipass automated gun technique. Clin Imaging. 1999 Nov-Dec;23(6):347-52. PMID: 10899415.

166. Stolier AJ. Stereotactic breast biopsy: a surgical series. J Am Coll Surg. 1997 Sep;185(3):224-8. PMID: 9291397.

167. Sutton S, Dahlstrom JE, Jain S. Stereotactic large-gauge core biopsy: its role in the diagnosis of non-palpable mammographic abnormalities presenting to a screening service. Australas Radiol. 1997 May;41(2):103-8. PMID: 9153803.

168. Tonegutti M, Girardi V. Stereotactic vacuum-assisted breast biopsy in 268 nonpalpable lesions. Radiol Med. 2008 Feb;113(1):65-75. PMID: 18338128.

169. Toth D, Sebo E, Sarkadi L, et al. Role of core needle biopsy in the treatment of radial scar. Breast. 2012 Dec;21(6):761-3. PMID: 22397896.

170. Tothova L, Rauova K, Valkovic L, et al. Stereotactic vacuum-assisted breast biopsy: our experience and comparison with stereotactic automated needle biopsy. Bratisl Lek Listy. 2013;114(2):71-7. PMID: 23331202.

171. Uematsu T, Kasami M, Yuen S. Usefulness and limitations of the Japan Mammography Guidelines for the categorization of microcalcifications. Breast Cancer. 2008;15(4):291-7. PMID: 18288569.

172. Uematsu T, Kasami M, Yuen S. A cluster of microcalcifications: women with high risk for breast cancer versus other women. Breast Cancer. 2009;16(4):307-14. PMID: 19350360.

173. Vag T, Pfleiderer SO, Bottcher J, et al. Ultrasound-guided breast biopsy using a 10-gauge self-contained vacuum-assisted device. Eur Radiol. 2007 Dec;17(12):3100-2. PMID: 17639409.

174. Vega A, Arrizabalaga R, Garijo F, et al. Nonpalpable breast lesion. Stereotaxic core needle aspiration biopsy with a single pass. Acta Radiol. 1995 Mar;36(2):117-21. PMID: 7710788.

175. Vega Bolivar A, Ortega Garcia E, Garijo Ayensa F. Stereotaxic core needle aspiration biopsy with multiple passes in nonpalpable breast lesions. Acta Radiol. 1998 Jul;39(4):389-94. PMID: 9685825.

176. Venkataraman S, Dialani V, Gilmore HL, et al. Stereotactic core biopsy: Comparison of 11 gauge with 8 gauge vacuum assisted breast biopsy. Eur J Radiol. 2012 Oct;81(10):2613-9. PMID: 22127375.

177. Verkooijen HM. Diagnostic accuracy of stereotactic large-core needle biopsy for nonpalpable breast disease: results of a multicenter prospective study with 95% surgical confirmation. Int J Cancer. 2002 Jun 20;99(6):853-9. PMID: 12115488.

178. Walker TM. Impalpable breast lesions: Stereotactic core biopsy with an 'add-on' unit. Breast. 1997 June;6(3):126-31.

179. Wang J, Kuo WH, Pan SL, et al. Use of Bayesian modeling to estimate the sensitivity of stereotactic directional vacuum-assisted breast biopsy when the gold standard is incomplete. Acad Radiol. 2009 Nov;16(11):1316-22. PMID: 19665906.

180. Ward SE, Taves DH, McCurdy LI. Stereotaxic core needle biopsy of breast microcalcifications obtained using a standard mammography table with an add-on unit. Can Assoc Radiol J. 2000 Feb;51(1):10-5. PMID: 10711288.

181. Weber WP, Zanetti R, Langer I, et al. Mammotome: less invasive than ABBI with similar accuracy for early breast cancer detection. World J Surg. 2005 Apr;29(4):495-9. PMID: 15770379.

182. Welle GJ, Clark M, Loos S, et al. Stereotactic breast biopsy: recumbent biopsy using add-on upright equipment. AJR Am J Roentgenol. 2000 Jul;175(1):59-63. PMID: 10882246.

183. White RR, Halperin TJ, Olson JA, Jr., et al. Impact of core-needle breast biopsy on the surgical management of mammographic abnormalities. Ann Surg. 2001 Jun;233(6):769-77. PMID: 11371735.

184. Whitman GJ, Kopans DB, McCarthy KA, et al. Coaxial core needle biopsy under mammographic guidance: indications and applications. AJR Am J Roentgenol. 1998 Jul;171(1):67-70. PMID: 9648766.

185. Wiratkapun C, Treesit T, Wibulpolprasert B, et al. Diagnostic accuracy of ultrasonography-guided core needle biopsy for breast lesions. Singapore Med J. 2012 Jan;53(1):40-5. PMID: 22252182.

186. Wong TE, Hisham AN. Core needle biopsy of palpable breast lump: the influence of needle size. Med J Malaysia. 2003 Aug;58(3):399-404. PMID: 14750380.

187. Wu YK, Huang YM, Chou ASB, et al. Management of breast fibroadenomas by ultrasound-guided vacuum-assisted biopsy-Three years experience. Tzu Chi Med J. 2005;17(6):405-8.

188. Wunderbaldinger P, Helbich TH, Partik B, et al. First experience with a new dedicated ultrasound system for computer-guided large-core breast biopsy. Eur Radiol. 2001;11(12):2460-4. PMID: 11734940.

189. Yeoman LJ, Michell MJ, Humphreys S, et al. Radiographically guided fine needle aspiration cytology and core biopsy in the assessment of impalpable breast lesions. The Breast. 1996;5:41-7.

190. Yeow KM, Lo YF, Wang CS, et al. Ultrasound-guided core needle biopsy as an initial diagnostic test for palpable breast masses. J Vasc Interv Radiol. 2001 Nov;12(11):1313-7. PMID: 11698631.

191. Youk JH, Kim EK, Kim MJ, et al. Sonographically guided 14-gauge core needle biopsy of breast masses: a review of 2,420 cases with long-term follow-up. AJR Am J Roentgenol. 2008 Jan;190(1):202-7. PMID: 18094312.

192. Zannis VJ, Aliano KM. The evolving practice pattern of the breast surgeon with disappearance of open biopsy for nonpalpable lesions. Am J Surg. 1998 Dec;176(6):525-8. PMID: 9926783.

193. Zografos G, Zagouri F, Sergentanis TN, et al. Vacuum-assisted breast biopsy in nonpalpable solid breast lesions without microcalcifications: the Greek experience. Diagn Interv Radiol. 2008 Sep;14(3):127-30. PMID: 18814132.

194. Zuiani C, Mazzarella F, Londero V, et al. Stereotactic vacuum-assisted breast biopsy: results, follow-up and correlation with radiological suspicion. Radiol Med. 2007 Mar;112(2):304-17. PMID: 17361368.

195. Awuah B, Martin IK, Takyi V, et al. Implementation of a percutaneous core needle biopsy training program: results from the University of Michigan-Komfo Anokye Teaching Hospital breast cancer research partnership. Ann Surg Oncol. 2011 Apr;18(4):957-60. PMID: 21104327.

196. Bi TQ, Ren CL, Chaudhary P, et al. Diagnosis and excision of breast multi-focal lesions by ultrasound-guided vacuum-assisted biopsy: A comparative evaluation. Journal of Xi'an Medical University. 2010(3):208-11.

197. Bleiweiss IJ, Nagi CS, Jaffer S. Axillary sentinel lymph nodes can be falsely positive due to iatrogenic displacement and transport of benign epithelial cells in patients with breast carcinoma. J Clin Oncol. 2006 May 1;24(13):2013-8. PMID: 16606970.

198. Brandon CJ, Mullan PB. Patients' perception of care during image-guided breast biopsy in a rural community breast center: communication matters. J Cancer Educ. 2011 Mar;26(1):156-60. PMID: 21188664.

199. Brenner RJ, Gordon LM. Malignant seeding following percutaneous breast biopsy: documentation with comprehensive imaging and clinical implications. Breast J. 2011 Nov-Dec;17(6):651-6. PMID: 21906209.

200. Carter BA, Jensen RA, Simpson JF, et al. Benign transport of breast epithelium into axillary lymph nodes after biopsy. Am J Clin Pathol. 2000 Feb;113(2):259-65. PMID: 10664628.

201. Chao C, Torosian MH, Boraas MC, et al. Local recurrence of breast cancer in the stereotactic core needle biopsy site: case reports and review of the literature. Breast J. 2001 Mar-Apr;7(2):124-7. PMID: 11328321.

202. Chen AM, Haffty BG, Lee CH. Local recurrence of breast cancer after breast conservation therapy in patients examined by means of stereotactic core-needle biopsy. Radiology. 2002 Dec;225(3):707-12. PMID: 12461249.

203. Chetlen AL, Kasales C, Mack J, et al. Hematoma formation during breast core needle biopsy in women taking antithrombotic therapy. AJR Am J Roentgenol. 2013 Jul;201(1):215-22. PMID: 23789678.

204. Chou CP, Wang YC, Chang SJ, et al. Evaluation of the Effects of Chitosan Hemostasis Dressings on Hemorrhage Caused by Breast Biopsy. Breast Care (Basel). 2012 Jun;7(3):220-4. PMID: 22872796.

205. Diaz LK, Wiley EL, Venta LA. Are malignant cells displaced by large-gauge needle core biopsy of the breast? AJR Am J Roentgenol. 1999 Nov;173(5):1303-13. PMID: 10541110.

206. Duchesne N, Parker SH, Klaus AJ, et al. Breast biopsy: multicenter study of radiofrequency introducer with US-guided handheld system--initial experience. Radiology. 2004 Jul;232(1):205-10. PMID: 15220503.

207. Faour I, Al-Salam S, El-Terifi H, et al. The use of a vacuum-assisted biopsy device (Mammotome) in the early detection of breast cancer in the United Arab Emirates. Ann N Y Acad Sci. 2008 Sep;1138:108-13. PMID: 18837890.

208. Fitzal F, Sporn EP, Draxler W, et al. Preoperative core needle biopsy does not increase local recurrence rate in breast cancer patients. Breast Cancer Res Treat. 2006 May;97(1):9-15. PMID: 16502019.

209. Frank LS, Frank JL, March D, et al. Does therapeutic touch ease the discomfort or distress of patients undergoing stereotactic core breast biopsy? A randomized clinical trial. Pain Med. 2007 Jul-Aug;8(5):419-24. PMID: 17661855.

210. Hansen NM, Ye X, Grube BJ, et al. Manipulation of the primary breast tumor and the incidence of sentinel node metastases from invasive breast cancer. Arch Surg. 2004 Jun;139(6):634-9; discussion 9-40. PMID: 15197090.

211. Harries R, Lawson S, Bruckers L. Assessment of microcalcifications with limited number of high-precision macrobiopsies. Eur J Cancer Prev. 2010 Sep;19(5):374-8. PMID: 20495463.

212. Harter LP, Curtis JS, Ponto G, et al. Malignant seeding of the needle track during stereotaxic core needle breast biopsy. Radiology. 1992 Dec;185(3):713-4. PMID: 1343569.

213. He Q, Fan X, Guan Y, et al. Percutaneous excisional biopsy of impalpable breast lesions under ultrasound visualization. Breast. 2008 Dec;17(6):666-70. PMID: 18835778.

214. Hertl K, Marolt-Music M, Kocijancic I, et al. Haematomas after percutaneus vacuum-assisted breast biopsy. Ultraschall Med. 2009 Feb;30(1):33-6. PMID: 18773386.

215. Hoorntje LE, Schipper ME, Kaya A, et al. Tumour cell displacement after 14G breast biopsy. Eur J Surg Oncol. 2004 Jun;30(5):520-5. PMID: 15135480.

216. Huber S, Wagner M, Medl M, et al. Benign breast lesions: minimally invasive vacuum-assisted biopsy with 11-gauge needles patient acceptance and effect on follow-up imaging findings. Radiology. 2003 Mar;226(3):783-90. PMID: 12616021.

217. Hyser MJ, Vanuno D, Mallesh A, et al. Changing patterns of care for occult breast lesions in a community teaching hospital. Am Surg. 2000 May;66(5):438-42; discussion 42-3. PMID: 10824743.

218. Ishizuna K, Ota D, Okamoto J, et al. A case of mucinous carcinoma of the breast in which needle tract seeding was diagnosed by preoperative diagnostic imaging. Breast Cancer. 2011 Oct;18(4):324-7. PMID: 19701680.

219. Kibil W, Hodorowicz-Zaniewska D, Kulig J. Mammotome biopsy under ultrasound control in the diagnostics and treatment of nodular breast lesions - own experience. Pol Przegl Chir. 2012 May 1;84(5):242-6. PMID: 22763299.

220. King TA, Hayes DH, Cederbom GJ, et al. Biopsy technique has no impact on local recurrence after breast-conserving therapy. Breast J. 2001 Jan-Feb;7(1):19-24. PMID: 11348411.

221. Knight R, Horiuchi K, Parker SH, et al. Risk of needle-track seeding after diagnostic image-guided core needle biopsy in breast cancer. JSLS. 2002 Jul-Sep;6(3):207-9. PMID: 12166757.

222. Koo JS, Jung WH, Kim H. Epithelial displacement into the lymphovascular space can be seen in breast core needle biopsy specimens. Am J Clin Pathol. 2010 May;133(5):781-7. PMID: 20395526.

223. Kubota K, Gomi N, Wakita T, et al. Magnetic resonance imaging of the metal clip in a breast: safety and its availability as a negative marker. Breast Cancer. 2004;11(1):55-9. PMID: 14718794.

224. Kwo S, Grotting JC. Does stereotactic core needle biopsy increase the risk of local recurrence of invasive breast cancer? Breast J. 2006 May-Jun;12(3):191-3. PMID: 16684313.

225. Lai JT, Burrowes P, MacGregor JH. Vacuum-assisted large-core breast biopsy: complications and their incidence. Can Assoc Radiol J. 2000 Aug;51(4):232-6. PMID: 10976242.

226. Lang EV, Berbaum KS, Faintuch S, et al. Adjunctive self-hypnotic relaxation for outpatient medical procedures: a prospective randomized trial with women undergoing large core breast biopsy. Pain. 2006 Dec 15;126(1-3):155-64. PMID: 16959427.

227. Liberman L, Vuolo M, Dershaw DD, et al. Epithelial displacement after stereotactic 11-gauge directional vacuum-assisted breast biopsy. AJR Am J Roentgenol. 1999 Mar;172(3):677-81. PMID: 10063859.

228. Lin JH, Kuo WH, Huang CS, et al. Ultrasound-guided mammotome biopsy of breast lesions in Taiwanese women. Journal of Medical Ultrasound. 2009;8(2):102-7.

229. Linebarger JH, Landercasper J, Ellis RL, et al. Core needle biopsy rate for new cancer diagnosis in an interdisciplinary breast center: evaluation of quality of care 2007-2008. Ann Surg. 2012 Jan;255(1):38-43. PMID: 22167007.

230. Michalopoulos NV, Zagouri F, Sergentanis TN, et al. Needle tract seeding after vacuum-assisted breast biopsy. Acta Radiol. 2008 Apr;49(3):267-70. PMID: 18365811.

231. Nakamura Y, Urashima M, Matsuura A, et al. Stereotactic directional vacuum-assisted breast biopsy using lateral approach. Breast Cancer. 2010 Oct;17(4):286-9. PMID: 19784717.

232. Newman EL, Kahn A, Diehl KM, et al. Does the method of biopsy affect the incidence of sentinel lymph node metastases? Breast J. 2006 Jan-Feb;12(1):53-7. PMID: 16409587.

233. Penco S, Rizzo S, Bozzini AC, et al. Stereotactic vacuum-assisted breast biopsy is not a therapeutic procedure even when all mammographically found calcifications are removed: analysis of 4,086 procedures. AJR Am J Roentgenol. 2010 Nov;195(5):1255-60. PMID: 20966337.

234. Peters-Engl C, Konstantiniuk P, Tausch C, et al. The impact of preoperative breast biopsy on the risk of sentinel lymph node metastases: analysis of 2502 cases from the Austrian Sentinel Node Biopsy Study Group. Br J Cancer. 2004 Nov 15;91(10):1782-6. PMID: 15477859.

235. Rissanen TJ, Makarainen HP, Mattila SI, et al. Wire localized biopsy of breast lesions: a review of 425 cases found in screening or clinical mammography. Clin Radiol. 1993 Jan;47(1):14-22. PMID: 8428412.

236. Rovera F, Dionigi G, Marelli M, et al. Breast cancer diagnosis: the role of stereotactic vacuum-assisted aspiration biopsy. Int J Surg. 2008;6 Suppl 1:S104-8. PMID: 19121611.

237. Schaefer FK, Order BM, Eckmann-Scholz C, et al. Interventional bleeding, hematoma and scar-formation after vacuum-biopsy under stereotactic guidance: Mammotome((R))-system 11 g/8 g vs. ATEC((R))-system 12 g/9 g. Eur J Radiol. 2012 May;81(5):e739-45. PMID: 22381441.

238. Sergentanis TN, Zagouri F, Domeyer P, et al. Biopsy method: a major predictor of adherence after benign breast biopsy? AJR Am J Roentgenol. 2009 Nov;193(5):W452-7. PMID: 19843727.

239. Seror JY, Lesieur B, Scheuer-Niro B, et al. Predictive factors for complete excision and underestimation of one-pass en bloc excision of non-palpable breast lesions with the Intact((R)) breast lesion excision system. Eur J Radiol. 2012 Apr;81(4):719-24. PMID: 21310570.

240. Stolier A, Skinner J, Levine EA. A prospective study of seeding of the skin after core biopsy of the breast. Am J Surg. 2000 Aug;180(2):104-7. PMID: 11044522.

241. Szynglarewicz B, Matkowski R, Kasprzak P, et al. Pain experienced by patients during minimal-invasive ultrasound-guided breast biopsy: vacuum-assisted vs core-needle procedure. Eur J Surg Oncol. 2011 May;37(5):398-403. PMID: 21367573.

242. Taplin SH, Abraham L, Geller BM, et al. Effect of previous benign breast biopsy on the interpretive performance of subsequent screening mammography. J Natl Cancer Inst. 2010 Jul 21;102(14):1040-51. PMID: 20601590.

243. Uematsu T, Kasami M. Risk of needle tract seeding of breast cancer: cytological results derived from core wash material. Breast Cancer Res Treat. 2008 Jul;110(1):51-5. PMID: 17674195.

244. Uematsu T, Kasami M. The use of positive core wash cytology to estimate potential risk of needle tract seeding of breast cancer: directional vacuum-assisted biopsy versus automated core needle biopsy. Breast Cancer. 2010;17(1):61-7. PMID: 19360459.

245. Uematsu T, Yuen S, Kasami M, et al. Dynamic contrast-enhanced MR imaging in screening detected microcalcification lesions of the breast: is there any value? Breast Cancer Res Treat. 2007 Jul;103(3):269-81. PMID: 17063274.

246. Uriburu JL, Vuoto HD, Cogorno L, et al. Local recurrence of breast cancer after skin-sparing mastectomy following core needle biopsy: case reports and review of the literature. Breast J. 2006 May-Jun;12(3):194-8. PMID: 16684314.

247. Ventrella V, Tufaro A, Zito FA, et al. Mammographic characteristics and vacuum-assisted breast biopsy (VABB) of non-palpable breast lesions. Acta Radiol. 2011 Jul 1;52(6):602-7. PMID: 21565889.

248. Viala J, Gignier P, Perret B, et al. Stereotactic vacuum-assisted biopsies on a digital breast 3D-tomosynthesis system. Breast J. 2013 Jan-Feb;19(1):4-9. PMID: 23252555.

249. Viehweg P, Bernerth T, Kiechle M, et al. MR-guided intervention in women with a family history of breast cancer. Eur J Radiol. 2006 Jan;57(1):81-9. PMID: 16364583.

250. Vitug AF, Newman LA. Complications in breast surgery. Surg Clin North Am. 2007 Apr;87(2):431-51, x. PMID: 17498536.

251. Wang ZL, Liu G, Huang Y, et al. Percutaneous excisional biopsy of clinically benign breast lesions with vacuum-assisted system: comparison of three devices. Eur J Radiol. 2012 Apr;81(4):725-30. PMID: 21300503.

252. Ward ST, Shepherd JA, Khalil H. Freehand versus ultrasound-guided core biopsies of the breast: reducing the burden of repeat biopsies in patients presenting to the breast clinic. Breast. 2010 Apr;19(2):105-8. PMID: 20074953.

253. Wei X, Li Y, Zhang S, et al. Experience in large-core needle biopsy in the diagnosis of 1431 breast lesions. Med Oncol. 2011 Jun;28(2):429-33. PMID: 20339957.

254. Wong CS, Chu YC, Wong KW, et al. Is ultrasonography-guided modified coaxial core biopsy of the breast a better technique? Hong Kong Med J. 2009 Aug;15(4):246-8. PMID: 19652229.

255. Yao F, Li J, Wan Y, et al. Sonographically guided vacuum-assisted breast biopsy for complete excision of presumed benign breast lesions. J Ultrasound Med. 2012 Dec;31(12):1951-7. PMID: 23197548.

256. Youngson BJ, Cranor M, Rosen PP. Epithelial displacement in surgical breast specimens following needling procedures. Am J Surg Pathol. 1994 Sep;18(9):896-903. PMID: 8067510.

257. Youngson BJ, Liberman L, Rosen PP. Displacement of carcinomatous epithelium in surgical breast specimens following stereotaxic core biopsy. Am J Clin Pathol. 1995 May;103(5):598-602. PMID: 7741106.

258. Zagouri F, Gounaris A, Liakou P, et al. Vacuum-assisted breast biopsy: more cores, more hematomas? In Vivo. 2011 Jul-Aug;25(4):703-5. PMID: 21709018.

259. Zografos GC, Zagouri F, Sergentanis TN, et al. Predictors of pain during open breast biopsy under local anesthesia: is there such a thing? Pain Pract. 2008 Mar-Apr;8(2):151. PMID: 18366472.

260. Zografos GC, Zagouri F, Sergentanis TN, et al. Minimizing underestimation rate of microcalcifications excised via vacuum-assisted breast biopsy: a blind study. Breast Cancer Res Treat. 2008 May;109(2):397-402. PMID: 17653855.

261. Zografos GC, Zagouri F, Sergentanis TN, et al. Hematoma after vacuum-assisted breast biopsy: are interleukins predictors? Onkologie. 2009 Jul;32(7):395-7. PMID: 19556816.

262. Arnaout A, Smylie J, Seely J, et al. Improving breast diagnostic services with a Rapid Access Diagnostic and Support (RADS) program. Ann Surg Oncol. 2013 Oct;20(10):3335-40. PMID: 23975290.

263. Berg WA, Arnoldus CL, Teferra E, et al. Biopsy of amorphous breast calcifications: pathologic outcome and yield at stereotactic biopsy. Radiology. 2001 Nov;221(2):495-503. PMID: 11687695.

264. Bleicher RJ, Ruth K, Sigurdson ER, et al. Preoperative delays in the US Medicare population with breast cancer. J Clin Oncol. 2012 Dec 20;30(36):4485-92. PMID: 23169513.

265. Brenner RJ, Fajardo L, Fisher PR, et al. Percutaneous core biopsy of the breast: effect of operator experience and number of samples on diagnostic accuracy. AJR Am J Roentgenol. 1996 Feb;166(2):341-6. PMID: 8553943.

266. Bugbee ME, Wellisch DK, Arnott IM, et al. Breast core-needle biopsy: clinical trial of relaxation technique versus medication versus no intervention for anxiety reduction. Radiology. 2005 Jan;234(1):73-8. PMID: 15564386.

267. Chang JM, Moon WK, Cho N, et al. Management of ultrasonographically detected benign papillomas of the breast at core needle biopsy. AJR Am J Roentgenol. 2011 Mar;196(3):723-9. PMID: 21343519.

268. Flory N, Lang EV. Distress in the radiology waiting room. Radiology. 2011 Jul;260(1):166-73. PMID: 21474702.

269. Gruber R, Walter E, Helbich TH. Cost comparison between ultrasound-guided 14-g large core breast biopsy and open surgical biopsy: an analysis for Austria. Eur J Radiol. 2010 Jun;74(3):519-24. PMID: 19427153.

270. Hahn M, Kagan KO, Siegmann KC, et al. Mammotome versus ATEC: a comparison of two breast vacuum biopsy techniques under sonographic guidance. Arch Gynecol Obstet. 2010 Feb;281(2):287-92. PMID: 19404655.

271. Hoover SJ, Berry MP, Rossick L, et al. Ultrasound-guided breast biopsy curriculum for surgical residents. Surg Innov. 2008 Mar;15(1):52-8. PMID: 18407929.

272. Landercasper J, Ellis RL, Mathiason MA, et al. A community breast center report card determined by participation in the national quality measures for breast centers program. Breast J. 2010 Sep-Oct;16(5):472-80. PMID: 20722650.

273. Landercasper J, Linebarger JH, Ellis RL, et al. A quality review of the timeliness of breast cancer diagnosis and treatment in an integrated breast center. J Am Coll Surg. 2010 Apr;210(4):449-55. PMID: 20347737.

274. Lee CH, Egglin TK, Philpotts L, et al. Cost-effectiveness of stereotactic core needle biopsy: analysis by means of mammographic findings. Radiology. 1997 Mar;202(3):849-54. PMID: 9051045.

275. Lee T. Comparison of Breast Cancer Screening Results in Korean Middle-Aged Women: A Hospital-based Prospective Cohort Study. Osong Public Health Res Perspect. 2013 Aug;4(4):197-202. PMID: 24159556.

276. Liao MN, Chen MF, Chen SC, et al. Uncertainty and anxiety during the diagnostic period for women with suspected breast cancer. Cancer Nurs. 2008 Jul-Aug;31(4):274-83. PMID: 18600114.

277. Lovrics P, Hodgson N, O'Brien MA, et al. The implementation of a surgeon-directed quality improvement strategy in breast cancer surgery. Am J Surg. 2013 Nov 8PMID: 24315382.

278. Michalopoulos NV, Maniou I, Zografos GC. Breast lesion excision system biopsy: the learning curve. AJR Am J Roentgenol. 2012 Nov;199(5):W667. PMID: 23096217.

279. Moran MS, Kaufman C, Burgin C, et al. What currently defines a breast center? Initial data from the national accreditation program for breast centers. J Oncol Pract. 2013 Mar;9(2):e62-70. PMID: 23814526.

280. Mosunjac M, Park J, Strauss A, et al. Time to treatment for patients receiving BCS in a public and a private university hospital in Atlanta. Breast J. 2012 Mar-Apr;18(2):163-7. PMID: 22239743.

281. Novy DM, Price M, Huynh PT, et al. Percutaneous core biopsy of the breast: correlates of anxiety. Acad Radiol. 2001 Jun;8(6):467-72. PMID: 11394538.

282. Park ER, Traeger L, Willett J, et al. A relaxation response training for women undergoing breast biopsy: exploring integrated care. Breast. 2013 Oct;22(5):799-805. PMID: 23587450.

283. Park HL, Min SY, Kwon SH, et al. Nationwide survey of use of vacuum-assisted breast biopsy in South Korea. Anticancer Res. 2012 Dec;32(12):5459-64. PMID: 23225452.

284. Rubin E, Mennemeyer ST, Desmond RA, et al. Reducing the cost of diagnosis of breast carcinoma: impact of ultrasound and imaging-guided biopsies on a clinical breast practice. Cancer. 2001 Jan 15;91(2):324-32. PMID: 11180078.

285. Sclafani LM, Bleznak A, Kelly T, et al. Training a new generation of breast surgeons: are we succeeding? Ann Surg Oncol. 2012 Jun;19(6):1856-61. PMID: 22219063.

286. Swan JS, Lawrence WF, Roy J. Process utility in breast biopsy. Med Decis Making. 2006 Jul-Aug;26(4):347-59. PMID: 16855124.

287. Szynglarewicz B, Kasprzak P, Kornafel J, et al. Duration time of vacuum-assisted biopsy for nonpalpable breast masses: comparison between stereotactic and ultrasound-guided procedure. Tumori. 2011 Jul-Aug;97(4):517-21. PMID: 21989443.

288. Walker MS, Farria D, Schmidt M, et al. Educational intervention for women undergoing image-guided breast biopsy: results of a randomized clinical trial. Cancer Control. 2007 Oct;14(4):380-7. PMID: 17914338.

289. Wallis MG, Cheung S, Kearins O, et al. Non-operative diagnosis--effect on repeat-operation rates in the UK breast screening programme. Eur Radiol. 2009 Feb;19(2):318-23. PMID: 18751983.

290. Wolf R, Quan G, Calhoun K, et al. Efficiency of Core Biopsy for BI-RADS-5 Breast Lesions. Breast J. 2008 Sep-Oct;14(5):471-5. PMID: 18821933.

291. van Breest Smallenburg V, Nederend J, Voogd AC, et al. Trends in breast biopsies for abnormalities detected at screening mammography: a population-based study in the Netherlands. Br J Cancer. 2013 Jul 9;109(1):242-8. PMID: 23695018.

292. Kulkarni D, Irvine T, Reyes RJ. The use of core biopsy imprint cytology in the 'one-stop' breast clinic. Eur J Surg Oncol. 2009 Oct;35(10):1037-40. PMID: 19268520.

293. de Roos MA, Pijnappel RM, Groote AD, et al. Ductal carcinoma in situ presenting as microcalcifications: the effect of stereotactic large-core needle biopsy on surgical therapy. Breast. 2004 Dec;13(6):461-7. PMID: 15563852.

294. Al-Sobhi SS, Helvie MA, Pass HA, et al. Extent of lumpectomy for breast cancer after diagnosis by stereotactic core versus wire localization biopsy. Ann Surg Oncol. 1999 Jun;6(4):330-5. PMID: 10379852.

295. Altomare V, Guerriero G, Giacomelli L, et al. Management of nonpalpable breast lesions in a modern functional breast unit. Breast Cancer Res Treat. 2005 Sep;93(1):85-9. PMID: 16184463.

296. Bloomston M, D'Angelo P, Galliano D, et al. One hundred consecutive advanced breast biopsy instrumentation procedures: complications, costs, and outcome. Ann Surg Oncol. 1999 Mar;6(2):195-9. PMID: 10082046.

297. Carmon M, Rivkin L, Abu-Dalo R, et al. Increased mammographic screening and use of percutaneous image-guided core biopsy in non-palpable breast cancer: impact on surgical treatment. Isr Med Assoc J. 2004 Jun;6(6):326-8. PMID: 15214456.

298. Chen SC, Yang HR, Hwang TL, et al. Intraoperative ultrasonographically guided excisional biopsy or vacuum-assisted core needle biopsy for nonpalpable breast lesions. Ann Surg. 2003 Nov;238(5):738-42. PMID: 14578737.

299. Chun K, Velanovich V. Patient-perceived cosmesis and satisfaction after breast biopsy: comparison of stereotactic incisional, excisional, and wire-localized biopsy techniques. Surgery. 2002 May;131(5):497-501. PMID: 12019401.

300. Collins LC, Connolly JL, Page DL, et al. Diagnostic agreement in the evaluation of image-guided breast core needle biopsies: results from a randomized clinical trial. Am J Surg Pathol. 2004 Jan;28(1):126-31. PMID: 14707874.

301. Deurloo EE, Gilhuijs K, Schultze Kool LJ, et al. Displacement of breast tissue and needle deviations during stereotactic procedures. Invest Radiol. 2001;36(6):347-53.

302. Diebold T, Hahn T, Solbach C, et al. Evaluation of the stereotactic 8G vacuum-assisted breast biopsy in the histologic evaluation of suspicious mammography findings (BI-RADS IV). Invest Radiol. 2005 Jul;40(7):465-71. PMID: 15973139.

303. Duchesne N, Parker SH, Lechner MC, et al. Multicenter evaluation of a new ultrasound-guided biopsy device: Improved ergonomics, sampling and rebiopsy rates. Breast J. 2007 Jan-Feb;13(1):36-43. PMID: 17214791.

304. Elliott RL, Haynes AE, Bolin JA, et al. Stereotaxic needle localization and biopsy of occult breast lesions: first year's experience. Am Surg. 1992 Feb;58(2):126-31. PMID: 1550304.

305. Fenoglio ME, Gallagher JQ, Joy N, et al. Stereotactic core breast biopsy versus needle localization breast biopsy—The effect of initial diagnostic modality on surgical therapy in patients with breast cancer. Minim Invasive Ther Allied Technol. 1997;6(3):225-7.

306. Fine RE, Whitworth PW, Kim JA, et al. Low-risk palpable breast masses removed using a vacuum-assisted hand-held device. Am J Surg. 2003 Oct;186(4):362-7. PMID: 14553851.

307. Florentine BD, Cobb CJ, Frankel K, et al. Core needle biopsy. A useful adjunct to fine-needle aspiration in select patients with palpable breast lesions. Cancer. 1997 Feb 25;81(1):33-9. PMID: 9100539.

308. Friese CR, Neville BA, Edge SB, et al. Breast biopsy patterns and outcomes in Surveillance, Epidemiology, and End Results-Medicare data. Cancer. 2009 Feb 15;115(4):716-24. PMID: 19152430.

309. Geller BM, Oppenheimer RG, Mickey RM, et al. Patient perceptions of breast biopsy procedures for screen-detected lesions. Am J Obstet Gynecol. 2004 Apr;190(4):1063-9. PMID: 15118643.

310. Golub RM, Bennett CL, Stinson T, et al. Cost minimization study of image-guided core biopsy versus surgical excisional biopsy for women with abnormal mammograms. J Clin Oncol. 2004 Jun 15;22(12):2430-7. PMID: 15197205.

311. Gukas ID, Nwana EJ, Ihezue CH, et al. Tru-cut biopsy of palpable breast lesions: a practical option for pre-operative diagnosis in developing countries. Cent Afr J Med. 2000 May;46(5):127-30. PMID: 11210334.

312. Handy RB, Fajardo LL, Innis CA, et al. Patient perceptions of stereotaxic large-core breast biopsy. Acad Radiol. 1996 Dec;3(12):1007-11. PMID: 9017015.

313. Hatmaker AR, Donahue RM, Tarpley JL, et al. Cost-effective use of breast biopsy techniques in a Veterans health care system. Am J Surg. 2006 Nov;192(5):e37-41. PMID: 17071179.

314. Hoffmann J. Analysis of surgical and diagnostic quality at a specialist breast unit. Breast. 2006 Aug;15(4):490-7. PMID: 16343904.

315. Holloway CM, Saskin R, Brackstone M, et al. Variation in the use of percutaneous biopsy for diagnosis of breast abnormalities in Ontario. Ann Surg Oncol. 2007 Oct;14(10):2932-9. PMID: 17619931.

316. Howisey RL, Acheson MB, Rowbotham RK, et al. A comparison of Medicare reimbursement and results for various imaging-guided breast biopsy techniques. Am J Surg. 1997 May;173(5):395-8. PMID: 9168074.

317. Hui JY, Chan LK, Chan RL, et al. Prone table stereotactic breast biopsy. Hong Kong Med J. 2002 Dec;8(6):447-51. PMID: 12459602.

318. Janes RH, Bouton MS. Initial 300 consecutive stereotactic core-needle breast biopsies by a surgical group. Am J Surg. 1994 Dec;168(6):533-6; discussion 6-7. PMID: 7977991.

319. Johnson JM, Dalton RR, Landercasper J, et al. Image-guided or needle-localized open biopsy of mammographic malignant-appearing microcalcifications? J Am Coll Surg. 1998 Dec;187(6):604-9. PMID: 9849733.

320. Kaufman CS, Delbecq R, Jacobson L. Excising the reexcision: stereotactic core-needle biopsy decreases need for reexcision of breast cancer. World J Surg. 1998 Oct;22(10):1023-7; discussion 8. PMID: 9747160.

321. Killebrew LK, Oneson RH. Comparison of the diagnostic accuracy of a vacuum-assisted percutaneous intact specimen sampling device to a vacuum-assisted core needle sampling device for breast biopsy: initial experience. Breast J. 2006 Jul-Aug;12(4):302-8. PMID: 16848839.

322. Krainick-Strobel U, Huber B, Majer I, et al. Complete extirpation of benign breast lesions with an ultrasound-guided vacuum biopsy system. Ultrasound Obstet Gynecol. 2007 Mar;29(3):342-6. PMID: 17167817.

323. Lehman CD, Deperi ER, Peacock S, et al. Clinical experience with MRI-guided vacuum-assisted breast biopsy. AJR Am J Roentgenol. 2005 Jun;184(6):1782-7. PMID: 15908530.

324. Liberman L, Dershaw DD, Rosen PP, et al. Stereotaxic core biopsy of impalpable spiculated breast masses. AJR Am J Roentgenol. 1995 Sep;165(3):551-4. PMID: 7645467.

325. Liberman L, Gougoutas CA, Zakowski MF, et al. Calcifications highly suggestive of malignancy: comparison of breast biopsy methods. AJR Am J Roentgenol. 2001 Jul;177(1):165-72. PMID: 11418420.

326. Liberman L, Holland AE, Marjan D, et al. Underestimation of atypical ductal hyperplasia at MRI-guided 9-gauge vacuum-assisted breast biopsy. AJR Am J Roentgenol. 2007 Mar;188(3):684-90. PMID: 17312054.

327. Liberman L, LaTrenta LR, Dershaw DD, et al. Impact of core biopsy on the surgical management of impalpable breast cancer. AJR Am J Roentgenol. 1997 Feb;168(2):495-9. PMID: 9016234.

328. Liberman L, Morris EA, Dershaw DD, et al. Fast MRI-guided vacuum-assisted breast biopsy: initial experience. AJR Am J Roentgenol. 2003 Nov;181(5):1283-93. PMID: 14573421.

329. Lind DS, Minter R, Steinbach B, et al. Stereotactic core biopsy reduces the reexcision rate and the cost of mammographically detected cancer. J Surg Res. 1998 Jul 15;78(1):23-6. PMID: 9733612.

330. Mainiero MB, Gareen IF, Bird CE, et al. Preferential use of sonographically guided biopsy to minimize patient discomfort and procedure time in a percutaneous image-guided breast biopsy program. J Ultrasound Med. 2002 Nov;21(11):1221-6. PMID: 12418763.

331. Mariotti C, Feliciotti F, Baldarelli M, et al. Digital stereotactic biopsies for nonpalpable breast lesion. Surg Endosc. 2003 Jun;17(6):911-7. PMID: 12632135.

332. Morrow M, Venta L, Stinson T, et al. Prospective comparison of stereotactic core biopsy and surgical excision as diagnostic procedures for breast cancer patients. Ann Surg. 2001 Apr;233(4):537-41. PMID: 11303136.

333. Orel SG, Rosen M, Mies C, et al. MR imaging-guided 9-gauge vacuum-assisted core-needle breast biopsy: initial experience. Radiology. 2006 Jan;238(1):54-61. PMID: 16304093.

334. Perlet C, Heywang-Kobrunner SH, Heinig A, et al. Magnetic resonance-guided, vacuum-assisted breast biopsy: results from a European multicenter study of 538 lesions. Cancer. 2006 Mar 1;106(5):982-90. PMID: 16456807.

335. Pijnappel RM, Peeters PH, van den Donk M, et al. Diagnostic strategies in non-palpable breast lesions. Eur J Cancer. 2002 Mar;38(4):550-5. PMID: 11872348.

336. Popiela TJ, Tabor J, Nowak W, et al. Detectability of pre-clinical breast pathologies in own experience. Pol Przegl Chir. 2002;74(1):36-43.

337. Rotenberg L, Verhille R, Schulz-Wendtland R, et al. Multicenter clinical experience with large core soft tissue biopsy without vacuum assistance. Eur J Cancer Prev. 2004 Dec;13(6):491-8. PMID: 15548942.

338. Schneider E, Rohling KW, Schnall MD, et al. An apparatus for MR-guided breast lesion localization and core biopsy: design and preliminary results. J Magn Reson Imaging. 2001 Sep;14(3):243-53. PMID: 11536401.

339. Shin S, Schneider HB, Cole FJ, Jr. , et al. Follow-up recommendations for benign breast biopsies. Breast J. 2006 Sep-Oct;12(5):413-7. PMID: 16958957.

340. Smith DN, Christian R, Meyer JE. Large-core needle biopsy of nonpalpable breast cancers. The impact on subsequent surgical excisions. Arch Surg. 1997 Mar;132(3):256-9; discussion 60. PMID: 9125023.

341. Soo MS, Kliewer MA, Ghate S, et al. Stereotactic breast biopsy of noncalcified lesions: a cost-minimization analysis comparing 14-gauge multipass automated core biopsy to 14- and 11-gauge vacuum-assisted biopsy. Clin Imaging. 2005 Jan-Feb;29(1):26-33. PMID: 15859015.

342. Strong JW, Worsham GF, Austin RM, et al. Stereotactic core biopsy of nonpalpable breast lesions. J S C Med Assoc. 1995 Dec;91(12):489-96. PMID: 8587312.

343. Uematsu T, Kasami M, Uchida Y, et al. Ultrasonographically guided 18-gauge automated core needle breast biopsy with post-fire needle position verification (PNPV). Breast Cancer. 2007;14(2):219-28. PMID: 17485909.

344. Verkooijen HM, Borel Rinkes IH, Peeters PH, et al. Impact of stereotactic large-core needle biopsy on diagnosis and surgical treatment of nonpalpable breast cancer. Eur J Surg Oncol. 2001 Apr;27(3):244-9. PMID: 11393185.

345. Whitten TM, Wallace TW, Bird RE, et al. Image-guided core biopsy has advantages over needle localization biopsy for the diagnosis of nonpalpable breast cancer. Am Surg. 1997 Dec;63(12):1072-7; discussion 7-8. PMID: 9393255.

346. Williams AB, Roberts JV, Michell MJ, et al. Prone stereotactic breast core biopsy: The impact on surgical management of nonpalpable breast cancers. Breast. 1999;8(1):12-5.

347. Wong TT, Cheung PS, Ma MK, et al. Experience of stereotactic breast biopsy using the vacuum-assisted core needle biopsy device and the advanced breast biopsy instrumentation system in Hong Kong women. Asian J Surg. 2005 Jan;28(1):18-23. PMID: 15691792.

348. Wunderbaldinger P, Wolf G, Turetschek K, et al. Comparison of sitting versus prone position for stereotactic large-core breast biopsy in surgically proven lesions. AJR Am J Roentgenol. 2002 May;178(5):1221-5. PMID: 11959735.

349. Yim JH, Barton P, Weber B, et al. Mammographically detected breast cancer. Benefits of stereotactic core versus wire localization biopsy. Ann Surg. 1996 Jun;223(6):688-97; discussion 97-700. PMID: 8645042.

350. Launders (editor). CER Breast Biopsy Project (ECRI Institute, Plymouth Meeting, PA). August 12, 2008.

351. Bossuyt PM, Reitsma JB, Bruns DE, et al. Towards complete and accurate reporting of studies of diagnostic accuracy: The STARD Initiative. Ann Intern Med. 2003 Jan 7;138(1):40-4. PMID: 12513043.

352. Brennan ME, Turner RM, Ciatto S, et al. Ductal carcinoma in situ at core-needle biopsy: meta-analysis of underestimation and predictors of invasive breast cancer. Radiology. 2011 Jul;260(1):119-28. PMID: 21493791.

353. Liebens F, Carly B, Cusumano P, et al. Breast cancer seeding associated with core needle biopsies: a systematic review. Maturitas. 2009 Feb 20;62(2):113-23. PMID: 19167175.

354. Schueller G, Schueller-Weidekamm C, Helbich TH. Accuracy of ultrasound-guided, large-core needle breast biopsy. Eur Radiol. 2008 Sep;18(9):1761-73. PMID: 18414872.

Appendix A. Search Strategy

Search strategy for CINAHL/Embase/Medline, adapted from the 2009 Comparative Effectiveness Review, "Comparative Effectiveness of Core Needle Biopsy and Open Surgical Biopsy for the Diagnosis of Breast Lesions"

Set Number	Concept	Search statement
1	Breast biopsy	(breast biopsy or stereotactic breast biopsy or directional vacuum assisted biopsy).de.
2	Breast	Breast
3	Breast diseases	Exp breast cancer/di or exp breast neoplasms/di or exp breast disease/di or exp breast diseases/di
4		(breast or mammar$) and (Papilloma or calcification$ or calcinosis or tum?or$ or lesion$ or cancer or carcinoma$ or lump$)
5	Combine sets	or/2-4
6	Biopsy	5 and ((Biopsy or tumor biopsy).de. or biops$)
7	Large core needle biopsy	6 and ((needle biopsy or biopsy needle or percutaneous biopsy).de. or (large core or needle or mammotome or mammatome or vacuum))
8	Open biopsy	6 and (breast/su or breast tumor/su)
9		6 and (su.fs. or open or excision$ or incision$ or surgical)
10	Combine sets	8 or 9
11	Combine sets	or/1,7,10
12	Limit by publication type	11 not ((letter or editorial or news or comment or case reports or note or conference paper).de. or (letter or editorial or news or comment or case reports).pt.)
13	Diagnostics filter	12 and (exp prediction and forecasting/ or (predictive value of tests or receiver operating characteristic or ROC curve or sensitivity and specificity or accuracy or diagnostic accuracy or precision or likelihood).de. or ((false or true) adj (positive or negative)))
14	Clinical trials filter	13 and ((Randomized controlled trials or random allocation or double-blind method or single-blind method or placebos or cross-over studies or crossover procedure or double blind procedure or single blind procedure or placebos or latin square design or crossover design or double-blind studies or single-blind studies or triple-blind studies or random assignment or exp controlled study/ or exp clinical trial/ or exp comparative study/ or cohort analysis or follow-up studies.de. or intermethod comparison or parallel design or control group or prospective study or retrospective study or case control study or major clinical study).de. or Case control studies/ or Cohort/ or Longitudinal studies/ or Evaluation studies/ or Follow-up studies/ or Prospective studies/ or Retrospective studies/ or Case control study/ or Cohort analysis/ or Longitudinal study/ or Follow up/ or Cohort analysis/ or Followup studies/ or random$.hw. or

		random$.ti. or placebo$.mp. or ((singl$ or doubl$ or tripl$ or trebl$) and (dummy or blind or sham or mask)).mp. or latin square.mp. or (time adj series) or (case adj (study or studies) or ISRCTN$.mp. or ACTRN$.mp. or (NCT$ not nctc$)))
15	Combine sets	13 or 14
16	Eliminate overlap	
17	Seeding	12 and seeding.ti,ab.
18	Patient satisfactionQOL	12 and ((patient satisfaction or pain measurement or pain assessment or visual analog scale or quality of life).de. or satisf$ or QOL or preference$)
19	Adverse events	12 and ((ae or co).fs. or cross infection or drainage or surgical wound infection).de.)
20	Disfiguration	12 and (disfigur$ or deform$)
21	Combine sets	Or/16-20

Appendix B. Excluded Studies

Reason for Exclusion	Excluded Studies (see list of references on the next page)
< 10 patients, no seeding	1-35
> 15% current or previous breast cancer	36-110
Case control or retrospective case study	111-260
Incomplete reference standard	261-315
Instrument no longer available	316
Less than 50% follow-up	317-372
No CNB or CNB not for diagnosis of breast cancer in women	373-573 574-769
No primary data	770-825
Non-English full text	826-914
Not outcome of interest (no KQ1, KQ2, KQ3)	915-1107 1108-1281 1282-1363 1364-1479
Selected on the basis of CNB or final outcomes	1480-1649 1650-1896 1897-2018 2019-2164

CNB = core-needle biopsy; KQ = Key Question.

Citations to Excluded Studies

1. . Idiopathic granulomatous mastitis in Hispanic women - Indiana, 2006-2008. MMWR Morb Mortal Wkly Rep. 2009 Dec 4;58(47):1317-21. PMID: 19959984.
2. Abrari A. Pseudoangiomatous stromal hyperplasia (PASH) tumour at the surgical scar site in a patient of carcinoma breast. BMJ Case Rep. 2011;2011PMID: 22688488.
3. Baker KS, Davey DD, Stelling CB. Ductal abnormalities detected with galactography: frequency of adequate excisional biopsy. AJR Am J Roentgenol. 1994 Apr;162(4):821-4. PMID: 8140998.
4. Beatty JS, Williams HT, Aldridge BA, et al. Incidental PET/CT findings in the cancer patient: how should they be managed? Surgery. 2009 Aug;146(2):274-81. PMID: 19628085.
5. Bitencourt AG, Cohen MP, Graziano L, et al. Pseudoaneurysm after ultrasound-guided vacuum-assisted core breast biopsy. Breast J. 2012 Mar-Apr;18(2):177-8. PMID: 22211950.
6. Chung A, Schoder H, Sampson M, et al. Incidental breast lesions identified by 18F-fluorodeoxyglucose-positron emission tomography. Ann Surg Oncol. 2010 Aug;17(8):2119-25. PMID: 20162459.
7. Dey D, Nicol A, Singer S. Benign phyllodes tumor of the breast with intracytoplasmic inclusion bodies identical to infantile digital fibromatosis. Breast J. 2008 Mar-Apr;14(2):198-9. PMID: 18266786.
8. Drubin D, Smith JS, Liu W, et al. Comparison of cryopreservation and standard needle biopsy for gene expression profiling of human breast cancer specimens. Breast Cancer Res Treat. 2005 Mar;90(1):93-6. PMID: 15770532.
9. Dutta Roy S, Kasipandian V, Scally J. Suspicious breast mass in an anticoagulated patient--is core biopsy safe? Int J Clin Pract. 2008 Oct;62(10):1632-4. PMID: 18822034.
10. Erdil I, Dursun M, Salmaslioglu A, et al. Pseudoaneurysm in the breast after core biopsy: doppler US and MRI findings. Breast J. 2010 Jul-Aug;16(4):427-9. PMID: 20545941.
11. Fischman AM, Epelboym Y, Siegelbaum RH, et al. Emergent embolization of arterial bleeding after vacuum-assisted breast biopsy. Cardiovasc Intervent Radiol. 2012 Feb;35(1):194-7. PMID: 21553162.
12. Fong CY, Mak WS, Lui CY, et al. Stereotactic biopsy of thin breasts: A previously unfeasible task. Hong Kong. 2011;14(1):4-9.
13. Kamer E, Unalp HR, Akguner T, et al. Thick-needle vacuum-assisted biopsy technique for inflammatory breast carcinoma diagnosis. Acta Cirurgica Brasileira. 2006;21(6):422-4.
14. Kamer E, Unalp HR, Akguner T, et al. [Thick-needle vacuum-assisted biopsy technique for inflammatory breast carcinoma diagnosis]. Acta Cir Bras. 2006 Nov-Dec;21(6):422-4. PMID: 17160256.
15. Kiyoto S, Sugawara Y, Inoue T, et al. False-positive (18)F-fluorodeoxyglucose positron emission tomography/computed tomography caused by incidental injury in a bulky intracystic carcinoma of the breast. Jpn J Radiol. 2010 May;28(4):305-8. PMID: 20512549.
16. Kuhl CK, Elevelt A, Leutner CC, et al. Interventional breast MR imaging: clinical use of a stereotactic localization and biopsy device. Radiology. 1997 Sep;204(3):667-75. PMID: 9280242.
17. Magro G. Epithelioid-cell myofibroblastoma of the breast: expanding the morphologic spectrum. Am J Surg Pathol. 2009 Jul;33(7):1085-92. PMID: 19390423.
18. Mendel JB, Long M, Slanetz PJ. CT-guided core needle biopsy of breast lesions visible only on MRI. AJR Am J Roentgenol. 2007 Jul;189(1):152-4. PMID: 17579165.

19. Nath ME, Robinson TM, Tobon H, et al. Automated large-core needle biopsy of surgically removed breast lesions: comparison of samples obtained with 14-, 16-, and 18-gauge needles. Radiology. 1995 Dec;197(3):739-42. PMID: 7480748.
20. O'Driscoll D, Britton P, Bobrow L, et al. Lobular carcinoma in situ on core biopsy-what is the clinical significance? Clin Radiol. 2001 Mar;56(3):216-20. PMID: 11247699.
21. Ogawa T, Tsuji E, Shirakawa K, et al. Primary non-Hodgkin's lymphoma of the breast treated nonsurgically: report of three cases. Breast Cancer. 2011 Jan;18(1):68-72. PMID: 19350354.
22. O'Sullivan-Mejia E, Idowu MO, Davis Masssey H, et al. Lymphoepithelioma-like carcinoma of the breast: diagnosis by core needle biopsy. Breast J. 2009 Nov-Dec;15(6):658-60. PMID: 19824996.
23. Romero-Guadarrama MB, Hernandez-Gonzalez MM, Duran-Padilla MA, et al. Primary lymphomas of the breast: a report on 5 cases studied in a period of 5 years at the Hospital General de Mexico. Ann Diagn Pathol. 2009 Apr;13(2):78-81. PMID: 19302954.
24. Roque DR, MacLaughlan S, Tejada-Berges T. Necrotizing infection of the breast after core needle biopsy. Breast J. 2013 Mar-Apr;19(2):201-2. PMID: 23294339.
25. Ruiz Tovar J, Reguero Callejas ME, Alaez Chillaron AB, et al. Mammary hamartoma. Clin Transl Oncol. 2006 Apr;8(4):290-3. PMID: 16648106.
26. Ruiz-Delgado ML, Lopez-Ruiz JA, Saiz-Lopez A. Abnormal mammography and sonography associated with foreign-body giant-cell reaction after stereotactic vacuum-assisted breast biopsy with carbon marking. Acta Radiol. 2008 Dec;49(10):1112-8. PMID: 18932053.
27. Samimi M, Bonneau C, Lebas P, et al. Mastectomies after vacuum core biopsy procedure for microcalcification clusters: value of clip. Eur J Radiol. 2009 Feb;69(2):296-9. PMID: 18178050.
28. Singh E, Selis JE. Ultrasound-guided percutaneous biopsy of the augmented breast using implant displacement: a new technique. Ultrasound Q. 2010 Sep;26(3):179-81. PMID: 20823752.
29. Soo MS, Walsh R, Patton J. Prone table stereotactic breast biopsy: facilitating biopsy of posterior lesions using the arm-through-the-hole technique. AJR Am J Roentgenol. 1998 Sep;171(3):615-7. PMID: 9725284.
30. Tilve A, Mallo R, Perez A, et al. Breast hemangiomas: correlation between imaging and pathologic findings. J Clin Ultrasound. 2012 Oct;40(8):512-7. PMID: 22434703.
31. Wahner-Roedler DL, Whaley DH, Brandt KR, et al. Vacuum-assisted breast biopsy device (mammotome) malfunction simulating microcalcifications. Breast J. 2005 Nov-Dec;11(6):474-5. PMID: 16297098.
32. Wang CF, Zhou Z, Yan YJ, et al. Clinical analyses of clustered microcalcifications after autologous fat injection for breast augmentation. Plast Reconstr Surg. 2011 Apr;127(4):1669-73. PMID: 21187809.
33. Wei H, Jiayi F, Qinping Z, et al. Ultrasound-guided vacuum-assisted breast biopsy system for diagnosis and minimally invasive excision of intraductal papilloma without nipple discharge. World J Surg. 2009 Dec;33(12):2579-81. PMID: 19777298.
34. Yalcin S, Ergul E, Ucar AE, et al. Glomus tumor of the breast: first report. Langenbecks Arch Surg. 2009 Mar;394(2):399-400. PMID: 18446361.
35. Yoshida M, Kinoshita T. A case of ductal carcinoma in situ of the breast. Jpn. J. Clin. Oncol. 2009;39(2):132.

36. Abe H, Schmidt RA, Shah RN, et al. MR-directed ("Second-Look") ultrasound examination for breast lesions detected initially on MRI: MR and sonographic findings. AJR Am J Roentgenol. 2010 Feb;194(2):370-7. PMID: 20093598.
37. Berg WA, Arnoldus CL, Teferra E, et al. Biopsy of Amorphous Breast Calcifications: Pathologic Outcome and Yield at Stereotactic Biopsy 1. Radiology. 2001;221(2):495-503.
38. Berg WA, Madsen KS, Schilling K, et al. Comparative effectiveness of positron emission mammography and MRI in the contralateral breast of women with newly diagnosed breast cancer. AJR Am J Roentgenol. 2012 Jan;198(1):219-32. PMID: 22194501.
39. Bernik SF, Troob S, Ying BL, et al. Papillary lesions of the breast diagnosed by core needle biopsy: 71 cases with surgical follow-up. Am J Surg. 2009 Apr;197(4):473-8. PMID: 18723154.
40. Brennan S, Liberman L, Dershaw DD, et al. Breast MRI screening of women with a personal history of breast cancer. AJR Am J Roentgenol. 2010 Aug;195(2):510-6. PMID: 20651211.
41. Brennan SB, Sung JS, Dershaw DD, et al. Cancellation of MR imaging-guided breast biopsy due to lesion nonvisualization: frequency and follow-up. Radiology. 2011 Oct;261(1):92-9. PMID: 21852565.
42. Britton PD, Provenzano E, Barter S, et al. Ultrasound guided percutaneous axillary lymph node core biopsy: how often is the sentinel lymph node being biopsied? Breast. 2009 Feb;18(1):13-6. PMID: 18993074.
43. Carbognin G, Girardi V, Brandalise A, et al. MR-guided vacuum-assisted breast biopsy in the management of incidental enhancing lesions detected by breast MR imaging. Radiol Med. 2011 Sep;116(6):876-85. PMID: 21293942.
44. Chae EY, Cha JH, Kim HH, et al. Evaluation of residual disease using breast MRI after excisional biopsy for breast cancer. AJR Am J Roentgenol. 2013 May;200(5):1167-73. PMID: 23617506.
45. Chan A, Morey A, Brown B, et al. A retrospective study investigating the rate of HER2 discordance between primary breast carcinoma and locoregional or metastatic disease. BMC Cancer. 2012;12:555. PMID: 23176370.
46. Choi HY, Kim SM, Jang M, et al. MRI-guided intervention for breast lesions using the freehand technique in a 3.0-T closed-bore MRI scanner: feasibility and initial results. Korean J Radiol. 2013 Mar-Apr;14(2):171-8. PMID: 23482868.
47. Crystal P, Sadaf A, Bukhanov K, et al. High-risk lesions diagnosed at MRI-guided vacuum-assisted breast biopsy: can underestimation be predicted? Eur Radiol. 2011 Mar;21(3):582-9. PMID: 20839000.
48. Davis KL, Barth RJ, Jr., Gui J, et al. Use of MRI in preoperative planning for women with newly diagnosed DCIS: risk or benefit? Ann Surg Oncol. 2012 Oct;19(10):3270-4. PMID: 22911365.
49. Demartini WB, Eby PR, Peacock S, et al. Utility of targeted sonography for breast lesions that were suspicious on MRI. AJR Am J Roentgenol. 2009 Apr;192(4):1128-34. PMID: 19304724.
50. DeMartini WB, Liu F, Peacock S, et al. Background parenchymal enhancement on breast MRI: impact on diagnostic performance. AJR Am J Roentgenol. 2012 Apr;198(4):W373-80. PMID: 22451576.
51. Destounis S, Arieno A, Somerville PA, et al. Community-based practice experience of unsuspected breast magnetic resonance imaging abnormalities evaluated with second-look sonography. J Ultrasound Med. 2009 Oct;28(10):1337-46. PMID: 19778880.

52. Deurloo EE, Sriram JD, Teertstra HJ, et al. MRI of the breast in patients with DCIS to exclude the presence of invasive disease. Eur Radiol. 2012 Jul;22(7):1504-11. PMID: 22367470.

53. Dogan BE, Le-Petross CH, Stafford JR, et al. MRI-guided vacuum-assisted breast biopsy performed at 3 T with a 9-gauge needle: preliminary experience. AJR Am J Roentgenol. 2012 Nov;199(5):W651-3. PMID: 23096211.

54. Eliahou R, Sella T, Allweis T, et al. Magnetic resonance-guided interventional procedures of the breast: initial experience. Isr Med Assoc J. 2009 May;11(5):275-9. PMID: 19637504.

55. Elmore L, Margenthaler JA. Breast MRI surveillance in women with prior curative-intent therapy for breast cancer. J Surg Res. 2010 Sep;163(1):58-62. PMID: 20605594.

56. Friedman P, Enis S, Pinyard J. Magnetic resonance imaging-guided vacuum-assisted breast biopsy: an initial experience in a community hospital. Can Assoc Radiol J. 2009 Oct;60(4):196-200. PMID: 19782886.

57. Ginter PS, Winant AJ, Hoda SA. Cystic apocrine hyperplasia is the most common finding in MRI detected breast lesions. J Clin Pathol. 2014 Feb;67(2):182-6. PMID: 24151291.

58. Grobmyer SR, Mortellaro VE, Marshall J, et al. Is there a role for routine use of MRI in selection of patients for breast-conserving cancer therapy? J Am Coll Surg. 2008 May;206(5):1045-50; discussion 50-2. PMID: 18471753.

59. Gutierrez RL, Demartini WB, Eby P, et al. Clinical indication and patient age predict likelihood of malignancy in suspicious breast MRI lesions. Acad Radiol. 2009 Oct;16(10):1281-5. PMID: 19733804.

60. Gutierrez RL, DeMartini WB, Eby PR, et al. BI-RADS lesion characteristics predict likelihood of malignancy in breast MRI for masses but not for nonmasslike enhancement. AJR Am J Roentgenol. 2009 Oct;193(4):994-1000. PMID: 19770321.

61. Han BK, Schnall MD, Orel SG, et al. Outcome of MRI-guided breast biopsy. AJR Am J Roentgenol. 2008 Dec;191(6):1798-804. PMID: 19020252.

62. Hauth EA, Jaeger HJ, Lubnau J, et al. MR-guided vacuum-assisted breast biopsy with a handheld biopsy system: clinical experience and results in postinterventional MR mammography after 24 h. Eur Radiol. 2008 Jan;18(1):168-76. PMID: 17609959.

63. He Q, Fan X, Guan Y, et al. Percutaneous excisional biopsy of impalpable breast lesions under ultrasound visualization. The Breast. 2008;17(6):666-70.

64. Heller SL, Moy L. Imaging features and management of high-risk lesions on contrast-enhanced dynamic breast MRI. AJR Am J Roentgenol. 2012 Feb;198(2):249-55. PMID: 22268165.

65. Johnson KS, Baker JA, Lee SS, et al. Suspicious breast lesions detected at 3.0 T magnetic resonance imaging: clinical and histological outcomes. Acad Radiol. 2012 Jun;19(6):667-74. PMID: 22459645.

66. Kalinyak JE, Schilling K, Berg WA, et al. PET-guided breast biopsy. Breast J. 2011 Mar-Apr;17(2):143-51. PMID: 21276128.

67. Lee JH, Kim EK, Oh JY, et al. US screening for detection of nonpalpable locoregional recurrence after mastectomy. Eur J Radiol. 2013 Mar;82(3):485-9. PMID: 23131395.

68. Lee JM, Kaplan JB, Murray MP, et al. Imaging histologic discordance at MRI-guided 9-gauge vacuum-assisted breast biopsy. AJR Am J Roentgenol. 2007 Oct;189(4):852-9. PMID: 17885056.

69. Lee JM, Kaplan JB, Murray MP, et al. Underestimation of DCIS at MRI-guided vacuum-assisted breast biopsy. AJR Am J Roentgenol. 2007 Aug;189(2):468-74. PMID: 17646475.

70. Lee J-M, Kaplan JB, Murray MP, et al. Imaging–histologic discordance at MRI-guided 9-gauge vacuum-assisted breast biopsy. American Journal of Roentgenology. 2007;189(4):852-9.
71. Liberman L, Bracero N, Morris E, et al. MRI-guided 9-gauge vacuum-assisted breast biopsy: initial clinical experience. AJR Am J Roentgenol. 2005 Jul;185(1):183-93. PMID: 15972421.
72. Liberman L, Dershaw DD, Durfee S, et al. Recurrent carcinoma after breast conservation: diagnosis with stereotaxic core biopsy. Radiology. 1995 Dec;197(3):735-8. PMID: 7480747.
73. Liberman L, Morris EA, Dershaw DD, et al. Fast MRI-guided vacuum-assisted breast biopsy: initial experience. American Journal of Roentgenology. 2003;181(5):1283-93.
74. Linda A, Zuiani C, Lorenzon M, et al. Hyperechoic lesions of the breast: not always benign. AJR Am J Roentgenol. 2011 May;196(5):1219-24. PMID: 21512095.
75. Malhaire C, El Khoury C, Thibault F, et al. Vacuum-assisted biopsies under MR guidance: results of 72 procedures. Eur Radiol. 2010 Jul;20(7):1554-62. PMID: 20119729.
76. Mameri CS, Kemp C, Goldman SM, et al. Impact of breast MRI on surgical treatment, axillary approach, and systemic therapy for breast cancer. Breast J. 2008 May-Jun;14(3):236-44. PMID: 18476882.
77. Masroor I, Afzal S, Shafqat G, et al. Comparison of stereotactic core breast biopsy and open surgical biopsy results at a tertiary care hospital in Pakistan. Int J Womens Health. 2011;3:193-6. PMID: 21792341.
78. Meeuwis C, Mann RM, Mus RD, et al. MRI-guided breast biopsy at 3T using a dedicated large core biopsy set: feasibility and initial results. Eur J Radiol. 2011 Aug;79(2):257-61. PMID: 20541338.
79. Meeuwis C, Veltman J, van Hall HN, et al. MR-guided breast biopsy at 3T: diagnostic yield of large core needle biopsy compared with vacuum-assisted biopsy. Eur Radiol. 2012 Feb;22(2):341-9. PMID: 21915606.
80. Meissnitzer M, Dershaw DD, Lee CH, et al. Targeted ultrasound of the breast in women with abnormal MRI findings for whom biopsy has been recommended. AJR Am J Roentgenol. 2009 Oct;193(4):1025-9. PMID: 19770325.
81. Noroozian M, Gombos EC, Chikarmane S, et al. Factors that impact the duration of MRI-guided core needle biopsy. AJR Am J Roentgenol. 2010 Feb;194(2):W150-7. PMID: 20093566.
82. Onega T, Weiss J, Diflorio R, et al. Evaluating surveillance breast imaging and biopsy in older breast cancer survivors. Int J Breast Cancer. 2012;2012:347646. PMID: 23097709.
83. Orel SG, Rosen M, Mies C, et al. MR Imaging–guided 9-gauge Vacuum-assisted Core-Needle Breast Biopsy: Initial Experience 1. Radiology. 2006;238(1):54-61.
84. Oxner CR, Vora L, Yim J, et al. Magnetic resonance imaging-guided breast biopsy in lesions not visualized by mammogram or ultrasound. Am Surg. 2012 Oct;78(10):1087-90. PMID: 23025947.
85. Parikh RP, Doren EL, Mooney B, et al. Differentiating fat necrosis from recurrent malignancy in fat-grafted breasts: an imaging classification system to guide management. Plast Reconstr Surg. 2012 Oct;130(4):761-72. PMID: 23018689.
86. Perlet C, Heinig A, Prat X, et al. Multicenter study for the evaluation of a dedicated biopsy device for MR-guided vacuum biopsy of the breast. Eur Radiol. 2002 Jun;12(6):1463-70. PMID: 12042955.
87. Perlet C, Heywang-Kobrunner SH, Heinig A, et al. Magnetic resonance-guided, vacuum-assisted breast biopsy. Cancer. 2006;106(5):982-90.

88. Perretta T, Pistolese CA, Bolacchi F, et al. MR imaging-guided 10-gauge vacuum-assisted breast biopsy: histological characterisation. Radiol Med. 2008 Sep;113(6):830-40. PMID: 18633687.

89. Pfleiderer SO, Marx C, Vagner J, et al. Magnetic resonance-guided large-core breast biopsy inside a 1.5-T magnetic resonance scanner using an automatic system: in vitro experiments and preliminary clinical experience in four patients. Invest Radiol. 2005 Jul;40(7):458-63. PMID: 15973138.

90. Pijnappel RM, Peeters PH, van den Donk M, et al. Diagnostic strategies in non-palpable breast lesions. Eur J Cancer. 2002 Mar;38(4):550-5. PMID: 11872348.

91. Pijnappel RM, van den Donk M, Holland R, et al. Diagnostic accuracy for different strategies of image-guided breast intervention in cases of nonpalpable breast lesions. Br J Cancer. 2004 Feb 9;90(3):595-600. PMID: 14760370.

92. Popiela TJ, Herman-Sucharska I, Kleinrok K, et al. Core breast biopsy under MR control - Preliminary results. Pol Przegl Radiol. 2007;72(2):15-24.

93. Rauch GM, Dogan BE, Smith TB, et al. Outcome analysis of 9-gauge MRI-guided vacuum-assisted core needle breast biopsies. AJR Am J Roentgenol. 2012 Feb;198(2):292-9. PMID: 22268171.

94. Raza S, Sekar M, Ong EM, et al. Small masses on breast MR: is biopsy necessary? Acad Radiol. 2012 Apr;19(4):412-9. PMID: 22277636.

95. Salem C, Sakr R, Chopier J, et al. Pain and complications of directional vacuum-assisted stereotactic biopsy: comparison of the Mammotome and Vacora techniques. Eur J Radiol. 2009 Nov;72(2):295-9. PMID: 18755562.

96. Salem C, Sakr R, Chopier J, et al. Accuracy of stereotactic vacuum-assisted breast biopsy with a 10-gauge hand-held system. Breast. 2009 Jun;18(3):178-82. PMID: 19364652.

97. Schneider JP, Schulz T, Horn LC, et al. MR-guided percutaneous core biopsy of small breast lesions: first experience with a vertically open 0.5T scanner. J Magn Reson Imaging. 2002 Apr;15(4):374-85. PMID: 11948826.

98. Schrading S, Simon B, Braun M, et al. MRI-guided breast biopsy: influence of choice of vacuum biopsy system on the mode of biopsy of MRI-only suspicious breast lesions. AJR Am J Roentgenol. 2010 Jun;194(6):1650-7. PMID: 20489109.

99. Sequeiros RB, Reinikainen H, Sequeiros AM, et al. MR-guided breast biopsy and hook wire marking using a low-field (0.23 T) scanner with optical instrument tracking. Eur Radiol. 2007 Mar;17(3):813-9. PMID: 17021710.

100. Slanetz PJ, Wu SP, Mendel JB. Percutaneous excision: a viable alternative to manage benign breast lesions. Can Assoc Radiol J. 2011 Nov;62(4):265-71. PMID: 20615659.

101. Sung JS, Malak SF, Bajaj P, et al. Screening breast MR imaging in women with a history of lobular carcinoma in situ. Radiology. 2011 Nov;261(2):414-20. PMID: 21900617.

102. Thompson MO, Lipson J, Daniel B, et al. Why are patients noncompliant with follow-up recommendations after MRI-guided core needle biopsy of suspicious breast lesions? AJR Am J Roentgenol. 2013 Dec;201(6):1391-400. PMID: 24261382.

103. Tozaki M, Yamashiro N, Sakamoto M, et al. Magnetic resonance-guided vacuum-assisted breast biopsy: results in 100 Japanese women. Jpn J Radiol. 2010 Aug;28(7):527-33. PMID: 20799018.

104. Tozaki M, Yamashiro N, Suzuki T, et al. MR-guided vacuum-assisted breast biopsy: is it an essential technique? Breast Cancer. 2009;16(2):121-5. PMID: 18807122.

105. van de Ven SM, Lin MC, Daniel BL, et al. Freehand MRI-guided preoperative needle localization of breast lesions after MRI-guided vacuum-assisted core needle biopsy without marker placement. J Magn Reson Imaging. 2010 Jul;32(1):101-9. PMID: 20575077.

106. van den Bosch MA, Daniel BL, Pal S, et al. MRI-guided needle localization of suspicious breast lesions: results of a freehand technique. Eur Radiol. 2006 Aug;16(8):1811-7. PMID: 16683117.

107. Wilhelm A, McDonough MD, DePeri ER. Malignancy rates of non-masslike enhancement on breast magnetic resonance imaging using American College of Radiology Breast Imaging Reporting and Data System descriptors. Breast J. 2012 Nov-Dec;18(6):523-6. PMID: 23009294.

108. Wiratkapun C, Fusuwankaya E, Wibulpholprasert B, et al. Diagnostic accuracy of vacuum-assisted stereotactic core needle biopsy for breast lesions. J Med Assoc Thai. 2010 Sep;93(9):1058-64. PMID: 20873078.

109. Zebic-Sinkovec M, Hertl K, Kadivec M, et al. Outcome of MRI-guided vacuum-assisted breast biopsy - initial experience at Institute of Oncology Ljubljana, Slovenia. Radiol Oncol. 2012 Jun;46(2):97-105. PMID: 23077445.

110. Zografos G, Zagouri F, Sergentanis TN, et al. Vacuum-assisted breast biopsy in nonpalpable solid breast lesions without microcalcifications: the Greek experience. Diagn Interv Radiol. 2008;14(3):127-30.

111. Acheson MB, Patton RG, Howisey RL, et al. Three- to six-year followup for 379 benign image-guided large-core needle biopsies of nonpalpable breast abnormalities. J Am Coll Surg. 2002 Oct;195(4):462-6. PMID: 12375750.

112. Agoff SN, Lawton TJ. Papillary lesions of the breast with and without atypical ductal hyperplasia: can we accurately predict benign behavior from core needle biopsy? Am J Clin Pathol. 2004 Sep;122(3):440-3. PMID: 15362376.

113. Arora N, Hill C, Hoda SA, et al. Clinicopathologic features of papillary lesions on core needle biopsy of the breast predictive of malignancy. Am J Surg. 2007 Oct;194(4):444-9. PMID: 17826053.

114. Arpino G, Allred DC, Mohsin SK, et al. Lobular neoplasia on core-needle biopsy--clinical significance. Cancer. 2004 Jul 15;101(2):242-50. PMID: 15241819.

115. Ashkenazi I, Ferrer K, Sekosan M, et al. Papillary lesions of the breast discovered on percutaneous large core and vacuum-assisted biopsies: reliability of clinical and pathological parameters in identifying benign lesions. Am J Surg. 2007 Aug;194(2):183-8. PMID: 17618801.

116. Baer HJ, Collins LC, Connolly JL, et al. Lobule type and subsequent breast cancer risk: results from the Nurses' Health Studies. Cancer. 2009 Apr 1;115(7):1404-11. PMID: 19170235.

117. Bauer VP, Ditkoff BA, Schnabel F, et al. The management of lobular neoplasia identified on percutaneous core breast biopsy. Breast J. 2003 Jan-Feb;9(1):4-9. PMID: 12558663.

118. Becker L, Trop I, David J, et al. Management of radial scars found at percutaneous breast biopsy. Can Assoc Radiol J. 2006 Apr;57(2):72-8. PMID: 16944680.

119. Bedei L, Falcini F, Sanna PA, et al. Atypical ductal hyperplasia of the breast: the controversial management of a borderline lesion: experience of 47 cases diagnosed at vacuum-assisted biopsy. Breast. 2006 Apr;15(2):196-202. PMID: 16055333.

120. Berg WA, Campassi CI, Ioffe OB. Cystic lesions of the breast: sonographic-pathologic correlation. Radiology. 2003 Apr;227(1):183-91. PMID: 12668745.

121. Berg WA, Mrose HE, Ioffe OB. Atypical lobular hyperplasia or lobular carcinoma in situ at core-needle breast biopsy. Radiology. 2001 Feb;218(2):503-9. PMID: 11161169.

122. Bode MK, Rissanen T, Apaja-Sarkkinen M. Ultrasonography and core needle biopsy in the differential diagnosis of fibroadenoma and tumor phyllodes. Acta Radiol. 2007 Sep;48(7):708-13. PMID: 17728999.

123. Bonnett M, Wallis T, Rossmann M, et al. Histopathologic analysis of atypical lesions in image-guided core breast biopsies. Mod Pathol. 2003 Feb;16(2):154-60. PMID: 12591968.

124. Bonnett M, Wallis T, Rossmann M, et al. Histologic and radiographic analysis of ductal carcinoma in situ diagnosed using stereotactic incisional core breast biopsy. Mod Pathol. 2002 Feb;15(2):95-101. PMID: 11850537.

125. Brem R, Tran K, Rapelyea J, et al. Percutaneous Biopsy of Papillary Lesions of the Breast: Accuracy of Pathologic Diagnosis. JOURNAL OF WOMENS IMAGING. 2005;7(4):157.

126. Brem RF, Behrndt VS, Sanow L, et al. Atypical ductal hyperplasia: histologic underestimation of carcinoma in tissue harvested from impalpable breast lesions using 11-gauge stereotactically guided directional vacuum-assisted biopsy. AJR Am J Roentgenol. 1999 May;172(5):1405-7. PMID: 10227526.

127. Brem RF, Lechner MC, Jackman RJ, et al. Lobular neoplasia at percutaneous breast biopsy: variables associated with carcinoma at surgical excision. AJR Am J Roentgenol. 2008 Mar;190(3):637-41. PMID: 18287433.

128. Brenner RJ, Jackman RJ, Parker SH, et al. Percutaneous core needle biopsy of radial scars of the breast: when is excision necessary? AJR Am J Roentgenol. 2002 Nov;179(5):1179-84. PMID: 12388495.

129. Buchbender S, Obenauer S, Mohrmann S, et al. Arterial spin labelling perfusion MRI of breast cancer using FAIR TrueFISP: initial results. Clin Radiol. 2013 Mar;68(3):e123-7. PMID: 23245275.

130. Burbank F. Stereotactic breast biopsy of atypical ductal hyperplasia and ductal carcinoma in situ lesions: improved accuracy with directional, vacuum-assisted biopsy. Radiology. 1997;202(3):843-7.

131. Carder PJ, Khan T, Burrows P, et al. Large volume "mammotome" biopsy may reduce the need for diagnostic surgery in papillary lesions of the breast. J Clin Pathol. 2008 Aug;61(8):928-33. PMID: 18495791.

132. Cawson JN, Malara F, Kavanagh A, et al. Fourteen-gauge needle core biopsy of mammographically evident radial scars: is excision necessary? Cancer. 2003 Jan 15;97(2):345-51. PMID: 12518358.

133. Chrzan R, Rudnicka L, Popiela T, Jr., et al. The problems with histopathological verification of breast microcalcification clusters in the stereotactic mammotome biopsy specimens. Pol J Pathol. 2006;57(3):133-5. PMID: 17219739.

134. Cox D, Bradley S, England D. The significance of mammotome core biopsy specimens without radiographically identifiable microcalcification and their influence on surgical management--a retrospective review with histological correlation. Breast. 2006 Apr;15(2):210-8. PMID: 16081287.

135. Crisi GM, Mandavilli S, Cronin E, et al. Invasive mammary carcinoma after immediate and short-term follow-up for lobular neoplasia on core biopsy. Am J Surg Pathol. 2003 Mar;27(3):325-33. PMID: 12604888.

136. Darling ML, Smith DN, Lester SC, et al. Atypical ductal hyperplasia and ductal carcinoma in situ as revealed by large-core needle breast biopsy: results of surgical excision. AJR Am J Roentgenol. 2000 Nov;175(5):1341-6. PMID: 11044038.

137. Das S, Sen S, Mukherjee A, et al. Risk factors of breast cancer among women in eastern India: a tertiary hospital based case control study. Asian Pac J Cancer Prev. 2012;13(10):4979-81. PMID: 23244094.

138. Day AC. Pilot study on the effect of smoking one cigarette on physiological postural tremors. Agressologie. 1977;18 Spec No:9-18. PMID: 900365.

139. de Mascarel I, Brouste V, Asad-Syed M, et al. All atypia diagnosed at stereotactic vacuum-assisted breast biopsy do not need surgical excision. Mod Pathol. 2011 Sep;24(9):1198-206. PMID: 21602816.

140. Deschryver K, Radford DM, Schuh ME. Pathology of large-caliber stereotactic biopsies in nonpalpable breast lesions. Semin Diagn Pathol. 1999 Aug;16(3):224-34. PMID: 10490199.

141. Destounis S, Hanson S, Morgan R, et al. Computer-aided detection of breast carcinoma in standard mammographic projections with digital mammography. Int J Comput Assist Radiol Surg. 2009 Jun;4(4):331-6. PMID: 20033580.

142. Dillon MF, McDermott EW, Hill AD, et al. Predictive value of breast lesions of "uncertain malignant potential" and "suspicious for malignancy" determined by needle core biopsy. Ann Surg Oncol. 2007 Feb;14(2):704-11. PMID: 17151788.

143. Dillon MF, McDermott EW, Quinn CM, et al. Predictors of invasive disease in breast cancer when core biopsy demonstrates DCIS only. J Surg Oncol. 2006 Jun 1;93(7):559-63. PMID: 16705731.

144. Dillon MF, Quinn CM, McDermott EW, et al. Needle core biopsy in the diagnosis of phyllodes neoplasm. Surgery. 2006 Nov;140(5):779-84. PMID: 17084721.

145. DiPiro PJ, Meyer JE, Denison CM, et al. Image-guided core breast biopsy of ductal carcinoma in situ presenting as a non-calcified abnormality. Eur J Radiol. 1999 Jun;30(3):231-6. PMID: 10452723.

146. Dmytrasz K, Tartter PI, Mizrachy H, et al. The significance of atypical lobular hyperplasia at percutaneous breast biopsy. Breast J. 2003 Jan-Feb;9(1):10-2. PMID: 12558664.

147. Doren E, Hulvat M, Norton J, et al. Predicting cancer on excision of atypical ductal hyperplasia. Am J Surg. 2008 Mar;195(3):358-61; discussion 61-2. PMID: 18206849.

148. Douglas-Jones AG, Denson JL, Cox AC, et al. Radial scar lesions of the breast diagnosed by needle core biopsy: analysis of cases containing occult malignancy. J Clin Pathol. 2007 Mar;60(3):295-8. PMID: 16731590.

149. Dupont WD, Breyer JP, Bradley KM, et al. Protein phosphatase 2A subunit gene haplotypes and proliferative breast disease modify breast cancer risk. Cancer. 2010 Jan 1;116(1):8-19. PMID: 19890961.

150. Easley S, Abdul-Karim FW, Klein N, et al. Segregation of radiographic calcifications in stereotactic core biopsies of breast: is it necessary? Breast J. 2007 Sep-Oct;13(5):486-9. PMID: 17760670.

151. Eby PR, Ochsner JE, DeMartini WB, et al. Is surgical excision necessary for focal atypical ductal hyperplasia found at stereotactic vacuum-assisted breast biopsy? Ann Surg Oncol. 2008 Nov;15(11):3232-8. PMID: 18696163.

152. Elsheikh TM, Silverman JF. Follow-up surgical excision is indicated when breast core needle biopsies show atypical lobular hyperplasia or lobular carcinoma in situ: a correlative study of 33 patients with review of the literature. Am J Surg Pathol. 2005 Apr;29(4):534-43. PMID: 15767810.

153. Ely KA, Carter BA, Jensen RA, et al. Core biopsy of the breast with atypical ductal hyperplasia: a probabilistic approach to reporting. Am J Surg Pathol. 2001 Aug;25(8):1017-21. PMID: 11474285.

154. Esserman LE, Lamea L, Tanev S, et al. Should the extent of lobular neoplasia on core biopsy influence the decision for excision? Breast J. 2007 Jan-Feb;13(1):55-61. PMID: 17214794.

155. Forgeard C, Benchaib M, Guerin N, et al. Is surgical biopsy mandatory in case of atypical ductal hyperplasia on 11-gauge core needle biopsy? A retrospective study of 300 patients. Am J Surg. 2008 Sep;196(3):339-45. PMID: 18585676.

156. Foster MC, Helvie MA, Gregory NE, et al. Lobular carcinoma in situ or atypical lobular hyperplasia at core-needle biopsy: is excisional biopsy necessary? Radiology. 2004 Jun;231(3):813-9. PMID: 15105449.

157. Foxcroft LM, Evans EB, Porter AJ. Difficulties in the pre-operative diagnosis of phyllodes tumours of the breast: a study of 84 cases. Breast. 2007 Feb;16(1):27-37. PMID: 16876413.

158. Gadzala DE, Cederbom GJ, Bolton JS, et al. Appropriate management of atypical ductal hyperplasia diagnosed by stereotactic core needle breast biopsy. Ann Surg Oncol. 1997 Jun;4(4):283-6. PMID: 9181225.

159. Gal-Gombos EC, Esserman LE, Recine MA, et al. Large-needle core biopsy in atypical intraductal epithelial hyperplasia including immunohistochemical expression of high molecular weight cytokeratin: analysis of results of a single institution. Breast J. 2002 Sep-Oct;8(5):269-74. PMID: 12199753.

160. Gatek J, Vrana D, Melichar B, et al. Significance of the resection margin and risk factors for close or positive resection margin in patients undergoing breast-conserving surgery. J BUON. 2012 Jul-Sep;17(3):452-6. PMID: 23033280.

161. Gendler LS, Feldman SM, Balassanian R, et al. Association of breast cancer with papillary lesions identified at percutaneous image-guided breast biopsy. Am J Surg. 2004 Oct;188(4):365-70. PMID: 15474427.

162. Georgian-Smith D, Kricun B, McKee G, et al. The mammary hamartoma: appreciation of additional imaging characteristics. J Ultrasound Med. 2004 Oct;23(10):1267-73. PMID: 15448315.

163. Grady I, Gorsuch H, Wilburn-Bailey S. Ultrasound-guided, vacuum-assisted, percutaneous excision of breast lesions: an accurate technique in the diagnosis of atypical ductal hyperplasia. J Am Coll Surg. 2005 Jul;201(1):14-7. PMID: 15978438.

164. Harvey JM, Sterrett GF, Frost FA. Atypical ductal hyperplasia and atypia of uncertain significance in core biopsies from mammographically detected lesions: correlation with excision diagnosis. Pathology. 2002 Oct;34(5):410-6. PMID: 12408338.

165. Harvey SC, Denison CM, Lester SC, et al. Fibrous nodules found at large-core needle biopsy of the breast: imaging features. Radiology. 1999 May;211(2):535-40. PMID: 10228539.

166. Hoorntje LE, Schipper ME, Peeters PH, et al. The finding of invasive cancer after a preoperative diagnosis of ductal carcinoma-in-situ: causes of ductal carcinoma-in-situ underestimates with stereotactic 14-gauge needle biopsy. Ann Surg Oncol. 2003;10(7):748-53.

167. Houssami N, Ciatto S, Bilous M, et al. Borderline breast core needle histology: predictive values for malignancy in lesions of uncertain malignant potential (B3). Br J Cancer. 2007 Apr 23;96(8):1253-7. PMID: 17438578.

168. Huo L, Sneige N, Hunt KK, et al. Predictors of invasion in patients with core-needle biopsy-diagnosed ductal carcinoma in situ and recommendations for a selective approach to

sentinel lymph node biopsy in ductal carcinoma in situ. Cancer. 2006 Oct 15;107(8):1760-8. PMID: 16977650.

169. Hwang H, Barke LD, Mendelson EB, et al. Atypical lobular hyperplasia and classic lobular carcinoma in situ in core biopsy specimens: routine excision is not necessary. Mod Pathol. 2008 Oct;21(10):1208-16. PMID: 18660792.

170. Ivan D, Selinko V, Sahin AA, et al. Accuracy of core needle biopsy diagnosis in assessing papillary breast lesions: histologic predictors of malignancy. Mod Pathol. 2004 Feb;17(2):165-71. PMID: 14631369.

171. Jackman RJ, Birdwell RL, Ikeda DM. Atypical ductal hyperplasia: can some lesions be defined as probably benign after stereotactic 11-gauge vacuum-assisted biopsy, eliminating the recommendation for surgical excision? Radiology. 2002 Aug;224(2):548-54. PMID: 12147855.

172. Jackman RJ, Burbank F, Parker SH, et al. Stereotactic breast biopsy of nonpalpable lesions: determinants of ductal carcinoma in situ underestimation rates. Radiology. 2001 Feb;218(2):497-502. PMID: 11161168.

173. Jang M, Cho N, Moon WK, et al. Underestimation of atypical ductal hyperplasia at sonographically guided core biopsy of the breast. AJR Am J Roentgenol. 2008 Nov;191(5):1347-51. PMID: 18941067.

174. Johnson JM, Dalton RR, Wester SM, et al. Histological correlation of microcalcifications in breast biopsy specimens. Arch Surg. 1999 Jul;134(7):712-5; discussion 5-6. PMID: 10401820.

175. Karabakhtsian RG, Johnson R, Sumkin J, et al. The clinical significance of lobular neoplasia on breast core biopsy. Am J Surg Pathol. 2007 May;31(5):717-23. PMID: 17460455.

176. Kil WH, Cho EY, Kim JH, et al. Is surgical excision necessary in benign papillary lesions initially diagnosed at core biopsy? Breast. 2008 Jun;17(3):258-62. PMID: 18054232.

177. Kim MJ, Kim EK, Kwak JY, et al. Nonmalignant papillary lesions of the breast at US-guided directional vacuum-assisted removal: a preliminary report. Eur Radiol. 2008 Sep;18(9):1774-83. PMID: 18446345.

178. Kim MY, Cho N, Yi A, et al. Sonoelastography in distinguishing benign from malignant complex breast mass and making the decision to biopsy. Korean J Radiol. 2013 Jul-Aug;14(4):559-67. PMID: 23901312.

179. King TA, Cederbom GJ, Champaign JL, et al. A core breast biopsy diagnosis of invasive carcinoma allows for definitive surgical treatment planning. Am J Surg. 1998 Dec;176(6):497-501. PMID: 9926778.

180. Kneeshaw PJ, Turnbull LW, Smith A, et al. Dynamic contrast enhanced magnetic resonance imaging aids the surgical management of invasive lobular breast cancer. Eur J Surg Oncol. 2003 Feb;29(1):32-7. PMID: 12559074.

181. Ko ES, Cho N, Cha JH, et al. Sonographically-guided 14-gauge core needle biopsy for papillary lesions of the breast. Korean J Radiol. 2007 May-Jun;8(3):206-11. PMID: 17554187.

182. Komenaka IK, El-Tamer M, Pile-Spellman E, et al. Core needle biopsy as a diagnostic tool to differentiate phyllodes tumor from fibroadenoma. Arch Surg. 2003 Sep;138(9):987-90. PMID: 12963656.

183. Kunju LP, Kleer CG. Significance of flat epithelial atypia on mammotome core needle biopsy: Should it be excised? Hum Pathol. 2007 Jan;38(1):35-41. PMID: 17095049.

184. Lam WW, Chu WC, Tse GM, et al. Role of fine needle aspiration and tru cut biopsy in diagnosis of mucinous carcinoma of breast--from a radiologist's perspective. Clin Imaging. 2006 Jan-Feb;30(1):6-10. PMID: 16377477.

185. Lavoue V, Graesslin O, Classe JM, et al. Management of lobular neoplasia diagnosed by core needle biopsy: study of 52 biopsies with follow-up surgical excision. Breast. 2007 Oct;16(5):533-9. PMID: 17629481.

186. Lee CH, Carter D, Philpotts LE, et al. Ductal carcinoma in situ diagnosed with stereotactic core needle biopsy: can invasion be predicted? Radiology. 2000 Nov;217(2):466-70. PMID: 11058647.

187. Leikola J, Heikkila P, Pamilo M, et al. Predicting invasion in patients with DCIS in the preoperative percutaneous biopsy. Acta Oncol. 2007;46(6):798-802. PMID: 17653903.

188. Liberman L, Bracero N, Vuolo MA, et al. Percutaneous large-core biopsy of papillary breast lesions. AJR Am J Roentgenol. 1999 Feb;172(2):331-7. PMID: 9930777.

189. Liberman L, Cohen MA, Dershaw DD, et al. Atypical ductal hyperplasia diagnosed at stereotaxic core biopsy of breast lesions: an indication for surgical biopsy. AJR Am J Roentgenol. 1995 May;164(5):1111-3. PMID: 7717215.

190. Liberman L, Dershaw D, Rosen P, et al. Stereotaxic core biopsy of impalpable spiculated breast masses. AJR Am J Roentgenol. 1995;165(3):551-4.

191. Liberman L, Drotman M, Morris EA, et al. Imaging-histologic discordance at percutaneous breast biopsy. Cancer. 2000 Dec 15;89(12):2538-46. PMID: 11135213.

192. Liberman L, Sama M, Susnik B, et al. Lobular carcinoma in situ at percutaneous breast biopsy: surgical biopsy findings. AJR Am J Roentgenol. 1999 Aug;173(2):291-9. PMID: 10430122.

193. Liberman L, Tornos C, Huzjan R, et al. Is surgical excision warranted after benign, concordant diagnosis of papilloma at percutaneous breast biopsy? AJR Am J Roentgenol. 2006 May;186(5):1328-34. PMID: 16632727.

194. Lim CN, Ho BC, Bay BH, et al. Nuclear morphometry in columnar cell lesions of the breast: is it useful? J Clin Pathol. 2006 Dec;59(12):1283-6. PMID: 16603646.

195. Lin PH, Clyde JC, Bates DM, et al. Accuracy of stereotactic core-needle breast biopsy in atypical ductal hyperplasia. Am J Surg. 1998 May;175(5):380-2. PMID: 9600282.

196. Londero V, Zuiani C, Furlan A, et al. Role of ultrasound and sonographically guided core biopsy in the diagnostic evaluation of ductal carcinoma in situ (DCIS) of the breast. Radiol Med. 2007 Sep;112(6):863-76. PMID: 17891529.

197. Londero V, Zuiani C, Linda A, et al. Lobular neoplasia: core needle breast biopsy underestimation of malignancy in relation to radiologic and pathologic features. Breast. 2008 Dec;17(6):623-30. PMID: 18619840.

198. Lopez-Medina A, Cintora E, Mugica B, et al. Radial scars diagnosed at stereotactic core-needle biopsy: surgical biopsy findings. Eur Radiol. 2006 Aug;16(8):1803-10. PMID: 16708220.

199. Lourenco AP, Mainiero MB, Lazarus E, et al. Stereotactic breast biopsy: comparison of histologic underestimation rates with 11- and 9-gauge vacuum-assisted breast biopsy. AJR Am J Roentgenol. 2007 Nov;189(5):W275-9. PMID: 17954625.

200. Maganini RO, Klem DA, Huston BJ, et al. Upgrade rate of core biopsy-determined atypical ductal hyperplasia by open excisional biopsy. Am J Surg. 2001 Oct;182(4):355-8. PMID: 11720670.

201. Makar AB, McMartin KE, Palese M, et al. Formate assay in body fluids: application in methanol poisoning. Biochem Med. 1975 Jun;13(2):117-26. PMID: 1.

202. Martel M, Barron-Rodriguez P, Tolgay Ocal I, et al. Flat DIN 1 (flat epithelial atypia) on core needle biopsy: 63 cases identified retrospectively among 1,751 core biopsies performed over an 8-year period (1992-1999). Virchows Arch. 2007 Nov;451(5):883-91. PMID: 17786469.

203. Masood S, Loya A, Khalbuss W. Is core needle biopsy superior to fine-needle aspiration biopsy in the diagnosis of papillary breast lesions? Diagn Cytopathol. 2003 Jun;28(6):329-34. PMID: 12768640.

204. McKian KP, Reynolds CA, Visscher DW, et al. Novel breast tissue feature strongly associated with risk of breast cancer. J Clin Oncol. 2009 Dec 10;27(35):5893-8. PMID: 19805686.

205. Mendez I, Andreu FJ, Saez E, et al. Ductal carcinoma in situ and atypical ductal hyperplasia of the breast diagnosed at stereotactic core biopsy. Breast J. 2001 Jan-Feb;7(1):14-8. PMID: 11348410.

206. Menon S, Porter GJ, Evans AJ, et al. The significance of lobular neoplasia on needle core biopsy of the breast. Virchows Arch. 2008 May;452(5):473-9. PMID: 18389278.

207. Mercado CL, Hamele-Bena D, Oken SM, et al. Papillary lesions of the breast at percutaneous core-needle biopsy. Radiology. 2006 Mar;238(3):801-8. PMID: 16424237.

208. Mercado CL, Hamele-Bena D, Singer C, et al. Papillary lesions of the breast: evaluation with stereotactic directional vacuum-assisted biopsy. Radiology. 2001 Dec;221(3):650-5. PMID: 11719659.

209. Middleton LP, Grant S, Stephens T, et al. Lobular carcinoma in situ diagnosed by core needle biopsy: when should it be excised? Mod Pathol. 2003 Feb;16(2):120-9. PMID: 12591964.

210. Miller KL, Marks LB, Barrier RC, Jr., et al. Increased sectioning of pathologic specimens with ductal carcinoma in situ of the breast: are there clinical consequences? Clin Breast Cancer. 2003 Aug;4(3):198-202. PMID: 14499013.

211. Millos J, Costas-Rodriguez M, Lavilla I, et al. Multielemental determination in breast cancerous and non-cancerous biopsies by inductively coupled plasma-mass spectrometry following small volume microwave-assisted digestion. Anal Chim Acta. 2008 Aug 1;622(1-2):77-84. PMID: 18602537.

212. Mitnick JS, Gianutsos R, Pollack AH, et al. Tubular carcinoma of the breast: sensitivity of diagnostic techniques and correlation with histopathology. AJR Am J Roentgenol. 1999 Feb;172(2):319-23. PMID: 9930775.

213. Mitnick JS, Gianutsos R, Pollack AH, et al. Comparative Value of Mammography, Fine-Needle Aspiration Biopsy, and Core Biopsy in the Diagnosis of Invasive Lobular Carcinoma. Breast J. 1998;4(2):75-83.

214. O'Hea B J, Tornos C. Mild ductal atypia after large-core needle biopsy of the breast: is surgical excision always necessary? Surgery. 2000 Oct;128(4):738-43. PMID: 11015109.

215. Pan J, Dogan BE, Carkaci S, et al. Comparing performance of the CADstream and the DynaCAD breast MRI CAD systems : CADstream vs. DynaCAD in breast MRI. J Digit Imaging. 2013 Oct;26(5):971-6. PMID: 23589186.

216. Philpotts LE, Lee CH, Horvath LJ, et al. Underestimation of breast cancer with II-gauge vacuum suction biopsy. AJR Am J Roentgenol. 2000 Oct;175(4):1047-50. PMID: 11000162.

217. Philpotts LE, Shaheen NA, Jain KS, et al. Uncommon high-risk lesions of the breast diagnosed at stereotactic core-needle biopsy: clinical importance. Radiology. 2000 Sep;216(3):831-7. PMID: 10966718.

218. Puglisi F, Zuiani C, Bazzocchi M, et al. Role of mammography, ultrasound and large core biopsy in the diagnostic evaluation of papillary breast lesions. Oncology. 2003;65(4):311-5. PMID: 14707450.

219. Rao A, Parker S, Ratzer E, et al. Atypical ductal hyperplasia of the breast diagnosed by 11-gauge directional vacuum-assisted biopsy. Am J Surg. 2002 Dec;184(6):534-7; discussion 7. PMID: 12488158.

220. Renshaw AA. Adequate histologic sampling of breast core needle biopsies. Arch Pathol Lab Med. 2001 Aug;125(8):1055-7. PMID: 11473457.

221. Renshaw AA. Can mucinous lesions of the breast be reliably diagnosed by core needle biopsy? Am J Clin Pathol. 2002 Jul;118(1):82-4. PMID: 12109860.

222. Renshaw AA, Cartagena N, Derhagopian RP, et al. Lobular neoplasia in breast core needle biopsy specimens is not associated with an increased risk of ductal carcinoma in situ or invasive carcinoma. Am J Clin Pathol. 2002 May;117(5):797-9. PMID: 12090431.

223. Renshaw AA, Cartagena N, Schenkman RH, et al. Atypical ductal hyperplasia in breast core needle biopsies. Correlation of size of the lesion, complete removal of the lesion, and the incidence of carcinoma in follow-up biopsies. Am J Clin Pathol. 2001 Jul;116(1):92-6. PMID: 11447758.

224. Renshaw AA, Derhagopian RP, Martinez P, et al. Lobular neoplasia in breast core needle biopsy specimens is associated with a low risk of ductal carcinoma in situ or invasive carcinoma on subsequent excision. Am J Clin Pathol. 2006 Aug;126(2):310-3. PMID: 16891208.

225. Renshaw AA, Derhagopian RP, Tizol-Blanco DM, et al. Papillomas and atypical papillomas in breast core needle biopsy specimens: risk of carcinoma in subsequent excision. Am J Clin Pathol. 2004 Aug;122(2):217-21. PMID: 15323138.

226. Renshaw AA, Gould EW. Comparison of disagreement and amendment rates by tissue type and diagnosis: identifying cases for directed blinded review. Am J Clin Pathol. 2006 Nov;126(5):736-9. PMID: 17050070.

227. Rizzo M, Lund MJ, Oprea G, et al. Surgical follow-up and clinical presentation of 142 breast papillary lesions diagnosed by ultrasound-guided core-needle biopsy. Ann Surg Oncol. 2008 Apr;15(4):1040-7. PMID: 18204989.

228. RJ GEaGJaPJ. Significance of extent of lobular neoplasia on breast core biopsy. J Womens Imaging.

229. Rosen EL, Bentley RC, Baker JA, et al. Imaging-guided core needle biopsy of papillary lesions of the breast. AJR Am J Roentgenol. 2002 Nov;179(5):1185-92. PMID: 12388496.

230. Rosen EL, Soo MS, Bentley RC. Focal fibrosis: a common breast lesion diagnosed at imaging-guided core biopsy. AJR Am J Roentgenol. 1999 Dec;173(6):1657-62. PMID: 10584816.

231. Rutstein LA, Johnson RR, Poller WR, et al. Predictors of residual invasive disease after core needle biopsy diagnosis of ductal carcinoma in situ. Breast J. 2007 May-Jun;13(3):251-7. PMID: 17461899.

232. Saxena A, Dhillon VS, Shahid M, et al. GSTP1 methylation and polymorphism increase the risk of breast cancer and the effects of diet and lifestyle in breast cancer patients. Exp Ther Med. 2012 Dec;4(6):1097-103. PMID: 23226781.

233. Shepherd JA, Kerlikowske K, Ma L, et al. Volume of mammographic density and risk of breast cancer. Cancer Epidemiol Biomarkers Prev. 2011 Jul;20(7):1473-82. PMID: 21610220.

234. Shin HJ, Kim HH, Kim SM, et al. Papillary lesions of the breast diagnosed at percutaneous sonographically guided biopsy: comparison of sonographic features and biopsy methods. AJR Am J Roentgenol. 2008 Mar;190(3):630-6. PMID: 18287432.

235. Shin SJ, Rosen PP. Excisional biopsy should be performed if lobular carcinoma in situ is seen on needle core biopsy. Arch Pathol Lab Med. 2002 Jun;126(6):697-701. PMID: 12033958.

236. Sie A, Bryan DC, Gaines V, et al. Multicenter evaluation of the breast lesion excision system, a percutaneous, vacuum-assisted, intact-specimen breast biopsy device. Cancer. 2006 Sep 1;107(5):945-9. PMID: 16874817.

237. Skandarajah AR, Field L, Yuen Larn Mou A, et al. Benign papilloma on core biopsy requires surgical excision. Ann Surg Oncol. 2008 Aug;15(8):2272-7. PMID: 18473143.

238. Sklair-Levy M, Samuels TH, Catzavelos C, et al. Stromal fibrosis of the breast. AJR Am J Roentgenol. 2001 Sep;177(3):573-7. PMID: 11517049.

239. Smetherman D, Dydynski P, Jackson P. Effect of breast core needle biopsy technique on detection of lobular intraepithelial neoplasia. Ochsner J. 2007 Fall;7(3):121-4. PMID: 21603526.

240. Sneige N, Lim SC, Whitman GJ, et al. Atypical ductal hyperplasia diagnosis by directional vacuum-assisted stereotactic biopsy of breast microcalcifications. Considerations for surgical excision. Am J Clin Pathol. 2003 Feb;119(2):248-53. PMID: 12579995.

241. Sohn V, Arthurs Z, Herbert G, et al. Atypical ductal hyperplasia: improved accuracy with the 11-gauge vacuum-assisted versus the 14-gauge core biopsy needle. Ann Surg Oncol. 2007 Sep;14(9):2497-501. PMID: 17564749.

242. Sohn VY, Arthurs ZM, Kim FS, et al. Lobular neoplasia: is surgical excision warranted? Am Surg. 2008 Feb;74(2):172-7. PMID: 18306873.

243. Sydnor MK, Wilson JD, Hijaz TA, et al. Underestimation of the presence of breast carcinoma in papillary lesions initially diagnosed at core-needle biopsy. Radiology. 2007 Jan;242(1):58-62. PMID: 17090707.

244. Tocino I, Garcia BM, Carter D. Surgical biopsy findings in patients with atypical hyperplasia diagnosed by stereotaxic core needle biopsy. Ann Surg Oncol. 1996 Sep;3(5):483-8. PMID: 8876891.

245. Tse GM, Law BK, Ma TK, et al. Hamartoma of the breast: a clinicopathological review. J Clin Pathol. 2002 Dec;55(12):951-4. PMID: 12461066.

246. Valdes EK, Tartter PI, Genelus-Dominique E, et al. Significance of papillary lesions at percutaneous breast biopsy. Ann Surg Oncol. 2006 Apr;13(4):480-2. PMID: 16474908.

247. Verkooijen HM, Hoorntje LE, Peeters PH. False-negative core needle biopsies of the breast: an analysis of clinical, radiologic, and pathologic findings in 27 consecutive cases of missed breast cancer. Cancer. 2004 Mar 1;100(5):1104-5; author reply 5-6. PMID: 14983508.

248. Winchester DJ, Bernstein JR, Jeske JM, et al. Upstaging of atypical ductal hyperplasia after vacuum-assisted 11-gauge stereotactic core needle biopsy. Arch Surg. 2003 Jun;138(6):619-22; discussion 22-3. PMID: 12799332.

249. Wiratkapun C, Wibulpholprasert B, Wongwaisayawan S, et al. Nondiagnostic core needle biopsy of the breast under imaging guidance: result of rebiopsy. J Med Assoc Thai. 2005 Mar;88(3):350-7. PMID: 15962643.

250. Won B, Reynolds H, Lazaridis C, et al. Stereotactic biopsy of ductal carcinoma in situ of the breast using an 11-gauge vacuum-assisted device: persistent underestimation of disease. AJR Am J Roentgenol. 1999;173(1):227-9.

251. Won B, Reynolds HE, Lazaridis CL, et al. Stereotactic biopsy of ductal carcinoma in situ of the breast using an 11-gauge vacuum-assisted device: persistent underestimation of disease. AJR Am J Roentgenol. 1999 Jul;173(1):227-9. PMID: 10397131.

252. Woolcott CG, SenGupta SK, Hanna WM, et al. Estrogen and progesterone receptor levels in nonneoplastic breast epithelium of breast cancer cases versus benign breast biopsy controls. BMC Cancer. 2008;8:130. PMID: 18466613.

253. Worsham MJ, Raju U, Lu M, et al. Risk factors for breast cancer from benign breast disease in a diverse population. Breast Cancer Res Treat. 2009 Nov;118(1):1-7. PMID: 18836828.

254. Xu HN, Tchou J, Li LZ. Redox imaging of human breast cancer core biopsies: a preliminary investigation. Acad Radiol. 2013 Jun;20(6):764-8. PMID: 23664401.

255. Yeh IT, Dimitrov D, Otto P, et al. Pathologic review of atypical hyperplasia identified by image-guided breast needle core biopsy. Correlation with excision specimen. Arch Pathol Lab Med. 2003 Jan;127(1):49-54. PMID: 12521366.

256. You JK, Kim EK, Kwak JY, et al. Focal fibrosis of the breast diagnosed by a sonographically guided core biopsy of nonpalpable lesions: imaging findings and clinical relevance. J Ultrasound Med. 2005 Oct;24(10):1377-84. PMID: 16179621.

257. Youk JH, Gweon HM, Son EJ, et al. Three-dimensional shear-wave elastography for differentiating benign and malignant breast lesions: comparison with two-dimensional shear-wave elastography. Eur Radiol. 2013 Jun;23(6):1519-27. PMID: 23212276.

258. Zagouri F, Sergentanis TN, Nonni A, et al. Vacuum-assisted breast biopsy: the value and limitations of cores with microcalcifications. Pathol Res Pract. 2007;203(8):563-6. PMID: 17611039.

259. Zhao L, Freimanis R, Bergman S, et al. Biopsy needle technique and the accuracy of diagnosis of atypical ductal hyperplasia for mammographic abnormalities. Am Surg. 2003 Sep;69(9):757-62; discussion 62. PMID: 14509322.

260. Zuiani C, Londero V, Bestagno A, et al. Proliferative high-risk lesions of the breast: contribution and limits of US-guided core biopsy. Radiol Med. 2005 Nov-Dec;110(5-6):589-602. PMID: 16437044.

261. Adrales G, Turk P, Wallace T, et al. Is surgical excision necessary for atypical ductal hyperplasia of the breast diagnosed by Mammotome? Am J Surg. 2000 Oct;180(4):313-5. PMID: 11113443.

262. Brem RF, Schoonjans JM, Goodman SN, et al. Nonpalpable Breast Cancer: Percutaneous Diagnosis with 11-and 8-gauge Stereotactic Vacuum-assisted Biopsy Devices 1. Radiology. 2001;219(3):793-6.

263. Burns RP, Brown JP, Roe SM, et al. Stereotactic core-needle breast biopsy by surgeons: minimum 2-year follow-up of benign lesions. Ann Surg. 2000 Oct;232(4):542-8. PMID: 10998652.

264. Caines JS, Chantziantoniou K, Wright BA, et al. Nova Scotia Breast Screening Program experience: use of needle core biopsy in the diagnosis of screening-detected abnormalities. Radiology. 1996 Jan;198(1):125-30. PMID: 8539363.

265. Caines JS, McPhee MD, Konok GP, et al. Stereotaxic needle core biopsy of breast lesions using a regular mammographic table with an adaptable stereotaxic device. AJR Am J Roentgenol. 1994 Aug;163(2):317-21. PMID: 8037022.

266. Cerwenka H, Hoff M, Rosanelli G, et al. Experience with a high speed biopsy gun in breast cancer diagnosis. Eur J Surg Oncol. 1997 Jun;23(3):206-7. PMID: 9236891.

267. Chen X, Lehman CD, Dee KE. MRI-guided breast biopsy: clinical experience with 14-gauge stainless steel core biopsy needle. AJR Am J Roentgenol. 2004 Apr;182(4):1075-80. PMID: 15039191.

268. Choo KS, Kwak HS, Tae Bae Y, et al. The value of a combination of wire localization and ultrasound-guided vacuum-assisted breast biopsy for clustered microcalcifications. Breast. 2008 Dec;17(6):611-6. PMID: 18653339.

269. Cilotti A, Iacconi C, Marini C, et al. Contrast-enhanced MR imaging in patients with BI-RADS 3-5 microcalcifications. Radiol Med. 2007 Mar;112(2):272-86. PMID: 17361370.

270. Costantini R, Sardellone A, Marino C, et al. Vacuum-assisted core biopsy (Mammotome) for the diagnosis of non-palpable breast lesions: four-year experience in an Italian center. Tumori. 2005 Jul-Aug;91(4):351-4. PMID: 16277103.

271. Crowe JP, Jr., Rim A, Patrick RJ, et al. Does core needle breast biopsy accurately reflect breast pathology? Surgery. 2003 Oct;134(4):523-6; discussion 6-8. PMID: 14605609.

272. Daniel BL, Birdwell RL, Butts K, et al. Freehand iMRI-guided large-gauge core needle biopsy: a new minimally invasive technique for diagnosis of enhancing breast lesions. J Magn Reson Imaging. 2001 Jun;13(6):896-902. PMID: 11382950.

273. Dronkers DJ. Stereotaxic core biopsy of breast lesions. Radiology. 1992 Jun;183(3):631-4. PMID: 1584909.

274. Evans AJ, Whitlock JP, Burrell HC, et al. A comparison of 14 and 12 gauge needles for core biopsy of suspicious mammographic calcification. Br J Radiol. 1999 Dec;72(864):1152-4. PMID: 10703470.

275. Fures R, Bukovic D, Lez C, et al. Large-gauge needle biopsy in diagnosing malignant breast neoplasia. Coll Antropol. 2003 Jun;27(1):259-62. PMID: 12974154.

276. Ghate SV, Rosen EL, Soo MS, et al. MRI-guided vacuum-assisted breast biopsy with a handheld portable biopsy system. AJR Am J Roentgenol. 2006 Jun;186(6):1733-6. PMID: 16714667.

277. Giardina C, Guerrieri A, Ingravallo G, et al. Mammary stereotaxic core-biopsy by Mammotome: an alternative to frozen section examination. Pathologica. 2002;94(4):182-9.

278. Giardina C, Guerrieri AM, Ingravallo G, et al. [The stereotaxic core breast biopsy using the Mammotome: an alternative to intraoperative examination]. Pathologica. 2002 Aug;94(4):182-9. PMID: 12325416.

279. Hirst C, Davis N. Core biopsy for microcalcifications in the breast. Aust N Z J Surg. 1997 Jun;67(6):320-4. PMID: 9193263.

280. Hoorntje LE, Peeters PH, Borel Rinkes IH, et al. Stereotactic large core needle biopsy for all nonpalpable breast lesions? Breast Cancer Res Treat. 2002 May;73(2):177-82. PMID: 12088119.

281. Israel PZ, Fine RE. Stereotactic needle biopsy for occult breast lesions: a minimally invasive alternative. Am Surg. 1995 Jan;61(1):87-91. PMID: 7832390.

282. Jackman RJ, Nowels KW, Shepard MJ, et al. Stereotaxic large-core needle biopsy of 450 nonpalpable breast lesions with surgical correlation in lesions with cancer or atypical hyperplasia. Radiology. 1994 Oct;193(1):91-5. PMID: 8090927.

283. Joshi M, Duva-Frissora A, Padmanabhan R, et al. Atypical ductal hyperplasia in stereotactic breast biopsies: enhanced accuracy of diagnosis with the mammotome. Breast J. 2001 Jul-Aug;7(4):207-13. PMID: 11678796.

284. Kikuchi M, Tsunoda-Shimizu H, Kawasaki T, et al. Indications for stereotactically-guided vacuum-assisted breast biopsy for patients with category 3 microcalcifications. Breast Cancer. 2007;14(3):285-91. PMID: 17690506.

285. Kim MJ, Kim EK, Park SY, et al. Imaging-histologic discordance at sonographically guided percutaneous biopsy of breast lesions. Eur J Radiol. 2008 Jan;65(1):163-9. PMID: 17466478.

286. Klar RM. National health insurance: the federal perspective. ASHA. 1975 Jun;17(6):388-91. PMID: 1137627.

287. Klem D, Jacobs HK, Jorgensen R, et al. Stereotactic breast biopsy in a community hospital setting. Am Surg. 1999 Aug;65(8):737-40; discussion 40-1. PMID: 10432083.

288. Kumaroswamy V, Liston J, Shaaban AM. Vacuum assisted stereotactic guided mammotome biopsies in the management of screen detected microcalcifications: experience of a large breast screening centre. J Clin Pathol. 2008 Jun;61(6):766-9. PMID: 18326021.

289. Lee JM, Kaplan JB, Murray MP, et al. Complete excision of the MRI target lesion at MRI-guided vacuum-assisted biopsy of breast cancer. AJR Am J Roentgenol. 2008 Oct;191(4):1198-202. PMID: 18806165.

290. Łuczyńska E, Kocurek A, Dyczek S, et al. Ultrasound-guided, vacuum-assisted biopsy in evaluation of breast lesions. NOWOTWORY. 2008;58.

291. Łuczyńska E, Skotnicki P, Kocurek A, et al. Vacuum mammotomy under ultrasound guidance. Polish Journal of Radiology. 2007;72(3):15-8.

292. McCombs MM, Bassett LW, Jahan R, et al. Imaging-Guided Core Biopsy of the Breast. The Breast Journal. 1995;1(1):9-16.

293. Mendez A, Cabanillas F, Echenique M, et al. Evaluation of Breast Imaging Reporting and Data System Category 3 mammograms and the use of stereotactic vacuum-assisted breast biopsy in a nonacademic community practice. Cancer. 2004 Feb 15;100(4):710-4. PMID: 14770425.

294. Morrow M, Schmidt R, Cregger B, et al. Preoperative evaluation of abnormal mammographic findings to avoid unnecessary breast biopsies. Arch Surg. 1994 Oct;129(10):1091-6. PMID: 7944941.

295. Newman MR, Frost FA, Sterrett GF, et al. Diagnosis of breast microcalcifications: a comparison of stereotactic FNA and core imprint cytology as adjuncts to core biopsy. Pathology. 2001 Nov;33(4):449-53. PMID: 11827411.

296. Nisbet AP, Borthwick-Clarke A, Scott N. 11-gauge vacuum assisted directional biopsy of breast calcifications, using upright stereotactic guidance. Eur J Radiol. 2000 Dec;36(3):144-6. PMID: 11091014.

297. Pillsbury SG, Jr., Haugen JA, Roux S. Reliability of multimodal evaluation of abnormal screening mammogram results. Am J Obstet Gynecol. 1996 Jun;174(6):1683-6; discussion 6-7. PMID: 8678127.

298. Rich PM, Michell MJ, Humphreys S, et al. Stereotactic 14G core biopsy of non-palpable breast cancer: what is the relationship between the number of core samples taken and the sensitivity for detection of malignancy? Clin Radiol. 1999 Jun;54(6):384-9. PMID: 10406340.

299. Schneider E, Rohling KW, Schnall MD, et al. An apparatus for MR-guided breast lesion localization and core biopsy: Design and preliminary results. Journal of Magnetic Resonance Imaging. 2001;14(3):243-53.

300. Senn Bahls E, Dupont Lampert V, Oelschlegel C, et al. Multitarget stereotactic core-needle breast biopsy (MSBB)--an effective and safe diagnostic intervention for non-palpable breast lesions: a large prospective single institution study. Breast. 2006 Jun;15(3):339-46. PMID: 16488609.

301. Seoudi H, Mortier J, Basile R, et al. Stereotactic core needle biopsy of nonpalpable breast lesions: initial experience with a promising technique. Arch Surg. 1998 Apr;133(4):366-72. PMID: 9565115.

302. Shin JH, Han BK, Ko EY, et al. Probably benign breast masses diagnosed by sonography: is there a difference in the cancer rate according to palpability? AJR Am J Roentgenol. 2009 Apr;192(4):W187-91. PMID: 19304679.

303. Smyczek-Gargya B, Krainick U, Muller-Schimpfle M, et al. Large-core needle biopsy for diagnosis and treatment of breast lesions. Arch Gynecol Obstet. 2002 Aug;266(4):198-200. PMID: 12192478.

304. Soo MS, Baker JA, Rosen EL, et al. Sonographically guided biopsy of suspicious microcalcifications of the breast: a pilot study. AJR Am J Roentgenol. 2002 Apr;178(4):1007-15. PMID: 11906892.

305. Taft R, Chao K, Dear P, et al. The role of core biopsy in the diagnosis of mammographically detected lesions. Aust N Z J Surg. 1996 Oct;66(10):664-7. PMID: 8855919.

306. Taourel P, Hoa D, Chaveron C, et al. Stereotactic vacuum biopsy of calcifications with a handheld portable biopsy system: a validation study. Eur Radiol. 2008 Jul;18(7):1319-25. PMID: 18351352.

307. Teh WL, Wilson AR, Evans AJ, et al. Ultrasound guided core biopsy of suspicious mammographic calcifications using high frequency and power Doppler ultrasound. Clin Radiol. 2000 May;55(5):390-4. PMID: 10816407.

308. Vega A, Garijo F, Ortega E. Core needle aspiration biopsy of palpable breast masses. Acta Oncol. 1995;34(1):31-4. PMID: 7865233.

309. Velanovich V, Lewis FR, Jr., Nathanson SD, et al. Comparison of mammographically guided breast biopsy techniques. Ann Surg. 1999 May;229(5):625-30; discussion 30-3. PMID: 10235520.

310. Wallace JE, Sayler C, McDowell NG, et al. The role of stereotactic biopsy in assessment of nonpalpable breast lesions. Am J Surg. 1996 May;171(5):471-3. PMID: 8651387.

311. Wong T-T, Cheung PS, Ma MK, et al. Experience of stereotactic breast biopsy using the vacuum-assisted core needle biopsy device and the advanced breast biopsy instrumentation system in Hong Kong women. Asian Journal of Surgery. 2005;28(1):18-23.

312. Woodcock NP, Glaves I, Morgan DR, et al. Ultrasound-guided Tru-cut biopsy of the breast. Ann R Coll Surg Engl. 1998 Jul;80(4):253-6. PMID: 9771224.

313. Zardawi IM. Fine needle aspiration cytology vs. core biopsy in a rural setting. Acta Cytol. 1998 Jul-Aug;42(4):883-7. PMID: 9684572.

314. Zografos GC, Zagouri F, Sergentanis TN, et al. Is zero underestimation feasible? Extended Vacuum-Assisted Breast Biopsy in solid lesions - a blind study. World J Surg Oncol. 2007;5:53. PMID: 17501997.

315. Zografos GC, Zagouri F, Sergentanis TN, et al. Pain during vacuum-assisted breast biopsy: are there any predictors? Breast. 2008 Dec;17(6):592-5. PMID: 18657974.

316. Lifrange E, Dondelinger RF, Quatresooz P, et al. Stereotactic breast biopsy with an 8-gauge, directional, vacuum-assisted probe: initial experience. Eur Radiol. 2002 Sep;12(9):2180-7. PMID: 12195467.

317. Abramovici G, Mainiero MB. Screening breast MR imaging: comparison of interpretation of baseline and annual follow-up studies. Radiology. 2011 Apr;259(1):85-91. PMID: 21285337.

318. Acheson MB, Patton RG, Howisey RL, et al. Histologic correlation of image-guided core biopsy with excisional biopsy of nonpalpable breast lesions. Arch Surg. 1997 Aug;132(8):815-8; discussion 9-21. PMID: 9267263.

319. Ahmed HG, Ali AS, Almobarak AO. Utility of fine-needle aspiration as a diagnostic technique in breast lumps. Diagn Cytopathol. 2009 Dec;37(12):881-4. PMID: 19760761.

320. Andreu FJ, Saez A, Sentis M, et al. Breast core biopsy reporting categories--An internal validation in a series of 3054 consecutive lesions. Breast. 2007 Feb;16(1):94-101. PMID: 16982194.

321. Aryal KR, Lengyel AJ, Purser N, et al. Nipple core biopsy for the deformed or scaling nipple. Breast. 2004 Aug;13(4):350-2. PMID: 15325673.

322. Berner A, Davidson B, Sigstad E, et al. Fine-needle aspiration cytology vs. core biopsy in the diagnosis of breast lesions. Diagn Cytopathol. 2003 Dec;29(6):344-8. PMID: 14648793.

323. Bick U, Engelken F, Diederichs G, et al. MRI of the breast as part of the assessment in population-based mammography screening. Rofo. 2013 Sep;185(9):849-56. PMID: 23740312.

324. Brancato B, Scialpi M, Pusiol T, et al. Needle core biopsy should replace fine needle aspiration cytology in ultrasound-guided sampling of breast lesions. Pathologica. 2011 Apr;103(2):52. PMID: 21797145.

325. Brunner AH, Sagmeister T, Kremer J, et al. The accuracy of frozen section analysis in ultrasound- guided core needle biopsy of breast lesions. BMC Cancer. 2009;9:341. PMID: 19778424.

326. Burak WE, Jr., Owens KE, Tighe MB, et al. Vacuum-assisted stereotactic breast biopsy: histologic underestimation of malignant lesions. Arch Surg. 2000 Jun;135(6):700-3. PMID: 10843367.

327. Carmichael AR, Berresford A, Sami A, et al. Imprint cytology of needle core-biopsy specimens of breast lesion: is it best of both worlds? Breast. 2004 Jun;13(3):232-4. PMID: 15177427.

328. Cupido BD, Vawda F, Sabri A, et al. Evaluation and correlation of mammographically suspicious lesions with histopathology at Addington Hospital, Durban. S Afr Med J. 2013 Apr;103(4):251-4. PMID: 23547702.

329. Duijm LE, Groenewoud JH, Roumen RM, et al. A decade of breast cancer screening in The Netherlands: trends in the preoperative diagnosis of breast cancer. Breast Cancer Res Treat. 2007 Nov;106(1):113-9. PMID: 17219049.

330. Duncan JL, 3rd, Cederbom GJ, Champaign JL, et al. Benign diagnosis by image-guided core-needle breast biopsy. Am Surg. 2000 Jan;66(1):5-9; discussion -10. PMID: 10651339.

331. Fotou M, Oikonomou V, Zagouri F, et al. Imprint cytology on microcalcifications excised by vacuum-assisted breast biopsy: a rapid preliminary diagnosis. World J Surg Oncol. 2007;5:40. PMID: 17407604.

332. Gebauer B, Bostanjoglo M, Moesta KT, et al. Magnetic resonance-guided biopsy of suspicious breast lesions with a handheld vacuum biopsy device. Acta Radiol. 2006 Nov;47(9):907-13. PMID: 17077039.

333. Green RS, Mathew S. The contribution of cytologic imprints of stereotactically guided core needle biopsies of the breast in the management of patients with mammographic abnormalities. Breast J. 2001 Jul-Aug;7(4):214-8. PMID: 11678797.

334. James JJ, Wilson AR, Evans AJ, et al. The use of a short-acting benzodiazepine to reduce the risk of syncopal episodes during upright stereotactic breast biopsy. Clin Radiol. 2005 Mar;60(3):394-6. PMID: 15710145.

335. Joulaee A, Kalantari M, Kadivar M, et al. Trucut biopsy of breast lesions: the first step toward international standards in developing countries. Eur J Cancer. 2012 Mar;48(5):648-54. PMID: 22244803.

336. Kam JK, Naidu P, Rose AK, et al. Five-year analysis of magnetic resonance imaging as a screening tool in women at hereditary risk of breast cancer. J Med Imaging Radiat Oncol. 2013 Aug;57(4):400-6. PMID: 23870334.

337. Kang SS, Ko EY, Han BK, et al. Breast US in patients who had microcalcifications with low concern of malignancy on screening mammography. Eur J Radiol. 2008 Aug;67(2):285-91. PMID: 17703906.

338. Kim MJ, Kim EK, Lee JY, et al. Breast lesions with imaging-histologic discordance during US-guided 14G automated core biopsy: can the directional vacuum-assisted removal replace the surgical excision? Initial findings. Eur Radiol. 2007 Sep;17(9):2376-83. PMID: 17361422.

339. Kumaraswamy V, Carder PJ. Examination of breast needle core biopsy specimens performed for screen-detected microcalcification. J Clin Pathol. 2007 Jun;60(6):681-4. PMID: 16882700.

340. Mak WS, Fong CY, Lui CY. Ultrasound-guided biopsy of solid breast lesions: Should fine-needle aspiration be replaced by core biopsy? Hong Kong. 2012;15(1):10-4.

341. Mohr Z, Hirche C, Klein T, et al. Vacuum-assisted minimally invasive biopsy of soft-tissue tumors. J Bone Joint Surg Am. 2012 Jan 18;94(2):103-9. PMID: 22257995.

342. Olaya W, Bae W, Wong J, et al. Accuracy and upgrade rates of percutaneous breast biopsy: the surgeon's role. Am Surg. 2010 Oct;76(10):1084-7. PMID: 21105615.

343. Parker SH, Klaus AJ, McWey PJ, et al. Sonographically guided directional vacuum-assisted breast biopsy using a handheld device. AJR Am J Roentgenol. 2001 Aug;177(2):405-8. PMID: 11461871.

344. Peter D, Grunhagen J, Wenke R, et al. False-negative results after stereotactically guided vacuum biopsy. Eur Radiol. 2008 Jan;18(1):177-82. PMID: 17637996.

345. Popiela TJ, Tabor J, Chrzan R, et al. Mammotome biopsy in the diagnostic management of non-palpable breast pathologies. Pol Przegl Radiol. 2006;71(3):48-56.

346. Sakamoto N, Tozaki M, Higa K, et al. False-negative ultrasound-guided vacuum-assisted biopsy of the breast: difference with US-detected and MRI-detected lesions. Breast Cancer. 2010 Apr;17(2):110-7. PMID: 19434473.

347. Sakamoto N, Tozaki M, Higa K, et al. Categorization of non-mass-like breast lesions detected by MRI. Breast Cancer. 2008;15(3):241-6. PMID: 18224381.

348. Sarff M, Schmidt K, Vetto JT. Targeted breast cancer screening in women younger than 40: results from a statewide program. Am J Surg. 2008 May;195(5):626-30; discussion 30. PMID: 18374894.

349. Schoonjans JM, Brem RF. Fourteen-gauge ultrasonographically guided large-core needle biopsy of breast masses. J Ultrasound Med. 2001 Sep;20(9):967-72. PMID: 11549157.

350. Schur EA, Elmore JE, Onega T, et al. The impact of obesity on follow-up after an abnormal screening mammogram. Cancer Epidemiol Biomarkers Prev. 2012 Feb;21(2):327-36. PMID: 22144503.

351. Sigal-Zafrani B, Muller K, El Khoury C, et al. Vacuum-assisted large-core needle biopsy (VLNB) improves the management of patients with breast microcalcifications - analysis of 1009 cases. Eur J Surg Oncol. 2008 Apr;34(4):377-81. PMID: 17604937.

352. Simon JR, Kalbhen CL, Cooper RA, et al. Accuracy and complication rates of US-guided vacuum-assisted core breast biopsy: initial results. Radiology. 2000 Jun;215(3):694-7. PMID: 10831686.

353. Smith GE, Burrows P. Ultrasound diagnosis of fibroadenoma - is biopsy always necessary? Clin Radiol. 2008 May;63(5):511-5; discussion 6-7. PMID: 18374713.

354. Sohn YM, Kim MJ, Kim EK, et al. Sonographic elastography combined with conventional sonography: how much is it helpful for diagnostic performance? J Ultrasound Med. 2009 Apr;28(4):413-20. PMID: 19321669.

355. Sonmez G, Cuce F, Mutlu H, et al. Value of diffusion-weighted MRI in the differentiation of benign and malign breast lesions. Wien Klin Wochenschr. 2011 Nov;123(21-22):655-61. PMID: 21922210.

356. Stijven S, Gielen E, Bevernage C, et al. Magnetic resonance imaging: value of diffusion-weighted imaging in differentiating benign from malignant breast lesions. Eur J Obstet Gynecol Reprod Biol. 2013 Feb;166(2):215-20. PMID: 23219320.

357. Sung JS, Lee CH, Morris EA, et al. Screening breast MR imaging in women with a history of chest irradiation. Radiology. 2011 Apr;259(1):65-71. PMID: 21325032.

358. Tabrizian P, Moezzi M, Menes TS. Synchronous benign-appearing calcifications in patients with ductal carcinoma in situ may not be benign. Breast Cancer. 2011 Oct;18(4):314-8. PMID: 20602184.

359. Tadwalkar RV, Rapelyea JA, Torrente J, et al. Breast-specific gamma imaging as an adjunct modality for the diagnosis of invasive breast cancer with correlation to tumour size and grade. Br J Radiol. 2012 Jun;85(1014):e212-6. PMID: 21712429.

360. Tozaki M. BI-RADS-MRI terminology and evaluation of intraductal carcinoma and ductal carcinoma in situ. Breast Cancer. 2013 Jan;20(1):13-20. PMID: 22109641.

361. Weigert JM, Bertrand ML, Lanzkowsky L, et al. Results of a multicenter patient registry to determine the clinical impact of breast-specific gamma imaging, a molecular breast imaging technique. AJR Am J Roentgenol. 2012 Jan;198(1):W69-75. PMID: 22194518.

362. Weinstein SP, Hanna LG, Gatsonis C, et al. Frequency of malignancy seen in probably benign lesions at contrast-enhanced breast MR imaging: findings from ACRIN 6667. Radiology. 2010 Jun;255(3):731-7. PMID: 20501712.

363. Whitlock JP, Evans AJ, Burrell HC, et al. Digital imaging improves upright stereotactic core biopsy of mammographic microcalcifications. Clin Radiol. 2000 May;55(5):374-7. PMID: 10816404.

364. Whitworth PW. Intact Percutaneous Excision (IPEX) for Definitive Diagnosis of High-Risk Breast Lesions. Ann Surg Oncol. 2011 Oct;18(11):3095. PMID: 21904961.

365. Wu YC, Chen DR, Kuo SJ. Personal experience of ultrasound-guided 14-gauge core biopsy of breast tumor. Eur J Surg Oncol. 2006 Sep;32(7):715-8. PMID: 16769196.

366. Xu H, Rao M, Varghese T, et al. Axial-shear strain imaging for differentiating benign and malignant breast masses. Ultrasound Med Biol. 2010 Nov;36(11):1813-24. PMID: 20800948.

367. Xu X, Gifford-Hollingsworth C, Sensenig R, et al. Breast tumor detection using piezoelectric fingers: first clinical report. J Am Coll Surg. 2013 Jun;216(6):1168-73. PMID: 23623223.

368. Yi A, Cho N, Chang JM, et al. Sonoelastography for 1,786 non-palpable breast masses: diagnostic value in the decision to biopsy. Eur Radiol. 2012 May;22(5):1033-40. PMID: 22116557.

369. Yoon JH, Jung HK, Lee JT, et al. Shear-wave elastography in the diagnosis of solid breast masses: what leads to false-negative or false-positive results? Eur Radiol. 2013 Sep;23(9):2432-40. PMID: 23673572.

370. Yoon JH, Kim EK, Kwak JY, et al. Is US-guided core needle biopsy (CNB) enough in probably benign nodules with interval growth? Ultraschall Med. 2012 Dec;33(7):E145-50. PMID: 23023453.

371. Yoon JH, Kim MJ, Moon HJ, et al. Subcategorization of ultrasonographic BI-RADS category 4: positive predictive value and clinical factors affecting it. Ultrasound Med Biol. 2011 May;37(5):693-9. PMID: 21458145.

372. Youk JH, Kim EK, Kim MJ, et al. Performance of hand-held whole-breast ultrasound based on BI-RADS in women with mammographically negative dense breast. Eur Radiol. 2011 Apr;21(4):667-75. PMID: 20853108.

373. . A mammographic screening pilot project in Victoria 1988-1990. The Essendon Breast X-ray Program Collaborative Group. Med J Aust. 1992 Nov 16;157(10):670-3. PMID: 1435408.

374. . Hereditary breast and ovarian cancer syndrome. Gynecol Oncol. 2009 Apr;113(1):6-11. PMID: 19309638.

375. National Guideline Clearinghouse (NGC). Guideline summary: American Society of Clinical Oncology/College of American Pathologists guideline recommendations for immunohistochemical testing of estrogen and progesterone receptors in breast cancer. In: National Guideline Clearinghouse (NGC) [Web site]. Rockville (MD): Agency for Healthcare Research and Quality (AHRQ); [cited 2013 June 25]. Available: http://www.guideline.gov.

376. National Guideline Clearinghouse (NGC). Guideline summary: Use of tumor markers in clinical practice: quality requirements. In: National Guideline Clearinghouse (NGC) [Web site]. Rockville (MD): Agency for Healthcare Research and Quality (AHRQ); [cited 2013 June 25]. Available: http://www.guideline.gov.

377. Abbas S, Miller G, Doyle T. Specimen Radiography Following Hook Wire Localization and Excision of Screen Detected Breast Abnormality. International Journal of Cancer Research. 2007;3(1):39-42.

378. Abe H, Schmidt RA, Kulkarni K, et al. Axillary lymph nodes suspicious for breast cancer metastasis: sampling with US-guided 14-gauge core-needle biopsy--clinical experience in 100 patients. Radiology. 2009 Jan;250(1):41-9. PMID: 18955508.

379. Abrahamson PE, Dunlap LA, Amamoo MA, et al. Factors predicting successful needle-localized breast biopsy. Acad Radiol. 2003 Jun;10(6):601-6. PMID: 12809412.

380. Abrahamsson A, Morad V, Saarinen NM, et al. Estradiol, tamoxifen, and flaxseed alter IL-1beta and IL-1Ra levels in normal human breast tissue in vivo. J Clin Endocrinol Metab. 2012 Nov;97(11):E2044-54. PMID: 22930784.

381. Acosta JA, Greenlee JA, Gubler KD, et al. Surgical margins after needle-localization breast biopsy. Am J Surg. 1995 Dec;170(6):643-5; discussion 5-6. PMID: 7492018.

382. Agodirin SO, Ojemakinde OM, Bello TO, et al. Ultrasound-guided wire localization of lesions detected on screening mammography in Osogbo, Nigeria and its impact on breast conservative surgery. Ann Afr Med. 2012 Apr-Jun;11(2):91-5. PMID: 22406668.

383. Aitken RJ, MacDonald HL, Kirkpatrick AE, et al. Outcome of surgery for non-palpable mammographic abnormalities. Br J Surg. 1990 Jun;77(6):673-6. PMID: 2383738.

384. Al Ayyan M, Bu Ali O, Al Sharri S, et al. Negative axillary ultrasonography with biopsy may predict non-involvement of the non-sentinel lymph nodes in operable breast cancer patients. Asia Pac J Clin Oncol. 2012 Nov 21PMID: 23167952.

385. Albert MP, Sachsse E, Coe NP, et al. Correlation between mammography and the pathology of nonpalpable breast lesions. J Surg Oncol. 1990 May;44(1):44-6. PMID: 2342374.

386. Alexander HR, Candela FC, Dershaw DD, et al. Needle-localized mammographic lesions. Results and evolving treatment strategy. Arch Surg. 1990 Nov;125(11):1441-4. PMID: 2241554.

387. Alhabshi SMI, Rahmat K, Abdul Halim N, et al. Semi-quantitative and qualitative assessment of breast ultrasound elastography in differentiating between malignant and benign lesions. Ultrasound Med Biol. 2013;39(4):568-78.

388. Al-Harethee W, Theodoropoulos G, Filippakis GM, et al. Complications of percutaneous stereotactic vacuum assisted breast biopsy system utilizing radio frequency. Eur J Radiol. 2013 Apr;82(4):623-6. PMID: 22227260.

389. Alicioglu B, Yucesoy C. A simple method to decrease surgical trauma in wire localization procedures. Diagn Interv Radiol. 2008 Sep;14(3):131-2. PMID: 18814133.

390. Al-Khawari H, Athyal R, Kovacs A, et al. Accuracy of the Fischer scoring system and the Breast Imaging Reporting and Data System in identification of malignant breast lesions. Ann Saudi Med. 2009 Jul-Aug;29(4):280-7. PMID: 19584584.

391. Allen SD, Nerurkar A, Della Rovere GU. The breast lesion excision system (BLES): a novel technique in the diagnostic and therapeutic management of small indeterminate breast lesions? Eur Radiol. 2011 May;21(5):919-24. PMID: 21240608.

392. Al-Thobhani AK, Raja'a YA, Noman TA, et al. Profile of breast lesions among women with positive biopsy findings in Yemen. East Mediterr Health J. 2006 Sep;12(5):599-604. PMID: 17333799.

393. Amitkumar K, Srigayathri S, Praburaj AR, et al. Immunohistochemical analysis and correlation of p53, Ki-67 and PCNA in core needle Biopsy specimens of carcinoma breast. Res. J. Pharm., Biol. Chem. Sci. 2012;3(4):1446-58.

394. Aoyama K, Kamio T, Hirano A, et al. Granular cell tumors: a report of six cases. World J Surg Oncol. 2012;10:204. PMID: 23021251.

395. Arambula Cosio F, Lira Berra E, Hevia Montiel N, et al. Computer assisted biopsy of breast tumors. Conf Proc IEEE Eng Med Biol Soc. 2010;2010:5995-8. PMID: 21097108.

396. Armstrong K, Handorf EA, Chen J, et al. Breast cancer risk prediction and mammography biopsy decisions: a model-based study. Am J Prev Med. 2013 Jan;44(1):15-22. PMID: 23253645.

397. Arora R, El Hameed AA, Al Ajrawi T, et al. The accuracy of abnormal cytology report in breast fine needle aspiration alone and in combination with clinical and imaging findings - a hospital based five year study in Kuwait. Gulf J Oncolog. 2008 Jul(4):33-8. PMID: 20084773.

398. Asadi M, Shobeiri H, Aliakbarian M, et al. Reproducibility of lymphoscintigraphy before and after excisional biopsy of primary breast lesions: a study using superficial peri-areolar injection of the radiotracer. Rev Esp Med Nucl Imagen Mol. 2013 May-Jun;32(3):152-5. PMID: 23044070.

399. Ashraf M, Biswas J, Gupta S, et al. Determinants of wound infections for breast procedures: assessment of the risk of wound infection posed by an invasive procedure for subsequent operation. Int J Surg. 2009 Dec;7(6):543-6. PMID: 19748602.

400. Asoglu O, Ozmen V, Karanlik H, et al. The role of sentinel lymph node biopsy with blue dye alone in breast cancer patients with excisional biopsy. Acta Chir Belg. 2005 May-Jun;105(3):291-6. PMID: 16018523.

401. Ball CG, Butchart M, MacFarlane JK. Effect on biopsy technique of the breast imaging reporting and data system (BI-RADS) for nonpalpable mammographic abnormalities. Can J Surg. 2002 Aug;45(4):259-63. PMID: 12174979.

402. Barbalaco Neto G, Rossetti C, Fonseca FL, et al. Ductal carcinoma in situ in core needle biopsies and its association with extensive in situ component in the surgical specimen. Int Arch Med. 2012;5(1):19. PMID: 22715888.

403. Bassiouny RH, Youssef T, Hassan O. Diagnostic performance of breast MRI with and without the addition of quantitative diffusion weighted imaging. Egypt. J. Radiol. Nucl. Med. 2012;43(2):311-23.

404. Bauer TL, Pandelidis SM, Rhoads JE, Jr., et al. Mammographically detected carcinoma of the breast. Surg Gynecol Obstet. 1991 Dec;173(6):482-6. PMID: 1948608.

405. Baute PB, Thibodeau ME, Newstead G. Improving the yield of biopsy for nonpalpable lesions of the breast. Surg Gynecol Obstet. 1992 Feb;174(2):93-6. PMID: 1734582.

406. Baykara M, Özkan Z, Gül Y, et al. Effectiveness of the Triple Test and Its Alternatives for Breast Mass Evaluation.

407. Bellantone R, Rossi S, Lombardi CP, et al. Excisional breast biopsy: when, why and how? Int Surg. 1995 Jan-Mar;80(1):75-8. PMID: 7657498.

408. Bender JS, Magnuson TH, Smith-Meek MA, et al. Will stereotactic breast biopsy achieve results as good as current techniques? Am Surg. 1996 Aug;62(8):637-9; discussion 9-40. PMID: 8712560.

409. Benedict S, Williams RD, Baron PL. Recalled anxiety: from discovery to diagnosis of a benign breast mass. Oncol Nurs Forum. 1994 Nov-Dec;21(10):1723-7. PMID: 7854934.

410. Benedict S, Williams RD, Baron PL. The effect of benign breast biopsy on subsequent breast cancer detection practices. Oncol Nurs Forum. 1994 Oct;21(9):1467-75. PMID: 7816674.

411. Benson SR, Harrison NJ, Lengyel J, et al. Combined image guidance excision of non-palpable breast lesions. Breast. 2004 Apr;13(2):110-4. PMID: 15019690.

412. Berkey CS, Willett WC, Frazier AL, et al. Prospective study of adolescent alcohol consumption and risk of benign breast disease in young women. Pediatrics. 2010 May;125(5):e1081-7. PMID: 20385629.

413. Berkey CS, Willett WC, Tamimi RM, et al. Dairy intakes in older girls and risk of benign breast disease in young women. Cancer Epidemiol Biomarkers Prev. 2013 Apr;22(4):670-4. PMID: 23542805.

414. Bianchini G, Qi Y, Alvarez RH, et al. Molecular anatomy of breast cancer stroma and its prognostic value in estrogen receptor-positive and -negative cancers. J Clin Oncol. 2010 Oct 1;28(28):4316-23. PMID: 20805453.

415. Bird D, Hart S. Early experience with needle localization and biopsy of mammographic lesions. Aust N Z J Surg. 1990 May;60(5):337-40. PMID: 2334355.

416. Bluvol N, Kornecki A, Shaikh A, et al. Freehand versus guided breast biopsy: comparison of accuracy, needle motion, and biopsy time in a tissue model. AJR Am J Roentgenol. 2009 Jun;192(6):1720-5. PMID: 19457840.

417. Bluvol N, Sheikh A, Kornecki A, et al. A needle guidance system for biopsy and therapy using two-dimensional ultrasound. Med Phys. 2008 Feb;35(2):617-28. PMID: 18383683.

418. Bohndiek SE, Royle GJ, Speller RD. An active pixel sensor x-ray diffraction (APXRD) system for breast cancer diagnosis. Phys Med Biol. 2009 Jun 7;54(11):3513-27. PMID: 19443951.

419. Bojia F, Demisse M, Dejane A, et al. Comparison of fine-needle aspiration cytology and excisional biopsy of breast lesions. East Afr Med J. 2001 May;78(5):226-8. PMID: 12002079.

420. Bosch AM, Beets GL, Kessels AG, et al. A needle-localised open-breast biopsy for nonpalpable breast lesions should not be performed for diagnosis. Breast. 2004 Dec;13(6):476-82. PMID: 15563854.

421. Bouton ME, Wilhelmson KL, Komenaka IK. Intraoperative ultrasound can facilitate the wire guided breast procedure for mammographic abnormalities. Am Surg. 2011 May;77(5):640-6. PMID: 21679601.

422. Bowa K, Jewel J, Mudenda V. Fine needle aspiration cytology in the investigation of breast lumps at the University Teaching Hospital in Lusaka, Zambia. Trop Doct. 2008 Oct;38(4):245-7. PMID: 18820201.

423. Brenner RJ. Lesions entirely removed during stereotactic biopsy: preoperative localization on the basis of mammographic landmarks and feasibility of freehand technique--initial experience. Radiology. 2000 Feb;214(2):585-90. PMID: 10671616.

424. Brenner RJ, Pfaff JM. Mammographic changes after excisional breast biopsy for benign disease. AJR Am J Roentgenol. 1996 Oct;167(4):1047-52. PMID: 8819410.

425. Brett J, Austoker J. Women who are recalled for further investigation for breast screening: psychological consequences 3 years after recall and factors affecting re-attendance. J Public Health Med. 2001 Dec;23(4):292-300. PMID: 11873891.

426. Brett J, Austoker J, Ong G. Do women who undergo further investigation for breast screening suffer adverse psychological consequences? A multi-centre follow-up study comparing different breast screening result groups five months after their last breast screening appointment. J Public Health Med. 1998 Dec;20(4):396-403. PMID: 9923945.

427. Budczies J, Weichert W, Noske A, et al. Genome-wide gene expression profiling of formalin-fixed paraffin-embedded breast cancer core biopsies using microarrays. J Histochem Cytochem. 2011 Feb;59(2):146-57. PMID: 21339180.

428. Burnside ES, Chhatwal J, Alagoz O. What is the optimal threshold at which to recommend breast biopsy? PLoS One. 2012;7(11):e48820. PMID: 23144986.

429. Burrell H, Murphy C, Wilson A, et al. Wire localization biopsies of non-palpable breast lesions: the use of the Nottingham localization device. The Breast. 1997;6(2):79-83.

430. Burrell HC, Pinder SE, Wilson AR, et al. The positive predictive value of mammographic signs: a review of 425 non-palpable breast lesions. Clin Radiol. 1996 Apr;51(4):277-81. PMID: 8617041.

431. Carswell H. Minimally invasive FNAB versus surgical biopsy. Diagn Imaging (San Franc). 1991 Jun;13(6):97-104. PMID: 10149914.

432. Castells X, Roman M, Romero A, et al. Breast cancer detection risk in screening mammography after a false-positive result. Cancer Epidemiol. 2013 Feb;37(1):85-90. PMID: 23142338.

433. Caya JG. Breast Frozen Section Outcome in the Community Hospital Setting A Detailed Analysis of 932 Cases. International Journal of Surgical Pathology. 1995;2(3):215-9.

434. Chadwick DR, Shorthouse AJ. Wire-directed localization biopsy of the breast: an audit of results and analysis of factors influencing therapeutic value in the treatment of breast cancer. Eur J Surg Oncol. 1997 Apr;23(2):128-33. PMID: 9158186.

435. Chang CB, Lvoff NM, Leung JW, et al. Solitary dilated duct identified at mammography: outcomes analysis. AJR Am J Roentgenol. 2010 Feb;194(2):378-82. PMID: 20093599.

436. Chen L, Abbey CK, Nosratieh A, et al. Anatomical complexity in breast parenchyma and its implications for optimal breast imaging strategies. Med Phys. 2012 Mar;39(3):1435-41. PMID: 22380376.

437. Chimenti F, Vomero S. [Synthesis of N-substituted isoindolines]. Farmaco Sci. 1975 Nov;30(11):884-90. PMID: 251.

438. Chinyama CN, Davies JD, Rayter Z, et al. Factors affecting surgical margin clearance in screen-detected breast cancer and the effect of cavity biopsies on residual disease. Eur J Surg Oncol. 1997 Apr;23(2):123-7. PMID: 9158185.

439. Chlebowski RT, Anderson G, Manson JE, et al. Estrogen alone in postmenopausal women and breast cancer detection by means of mammography and breast biopsy. J Clin Oncol. 2010 Jun 1;28(16):2690-7. PMID: 20439627.

440. Ciatto S, Bonardi R, Ravaioli A, et al. Benign breast surgical biopsies: are they always justified? Tumori. 1998 Sep-Oct;84(5):521-4. PMID: 9862509.

441. Cleverley JR, Jackson AR, Bateman AC. Pre-operative localization of breast microcalcification using high-frequency ultrasound. Clin Radiol. 1997 Dec;52(12):924-6. PMID: 9413966.

442. Coady MS, Benson EA, Hartley MN. Provision and acceptability of day case breast biopsy: an audit of current practice. Ann R Coll Surg Engl. 1993 Jul;75(4):281-4; discussion 5. PMID: 8379634.

443. Colbert ST, O'Hanlon DM, McDonnell C, et al. Analgesia in day case breast biopsy--the value of pre-emptive tenoxicam. Can J Anaesth. 1998 Mar;45(3):217-22. PMID: 9579258.

444. Collins JC, Liao S, Wile AG. Surgical management of breast masses in pregnant women. J Reprod Med. 1995 Nov;40(11):785-8. PMID: 8592313.

445. Cooper RA. Dual technique for preoperative localization of nonpalpable breast lesions. Can Assoc Radiol J. 1991 Dec;42(6):439-40. PMID: 1751909.

446. Coskun G, Dogan L, Karaman N, et al. Value of sentinel lymph node biopsy in breast cancer patients with previous excisional biopsy. J Breast Cancer. 2012 Mar;15(1):87-90. PMID: 22493633.

447. Cox CE, Reintgen DS, Nicosia SV, et al. Analysis of residual cancer after diagnostic breast biopsy: an argument for fine-needle aspiration cytology. Ann Surg Oncol. 1995 May;2(3):201-6. PMID: 7641015.

448. Cox G, Didlake R, Powers C, et al. Choice of anesthetic technique for needle localized breast biopsy. Am Surg. 1991 Jul;57(7):414-8. PMID: 1647712.

449. Crawford MD, Biankin AV, Rickard MT, et al. The operative management of screen-detected breast cancers. Aust N Z J Surg. 2000 Mar;70(3):168-73. PMID: 10765897.

450. D'Alfonso TM, Liu YF, Chen Z, et al. SP3, a reliable alternative to HercepTest in determining HER-2/neu status in breast cancer patients. J Clin Pathol. 2013 May;66(5):409-14. PMID: 23386665.

451. Davies AH, Cowan A, Jones P, et al. Ultrasound localization of screen detected impalpable breast tumours. J R Coll Surg Edinb. 1994 Dec;39(6):353-4. PMID: 7869290.

452. Davies RJ, A'Hern RP, Parsons CA, et al. Mammographic accuracy and patient age: a study of 297 patients undergoing breast biopsy. Clin Radiol. 1993 Jan;47(1):23-5. PMID: 8280193.

453. Day JC, Stone N. A subcutaneous Raman needle probe. Appl Spectrosc. 2013 Mar;67(3):349-54. PMID: 23452501.

454. Dayal S, Murray J, Wilson K, et al. Imprint cytology from core biopsies increases the sensitivity of fine needle aspiration (FNA) in breast cancer patients. Magy Seb. 2011 Apr;64(2):59-62. PMID: 21504853.

455. De Koning HJ, Fracheboud J, Boer R, et al. Nation-wide breast cancer screening in The Netherlands: support for breast-cancer mortality reduction. National Evaluation Team for Breast Cancer Screening (NETB). Int J Cancer. 1995 Mar 16;60(6):777-80. PMID: 7896444.

456. Deane KA, Degner LF. Information needs, uncertainty, and anxiety in women who had a breast biopsy with benign outcome. Cancer Nurs. 1998 Apr;21(2):117-26. PMID: 9556938.

457. Degnim AC, Miller J, Hoskin TL, et al. A prospective study of breast lymphedema: frequency, symptoms, and quality of life. Breast Cancer Res Treat. 2012 Aug;134(3):915-22. PMID: 22415476.

458. della Rovere GQ, Benson JR, Morgan M, et al. Localization of impalpable breast lesions--a surgical approach. Eur J Surg Oncol. 1996 Oct;22(5):478-82. PMID: 8903489.

459. Di Giorgio A, Alessi G, Arnone P, et al. Ultrasonographically guided excisional biopsy of non-palpable breast lesions. Br J Surg. 1996 Jan;83(1):103. PMID: 8653327.

460. Diepstraten SC, Verkooijen HM, van Diest PJ, et al. Radiofrequency-assisted intact specimen biopsy of breast tumors: critical evaluation according to the IDEAL recommendations. Cancer Imaging. 2011;11:247-52. PMID: 22201702.

461. Domanski AM, Monsef N, Domanski HA, et al. Comparison of the oestrogen and progesterone receptor status in primary breast carcinomas as evaluated by immunohistochemistry and immunocytochemistry: a consecutive series of 267 patients. Cytopathology. 2013 Feb;24(1):21-5. PMID: 22783929.

462. Dominguez WG, Nardi H, Montero H, et al. HER2/neu protein expression and fine needle breast aspiration from Argentinean patients with non-palpable breast lesions. Exp Ther Med. 2010 Jul;1(4):597-602. PMID: 22993582.

463. Dowlatshahi K, Jokich PM, Kluskens LF, et al. A prospective study of double diagnosis of nonpalpable lesions of the breast. Surg Gynecol Obstet. 1991 Feb;172(2):121-4. PMID: 1846452.

464. Drosos Y, Kouloukoussa M, Ostvold AC, et al. NUCKS overexpression in breast cancer. Cancer Cell Int. 2009;9:19. PMID: 19664271.

465. Du J, Wang L, Wan CF, et al. Differentiating benign from malignant solid breast lesions: combined utility of conventional ultrasound and contrast-enhanced ultrasound in comparison with magnetic resonance imaging. Eur J Radiol. 2012 Dec;81(12):3890-9. PMID: 23062280.

466. Dyess DL, Lorino CO, Grieco A, et al. Selective nonoperative management of solid breast masses. Am Surg. 1992 Jul;58(7):435-40. PMID: 1616189.

467. Ebeed SA, Abd El-Moneim NA, Saad A, et al. Diagnostic and prognostic value of circulating tumor cells in female breast cancer patients. Alex. J. Med. 2012;48(3):197-206.

468. Egyed Z, Pentek Z, Jaray B, et al. Radial scar-significant diagnostic challenge. Pathol Oncol Res. 2008 Jun;14(2):123-9. PMID: 18409019.

469. Erguvan-Dogan B, Whitman GJ, Nguyen VA, et al. Specimen radiography in confirmation of MRI-guided needle localization and surgical excision of breast lesions. AJR Am J Roentgenol. 2006 Aug;187(2):339-44. PMID: 16861535.

470. Estourgie SH, Valdes Olmos RA, Nieweg OE, et al. Excision biopsy of breast lesions changes the pattern of lymphatic drainage. Br J Surg. 2007 Sep;94(9):1088-91. PMID: 17514636.

471. Ezer SS, Oguzkurt P, Ince E, et al. Surgical treatment of the solid breast masses in female adolescents. J Pediatr Adolesc Gynecol. 2013 Feb;26(1):31-5. PMID: 23158756.

472. Fedoruk LM, Bojm MA, Bugis SP. Fine-wire localization for nonpalpable mammographic abnormalities. Can J Surg. 1995 Apr;38(2):173-7. PMID: 7728673.

473. Feng XZ, Song YH, Zhang FX, et al. Diagnostic accuracy of fiberoptic ductoscopy plus in vivo iodine staining for intraductal proliferative lesions. Chin Med J (Engl). 2013 Aug;126(16):3124-9. PMID: 23981624.

474. Feoli F, Ameye L, Van Eeckhout P, et al. Liquid-based cytology of the breast: pitfalls unrecognized before specific liquid-based cytology training - proposal for a modification of the diagnostic criteria. Acta Cytol. 2013;57(4):369-76. PMID: 23860126.

475. Ferno M, Baldetorp B, Fallenius G, et al. Preoperative fine needle aspiration from human breast cancer is a valuable sampling material for progesterone receptor and cytometric DNA analysis. Acta Oncol. 1996;35 Suppl 8:19-25. PMID: 9073045.

476. Ferreiro JA, Gisvold JJ, Bostwick DG. Accuracy of frozen-section diagnosis of mammographically directed breast biopsies. Results of 1,490 consecutive cases. Am J Surg Pathol. 1995 Nov;19(11):1267-71. PMID: 7573688.

477. Flanagan JJ, Conry BG, Rubin G, et al. Short communication: Prospective assessment of a new graduated hookwire for the localization of impalpable breast lesions. Br J Radiol. 1996 Apr;69(820):341-3. PMID: 8665134.

478. Fleury Ede F, Fleury JC, Piato S, et al. New elastographic classification of breast lesions during and after compression. Diagn Interv Radiol. 2009 Jun;15(2):96-103. PMID: 19517379.

479. Florentine BD, Kirsch D, Carroll-Johnson RM, et al. Conservative excision of wire-bracketed breast carcinomas: a community hospital's experience. Breast J. 2004 Sep-Oct;10(5):398-404. PMID: 15327492.

480. Franceschi D, Crowe J, Zollinger R, et al. Biopsy of the breast for mammographically detected lesions. Surg Gynecol Obstet. 1990 Dec;171(6):449-55. PMID: 2244276.

481. Frank JL, Lynch K, Barrows G. Nipple smear cytology is of no value in the management of women with nipple discharge. Conn Med. 2010 Apr;74(4):207-10. PMID: 20441001.

482. Frattini V, Ghisoni L, Teodoro A, et al. Clinical approach with optical imaging instrument. perspective analysis on 617 young females: Studio clinico mediante dinamica ottica mammaria per immagini. analisi prospettica in 617 donne con eta inferiore a 40 anni. Ital. J. Gynaecol. Obstet. 2011;23(2-3):101-6.

483. Fukutomi T, Yamamoto H, Nanasawa T, et al. Prognostic factors for local recurrence in breast conservation therapy: residual cancers after lumpectomy. Surg Today. 1993;23(5):402-6. PMID: 8324333.

484. Garcia-Ortega MJ, Benito MA, Vahamonde EF, et al. Pretreatment axillary ultrasonography and core biopsy in patients with suspected breast cancer: diagnostic accuracy and impact on management. Eur J Radiol. 2011 Jul;79(1):64-72. PMID: 20047809.

485. Garcia-Vilanova-Comas A, Fuster-Diana C, Cubells-Parrilla M, et al. Nicolau syndrome after lidocaine injection and cold application: a rare complication of breast core needle biopsy. Int J Dermatol. 2011 Jan;50(1):78-80. PMID: 21182507.

486. Geelhoed GW, Barr HM, Curtis DJ, et al. Radiologic recommendation for breast biopsy on screening mammography reports. Am Surg. 1991 Jul;57(7):419-24. PMID: 2058848.

487. Giacalone PL, Bourdon A, Trinh PD, et al. Radioguided occult lesion localization plus sentinel node biopsy (SNOLL) versus wire-guided localization plus sentinel node detection: a case control study of 129 unifocal pure invasive non-palpable breast cancers. Eur J Surg Oncol. 2012 Mar;38(3):222-9. PMID: 22231127.

488. Giagounidis EM, Markus R, Josef L, et al. CT-guided preoperative needle localization of MRI-detected breast lesions. Eur J Radiol. 2001 Aug;39(2):100-3. PMID: 11522418.

489. Goedde TA, Frykberg ER, Crump JM, et al. The impact of mammography on breast biopsy. Am Surg. 1992 Nov;58(11):661-6. PMID: 1485695.

490. Goff JM, Molloy M, Debbas MT, et al. Long-term impact of previous breast biopsy on breast cancer screening modalities. J Surg Oncol. 1995 May;59(1):18-20. PMID: 7745971.

491. Goldberg JA, Scott RN, Davidson PM, et al. Psychological morbidity in the first year after breast surgery. Eur J Surg Oncol. 1992 Aug;18(4):327-31. PMID: 1521623.

492. Gossmann A, Bangard C, Warm M, et al. Real-time MR-guided wire localization of breast lesions by using an open 1.0-T imager: initial experience. Radiology. 2008 May;247(2):535-42. PMID: 18349317.

493. Gouin F, Tournigand T, Moisan D, et al. [Preparation of the patient for reoperation]. Ann Anesthesiol Fr. 1975 Jul;16(4):237-40. PMID: 2040.

494. Grannan KJ, Lamping K. Impact of method of anesthesia on the accuracy of needle-localized breast biopsies. Am J Surg. 1993 Feb;165(2):218-20. PMID: 8427399.

495. Gray RJ, Salud C, Nguyen K, et al. Randomized prospective evaluation of a novel technique for biopsy or lumpectomy of nonpalpable breast lesions: radioactive seed versus wire localization. Ann Surg Oncol. 2001 Oct;8(9):711-5. PMID: 11597011.

496. Green B, Dowley A, Turnbull LS, et al. Impact of fine-needle aspiration cytology, ultrasonography and mammography on open biopsy rate in patients with benign breast disease. Br J Surg. 1995 Nov;82(11):1509-11. PMID: 8535805.

497. Griffen MM, Welling RE. Needle-localized biopsy of the breast. Surg Gynecol Obstet. 1990 Feb;170(2):145-8. PMID: 2154039.

498. Guarneri V, Barbieri E, Piacentini F, et al. Predictive and prognostic role of p53 according to tumor phenotype in breast cancer patients treated with preoperative chemotherapy: a single-institution analysis. Int J Biol Markers. 2010 Apr-Jun;25(2):104-11. PMID: 20544688.

499. Gupta A, Subhas G, Dubay L, et al. Review of re-excision for narrow or positive margins of invasive and intraductal carcinoma. Am Surg. 2010 Jul;76(7):731-4. PMID: 20698380.

500. Gwin JL, Jr., King B, Hudson KB, et al. Interval mammography after needle localization biopsy of breast abnormalities that are pathologically benign. Am J Surg. 1995 Oct;170(4):323-6. PMID: 7573722.

501. Hall JA, Murphy DC, Hall BR, et al. Open surgical biopsy for nonpalpable mammographic abnormalities: still an option compared with core needle biopsy. Am J Obstet Gynecol. 1998 Jun;178(6):1245-50. PMID: 9662308.

502. Halladay JR, Yankaskas BC, Bowling JM, et al. Positive predictive value of mammography: comparison of interpretations of screening and diagnostic images by the same radiologist and by different radiologists. AJR Am J Roentgenol. 2010 Sep;195(3):782-5. PMID: 20729460.

503. Hamby LS, McGrath PC, Stelling CB, et al. Management of mammographic indeterminate lesions. First place winner of the Conrad Jobst Award in the Gold Medal paper competition. Am Surg. 1993 Jan;59(1):4-8. PMID: 8386912.

504. Hashemzadeh SH, Kumar PV, Malekpour N, et al. Diagnostic accuracy of fine needle aspiration cytology: Comparison of results in Tabriz Imam Khomeini Hospital and Shiraz University of Medical Sciences. Iran. J. Cancer Prev. 2009;2(3):133-6.

505. Hasselgren PO, Hummel RP, Georgian-Smith D, et al. Breast biopsy with needle localization: accuracy of specimen x-ray and management of missed lesions. Surgery. 1993 Oct;114(4):836-40; discussion 40-2. PMID: 8211702.

506. Haupt LM, Irving RE, Weinstein SR, et al. Matrix metalloproteinase localisation by in situ-RT-PCR in archival human breast biopsy material. Mol Cell Probes. 2008 Apr;22(2):83-9. PMID: 17669621.

507. Hewes JC, Imkampe A, Haji A, et al. Importance of routine cavity sampling in breast conservation surgery. Br J Surg. 2009 Jan;96(1):47-53. PMID: 19108003.

508. Higgins G, Abdulkareen A, Loutfi A, et al. Productivity of needle localization to facilitate excision of nonpalpable, mammographically suspicious lesions. Can J Surg. 1991 Jun;34(3):287-9. PMID: 2054762.

509. Hizukuri A, Nakayama R, Kashikura Y, et al. Computerized determination scheme for histological classification of breast mass using objective features corresponding to clinicians' subjective impressions on ultrasonographic images. J Digit Imaging. 2013 Oct;26(5):958-70. PMID: 23546774.

510. Homer MJ. Nonpalpable breast microcalcifications: frequency, management, and results of incisional biopsy. Radiology. 1992 Nov;185(2):411-3. PMID: 1410347.

511. Hong JY, Kang YS, Kil HK. Anaesthesia for day case excisional breast biopsy: propofol-remifentanil compared with sevoflurane-nitrous oxide. Eur J Anaesthesiol. 2008 Jun;25(6):460-7. PMID: 18298873.

512. Howe JR, Monsees B, Destouet J, et al. Needle localization breast biopsy: a model for multidisciplinary quality assurance. J Surg Oncol. 1995 Apr;58(4):233-9. PMID: 7723366.

513. Hubbard R, Kerlikowske K, Buist D, et al. Evaluation of breast cancer screening strategies must be based on comparison of harms and benefits. AJR Am J Roentgenol. 2011 Oct;197(4):W793; author reply 4. PMID: 21940562.

514. Hughes JH, Mason MC, Gray RJ, et al. A multi-site validation trial of radioactive seed localization as an alternative to wire localization. Breast J. 2008 Mar-Apr;14(2):153-7. PMID: 18248562.

515. Iggo R, Rudewicz J, Monceau E, et al. Validation of a yeast functional assay for p53 mutations using clonal sequencing. J Pathol. 2013 Dec;231(4):441-8. PMID: 23897043.

516. Irabor D, Okolo C. An audit of 149 consecutive breast biopsies in Ibadan, Nigeria. PAKISTAN JOURNAL OF MEDICAL SCIENCES. 2008;24(2):257.

517. Jacquemier J, Spyratos F, Esterni B, et al. SISH/CISH or qPCR as alternative techniques to FISH for determination of HER2 amplification status on breast tumors core needle biopsies: a multicenter experience based on 840 cases. BMC Cancer. 2013;13:351. PMID: 23875536.

518. Jardines L, Fowble B, Schultz D, et al. Factors associated with a positive reexcision after excisional biopsy for invasive breast cancer. Surgery. 1995 Nov;118(5):803-9. PMID: 7482265.

519. Javid SH, Carlson JW, Garber JE, et al. Breast MRI wire-guided excisional biopsy: specimen size as compared to mammogram wire-guided excisional biopsy and implications for use. Ann Surg Oncol. 2007 Dec;14(12):3352-8. PMID: 17849165.

520. Javid SH, Kirstein LJ, Rafferty E, et al. Outcome of multiple-wire localization for larger breast cancers: do multiple wires translate into additional imaging, biopsies, and recurrences? Am J Surg. 2009 Sep;198(3):368-72. PMID: 19716884.

521. Jeter DD, Vest GR, Buday SJ. Mammographic guidewire localization of nonpalpable breast lesions. Am Surg. 1991 Jul;57(7):431-3. PMID: 1647713.

522. Johnston JA, Clee CZ. Analysis of 308 localisation breast biopsies in a New Zealand hospital. Australas Radiol. 1991 May;35(2):148-51. PMID: 1930011.

523. Johnston S, Trudeau M, Kaufman B, et al. Phase II study of predictive biomarker profiles for response targeting human epidermal growth factor receptor 2 (HER-2) in advanced inflammatory breast cancer with lapatinib monotherapy. J Clin Oncol. 2008 Mar 1;26(7):1066-72. PMID: 18212337.

524. Johnstone AJ, John TG, Thompson AM, et al. PDS II (polydioxanone) is the monofilament suture of choice for subcuticular wound closure following breast biopsy. J R Coll Surg Edinb. 1992 Apr;37(2):94-6. PMID: 1377271.

525. Johnstone AJ, Thompson AM, Charles M, et al. Wound compression pads are of no value after local anaesthetic breast biopsy. Ann R Coll Surg Engl. 1991 Sep;73(5):303-4. PMID: 1929132.

526. Joo JD, In JH, Kim DW, et al. The comparison of sedation quality, side effect and recovery profiles on different dosage of remifentanil patient-controlled sedation during breast biopsy surgery. Korean J Anesthesiol. 2012 Nov;63(5):431-5. PMID: 23198037.

527. Kaelin CM, Smith TJ, Homer MJ, et al. Safety, accuracy, and diagnostic yield of needle localization biopsy of the breast performed using local anesthesia. J Am Coll Surg. 1994 Sep;179(3):267-72. PMID: 8069420.

528. Kalu ON, Chow C, Wheeler A, et al. The diagnostic value of nipple discharge cytology: breast imaging complements predictive value of nipple discharge cytology. J Surg Oncol. 2012 Sep 15;106(4):381-5. PMID: 22396104.

529. Kanchwala SK, Bucky LP. Precision transverse rectus abdominis muscle flap breast reconstruction: a reliable technique for efficient preoperative planning. Ann Plast Surg. 2008 May;60(5):521-6. PMID: 18434826.

530. Kanjer K, Tatic S, Neskovic-Konstantinovic Z, et al. Treatment response to preoperative anthracycline-based chemotherapy in locally advanced breast cancer: the relevance of proliferation and apoptosis rates. Pathol Oncol Res. 2013 Jul;19(3):577-88. PMID: 23526163.

531. Kapp JM, Walker R, Haneuse S, et al. Are there racial/ethnic disparities among women younger than 40 undergoing mammography? Breast Cancer Res Treat. 2010 Nov;124(1):213-22. PMID: 20204501.

532. Karp G, Abu-Ghanem S, Novack V, et al. Localization of PKCeta in cell membranes as a predictor for breast cancer response to treatment. Onkologie. 2012;35(5):260-6. PMID: 22868505.

533. Kaviani A, Fateh M, Ataie-Fashtami L, et al. Comparison of carbon dioxide laser and scalpel for breast lumpectomy: a randomized controlled trial. Photomed Laser Surg. 2008 Jun;26(3):257-62. PMID: 18588441.

534. Kearney TJ, Morrow M. Effect of reexcision on the success of breast-conserving surgery. Ann Surg Oncol. 1995 Jul;2(4):303-7. PMID: 7552618.

535. Kelly P, Winslow EH. Needle wire localization for nonpalpable breast lesions: sensations, anxiety levels, and informational needs. Oncol Nurs Forum. 1996 May;23(4):639-45. PMID: 8735322.

536. Kim J, Lee J, Chang E, et al. Selective Sentinel Node Plus Additional Non-Sentinel Node Biopsy Based on an FDG-PET/CT Scan in Early Breast Cancer Patients: Single Institutional Experience. World J Surg. 2009 May;33(5):943-9. PMID: 19259728.

537. Kim JA, Son EJ, Kim EK, et al. Postexcisional breast magnetic resonance imaging in patients with breast cancer: predictable findings of residual cancer. J Comput Assist Tomogr. 2009 Nov-Dec;33(6):940-5. PMID: 19940664.

538. Kinsella MD, Nassar A, Siddiqui MT, et al. Estrogen receptor (ER), progesterone receptor (PR), and HER2 expression pre- and post- neoadjuvant chemotherapy in primary breast carcinoma: a single institutional experience. Int J Clin Exp Pathol. 2012;5(6):530-6. PMID: 22949935.

539. Kishen R, Bartlett JM, Dixon JM, et al. Constructing tissue microarrays from core needle biopsies of breast cancers. Histopathology. 2011 Oct;59(4):794-6. PMID: 21906129.

540. Klimberg VS, Westbrook KC, Korourian S. Use of touch preps for diagnosis and evaluation of surgical margins in breast cancer. Ann Surg Oncol. 1998 Apr-May;5(3):220-6. PMID: 9607622.

541. Knutzen AM, Gisvold JJ. Likelihood of malignant disease for various categories of mammographically detected, nonpalpable breast lesions. Mayo Clin Proc. 1993 May;68(5):454-60. PMID: 8479209.

542. Ko ES, Han H, Lee BH, et al. Sonographic changes after removing all benign breast masses with sonographically guided vacuum-assisted biopsy. Acta Radiol. 2009 Nov;50(9):968-74. PMID: 19863404.

543. Kochli OR. Available stereotactic systems for breast biopsy. Recent Results Cancer Res. 2009;173:105-13. PMID: 19763450.

544. Kombar OR, Fahmy DM, Brown MV, et al. Sonomammographic characteristics of invasive lobular carcinoma. Breast Cancer: Target Ther. 2012;4:115-24.

545. Kowal M, Filipczuk P, Obuchowicz A, et al. Computer-aided diagnosis of breast cancer based on fine needle biopsy microscopic images. Comput Biol Med. 2013 Oct 1;43(10):1563-72. PMID: 24034748.

546. Kruger JM, Thomas M, Korn R, et al. Detection of truncated HER2 forms in formalin-fixed, paraffin-embedded breast cancer tissue captures heterogeneity and is not affected by HER2-targeted therapy. Am J Pathol. 2013 Aug;183(2):336-43. PMID: 23727348.

547. Kumar N, Sayed S, Moloo Z, et al. Fine-needle aspiration in suspected inflammatory breast cancer: case series with emphasis on approach to specimen adequacy. Acta Cytol. 2011;55(3):239-44. PMID: 21525734.

548. Kuo SJ. Evaluation of the CO2 laser in performance of breast surgery. Zhonghua Yi Xue Za Zhi (Taipei). 1994 May;53(5):288-92. PMID: 8039042.

549. Kyle DJ, Harvey AG, Shih B, et al. Identification of molecular phenotypic descriptors of breast capsular contracture formation using informatics analysis of the whole genome transcriptome. Wound Repair Regen. 2013 Sep-Oct;21(5):762-9. PMID: 23941504.

550. Lai YC, Huang YS, Wang DW, et al. Computer-aided diagnosis for 3-d power Doppler breast ultrasound. Ultrasound Med Biol. 2013 Apr;39(4):555-67. PMID: 23384464.

551. Laird-Fick HS, Gardiner JC, Tokala H, et al. HER2 status in elderly women with breast cancer. Journal of geriatric oncology. 2013;4(4):362-7.

552. Landheer ML, Klinkenbijl JH, Pasker-de Jong PC, et al. Residual disease after excision of non-palpable breast tumours: analysis of tumour characteristics. Eur J Surg Oncol. 2004 Oct;30(8):824-8. PMID: 15336726.

553. Landheer ML, Veltman J, van Eekeren R, et al. MRI-guided preoperative wire localization of nonpalpable breast lesions. Clin Imaging. 2006 Jul-Aug;30(4):229-33. PMID: 16814136.

554. Langlois SL, Carter ML. Carbon localisation of impalpable mammographic abnormalities. Australas Radiol. 1991 Aug;35(3):237-41. PMID: 1763986.

555. Lantsberg L, Kirshtein B, Koretz M, et al. Role of wire-guided breast biopsy for diagnosis of malignant nonpalpable mammographic lesions. World J Surg. 1999 Dec;23(12):1279-81. PMID: 10552121.

556. Law MT, Bennett IC. Structured ultrasonography workshop for breast surgeons: is it an effective training tool? World J Surg. 2010 Mar;34(3):549-54. PMID: 20054545.

557. Law NW, Johnson CD, Lamont PM, et al. Drainage or suture of the cavity after breast biopsy. Ann R Coll Surg Engl. 1990 Jan;72(1):11-3. PMID: 2405764.

558. Lay SF, Crump JM, Frykberg ER, et al. Breast biopsy. Changing patterns during a five-year period. Am Surg. 1990 Feb;56(2):79-85. PMID: 2306056.

559. Layfield LJ, Chrischilles EA, Cohen MB, et al. The palpable breast nodule. A cost-effectiveness analysis of alternate diagnostic approaches. Cancer. 1993 Sep 1;72(5):1642-51. PMID: 8348496.

560. Lazarus E, Mainiero MB, Gareen IF. Effect of referring physician specialty and practice type on referral for image-guided breast biopsy. J Am Coll Radiol. 2005 Jun;2(6):488-93. PMID: 17411865.

561. Lee AH, Hodi Z, Ellis IO. False-negative assessment of oestrogen receptor on needle core biopsy of invasive carcinoma of the breast. J Clin Pathol. 2008 Feb;61(2):239-40. PMID: 18223101.

562. Lee CH, Carter D. Detecting residual tumor after excisional biopsy of impalpable breast carcinoma: efficacy of comparing preoperative mammograms with radiographs of the biopsy specimen. AJR Am J Roentgenol. 1995 Jan;164(1):81-6. PMID: 7998574.

563. Lee EJ, Oh SM. The efficacy of stereotactic vacuum-assisted biopsy and needle localization vacuum-assisted biopsy for diagnosing breast microcalcification. J. Breast Cancer. 2010;13(1):53-8.

564. Lehr HA, Rochat C, Schaper C, et al. Mitotic figure counts are significantly overestimated in resection specimens of invasive breast carcinomas. Mod Pathol. 2013 Mar;26(3):336-42. PMID: 23041831.

565. Lein BC, Alex WR, Zebley DM, et al. Results of needle localized breast biopsy in women under age 50. Am J Surg. 1996 Mar;171(3):356-9. PMID: 8615472.

566. Leung TK, Huang PJ, Liang HH, et al. Retrospective Study of False-positive Breast Magnetic Resonance Images and Pathological Results in Taiwan. J. Exp. Clin. Med. 2012;4(5):284-8.

567. Liberman L, Mason G, Morris EA, et al. Does size matter? Positive predictive value of MRI-detected breast lesions as a function of lesion size. AJR Am J Roentgenol. 2006 Feb;186(2):426-30. PMID: 16423948.

568. Linda A, Zuiani C, Londero V, et al. Magnetic resonance imaging of radial sclerosing lesions (radial scars) of the breast. Eur J Radiol. 2012 Nov;81(11):3201-7. PMID: 22386132.

569. Liu X, Li L, Chen F, et al. An intraoperative localization technique for a postexcision specimen of nonpalpable breast calcifications: a pilot study. Am Surg. 2011 Nov;77(11):1467-71. PMID: 22196659.

570. London SJ, Connolly JL, Schnitt SJ, et al. A prospective study of benign breast disease and the risk of breast cancer. JAMA. 1992 Feb 19;267(7):941-4. PMID: 1734106.

571. Lopes-Costa PV, dos Santos AR, da Silva BB. The effect of raloxifene on Bax protein expression in breast carcinomas of postmenopausal women. Diagn Cytopathol. 2012 Jul;40(7):570-4. PMID: 22707322.

572. Lorenzen J, Finck-Wedel AK, Lisboa B, et al. Second opinion assessment in diagnostic mammography at a breast cancer centre. Geburtshilfe Frauenheilkd. 2012;72(8):734-9.

573. Loubeyre P, Bodmer A, Tille JC, et al. Concordance between core needle biopsy and surgical excision specimens for tumour hormone receptor profiling according to the 2011 St. Gallen Classification, in clinical practice. Breast J. 2013 Nov-Dec;19(6):605-10. PMID: 24165313.

574. Loukas C, Kostopoulos S, Tanoglidi A, et al. Breast cancer characterization based on image classification of tissue sections visualized under low magnification. Comput Math Methods Med. 2013;2013:829461. PMID: 24069067.

575. Lu P, Zhu XQ, Xu ZL, et al. Increased infiltration of activated tumor-infiltrating lymphocytes after high intensity focused ultrasound ablation of human breast cancer. Surgery. 2009 Mar;145(3):286-93. PMID: 19231581.

576. Luciani ML, Pediconi F, Telesca M, et al. Incidental enhancing lesions found on preoperative breast MRI: management and role of second-look ultrasound. Radiol Med. 2011 Sep;116(6):886-904. PMID: 21293943.

577. Luini A, Sacchini V, Galimberti V, et al. Preoperative localization and surgical approach in 344 cases of non-palpable breast lesions. Eur J Surg Oncol. 1991 Oct;17(5):480-4. PMID: 1936294.

578. Luo HJ, Chen X, Tu G, et al. Therapeutic application of ultrasound-guided 8-gauge Mammotome system in presumed benign breast lesions. Breast J. 2011 Sep-Oct;17(5):490-7. PMID: 21762243.

579. Lyng MB, Laenkholm AV, Pallisgaard N, et al. Identification of genes for normalization of real-time RT-PCR data in breast carcinomas. BMC Cancer. 2008;8:20. PMID: 18211679.

580. Ma K, Fenster A, Kornecki A, et al. A new lateral guidance device for stereotactic breast biopsy using an add-on unit to an upright mammography system. Conf Proc IEEE Eng Med Biol Soc. 2008;2008:3653-6. PMID: 19163502.

581. Madeira M, Mattar A, Logullo AF, et al. Estrogen receptor alpha/beta ratio and estrogen receptor beta as predictors of endocrine therapy responsiveness-a randomized neoadjuvant trial comparison between anastrozole and tamoxifen for the treatment of postmenopausal breast cancer. BMC Cancer. 2013;13:425. PMID: 24047421.

582. Mallapragada VG, Sarkar N, Podder TK. Robotic system for tumor manipulation and ultrasound image guidance during breast biopsy. Conf Proc IEEE Eng Med Biol Soc. 2008;2008:5589-92. PMID: 19163984.

583. Mansour SM, Abolfotooh A. Does MRI help in the assessment of inflammatory breast disorders? The Egyptian Journal of Radiology and Nuclear Medicine. 2012;43(3):487-97.

584. Markopoulos C, Kakisis J, Kouskos S, et al. Management of nonpalpable, mammographically detectable breast lesions. World J Surg. 1999 May;23(5):434-8. PMID: 10085389.

585. Markopoulos C, Kouskos E, Revenas K, et al. Open surgical biopsy for nonpalpable breast lesions detected on screening mammography. Eur J Gynaecol Oncol. 2005;26(3):311-4. PMID: 15991535.

586. Masroor I, Afzal S, Sakhawat S, et al. Negative predictive value of mammography and sonography in mastalgia with negative physical findings. J Pak Med Assoc. 2009 Sep;59(9):598-601. PMID: 19750852.

587. Masroor I, Afzal S, Shafqat G, et al. Usefulness of hook wire localization biopsy under imaging guidance for nonpalpable breast lesions detected radiologically. Int J Womens Health. 2012;4:445-9. PMID: 23071414.

588. Maxwell AJ. Ultrasound-guided vacuum-assisted excision of breast papillomas: review of 6-years experience. Clin Radiol. 2009 Aug;64(8):801-6. PMID: 19589419.

589. Maxwell AJ, Pearson JM, Bishop HM. Crude open biopsy rates for benign screen detected lesions no longer reflect breast screening quality--time to change the standard. J Med Screen. 2002;9(2):83-5. PMID: 12133928.

590. McCreery BR, Frankl G, Frost DB. An analysis of the results of mammographically guided biopsies of the breast. Surg Gynecol Obstet. 1991 Mar;172(3):223-6. PMID: 1847244.

591. McGhan LJ, McKeever SC, Pockaj BA, et al. Radioactive seed localization for nonpalpable breast lesions: review of 1,000 consecutive procedures at a single institution. Ann Surg Oncol. 2011 Oct;18(11):3096-101. PMID: 21947587.

592. McMahon MA, James JJ, Cornford EJ, et al. Does the insertion of a gel-based marker at stereotactic breast biopsy allow subsequent wire localizations to be carried out under ultrasound guidance? Clin Radiol. 2011 Sep;66(9):840-4. PMID: 21658688.

593. McManus V, Desautels JE, Benediktsson H, et al. Enhancement of true-positive rates for nonpalpable carcinoma of the breast through mammographic selection. Surg Gynecol Obstet. 1992 Sep;175(3):212-8. PMID: 1514155.

594. Medjhoul A, Canale S, Mathieu MC, et al. Breast lesion excision sample (BLES biopsy) combining stereotactic biopsy and radiofrequency: is it a safe and accurate procedure in case of BIRADS 4 and 5 breast lesions? Breast J. 2013 Nov-Dec;19(6):590-4. PMID: 24102869.

595. Meeuwis C, Peters NH, Mali WP, et al. Targeting difficult accessible breast lesions: MRI-guided needle localization using a freehand technique in a 3.0 T closed bore magnet. Eur J Radiol. 2007 May;62(2):283-8. PMID: 17218074.

596. Melanson GF, Otchy DP, Walters MJ, et al. The importance of stabilizing the specimen taken at needle localized biopsy of the breast for microcalcifications. Surg Gynecol Obstet. 1992 May;174(5):376-8. PMID: 1570614.

597. Memis A, Ustun EE, Orguc S. Mammographic and ultrasonographic evaluation of breast after excisional biopsy. European journal of ultrasound. 1997;5(1):47-51.

598. Menet E, Becette V, Briffod M. Cytologic diagnosis of lobular carcinoma of the breast: experience with 555 patients in the Rene Huguenin Cancer Center. Cancer. 2008 Apr 25;114(2):111-7. PMID: 18300231.

599. Meng W, Zhang G, Wu C, et al. Preliminary results of acoustic radiation force impulse (ARFI) ultrasound imaging of breast lesions. Ultrasound Med Biol. 2011 Sep;37(9):1436-43. PMID: 21767903.

600. Meyer JE, Eberlein TJ, Stomper PC, et al. Biopsy of occult breast lesions. Analysis of 1261 abnormalities. JAMA. 1990 May 2;263(17):2341-3. PMID: 2157903.

601. Meyer JE, Kopans DB. Analysis of mammographically obvious carcinomas of the breast with benign results upon initial biopsy. Surg Gynecol Obstet. 1981 Oct;153(4):570-2. PMID: 6269239.

602. Meyer JE, Smith DN, Kaelin C, et al. Surgical breast biopsy after wire localization: The impact of large core needle biopsy. JOURNAL OF WOMENS IMAGING. 2004;6(3):125-31.

603. Miller RS, Adelman RW, Espinosa MH, et al. The early detection of nonpalpable breast carcinoma with needle localization. Experience with 500 patients in a community hospital. Am Surg. 1992 Mar;58(3):193-8. PMID: 1313665.

604. Mok PM, Keepin Y. Stereotactic breast biopsies for lesions discovered on routine mammography: experience at the North Shore Hospital. N Z Med J. 2000 Jul 14;113(1113):273-4. PMID: 10935565.

605. Mokbel K, Ahmed M, Nash A, et al. Re-excision operations in nonpalpable breast cancer. J Surg Oncol. 1995 Apr;58(4):225-8; discussion 9-32. PMID: 7723365.

606. Monostori Z, Herman PG, Carmody DP, et al. Limitations in distinguishing malignant from benign lesions of the breast by systematic review of mammograms. Surg Gynecol Obstet. 1991 Dec;173(6):438-42. PMID: 1948599.

607. Montgomery GH, Weltz CR, Seltz M, et al. Brief presurgery hypnosis reduces distress and pain in excisional breast biopsy patients. Int J Clin Exp Hypn. 2002 Jan;50(1):17-32. PMID: 11778705.

608. Montrey JS, Levy JA, Brenner RJ. Wire fragments after needle localization. AJR Am J Roentgenol. 1996 Nov;167(5):1267-9. PMID: 8911193.

609. Moreno M, Wiltgen JE, Bodanese B, et al. Radioguided breast surgery for occult lesion localization - correlation between two methods. J Exp Clin Cancer Res. 2008;27:29. PMID: 18706096.

610. Morris EA, Liberman L, Dershaw DD, et al. Preoperative MR imaging-guided needle localization of breast lesions. AJR Am J Roentgenol. 2002 May;178(5):1211-20. PMID: 11959734.

611. Morris KT, Pommier RF, Vetto JT. Office-based wire-guided open breast biopsy under local anesthesia is accurate and cost effective. Am J Surg. 2000 May;179(5):422-5. PMID: 10930494.

612. Mueller X, Amery A, Lallemand RC. Biopsy of mammographically-detected breast lesions in a district hospital. Eur J Surg Oncol. 1993 Oct;19(5):415-9. PMID: 8405476.

613. Mujtaba S, Haroon S, Faridi N, et al. Correlation of human epidermal growth factor receptor 2 (HER-2/neu) receptor status with hormone receptors Oestrogen Receptor, Progesterone Receptor status and other prognostic markers in breast cancer: an experience at tertiary care hospital in Karachi. J Pak Med Assoc. 2013 Jul;63(7):854-8. PMID: 23901708.

614. Murgo S, Wyshoff H, Faverly D, et al. Computed tomography-guided localization of breast lesions. Breast J. 2008 Mar-Apr;14(2):169-75. PMID: 18248560.

615. Muslumanoglu M, Dolay K, Ozmen V, et al. Comparison of fine needle aspiration cytology and excisional biopsy in palpable breast cancers. Radiol Med. 1995 Mar;89(3):225-8. PMID: 7754112.

616. Nair A, Jaleel S, Sathya V, et al. The role of freehand needle core biopsy in the diagnosis of isolated axillary lymphadenopathy. Breast. 2009 Jun;18(3):175-7. PMID: 19362840.

617. Nassar A, Radhakrishnan A, Cabrero IA, et al. Intratumoral heterogeneity of immunohistochemical marker expression in breast carcinoma: a tissue microarray-based study. Appl Immunohistochem Mol Morphol. 2010 Oct;18(5):433-41. PMID: 20485156.

618. National Guideline Clearinghouse (NGC). Guideline summary: Advanced breast cancer. Diagnosis and treatment. In: National Guideline Clearinghouse (NGC) [Web site]. Rockville (MD): Agency for Healthcare Research and Quality (AHRQ); [cited 2013 June 25]. Available: http://www.guideline.gov.

619. National Guideline Clearinghouse (NGC). Guideline summary: Staging. In: Management of early breast cancer. In: National Guideline Clearinghouse (NGC) [Web site]. Rockville (MD): Agency for Healthcare Research and Quality (AHRQ); [cited 2013 June 25]. Available: http://www.guideline.gov.

620. National Guideline Clearinghouse (NGC). Guideline summary: Use of tumor markers in testicular, prostate, colorectal, breast, and ovarian cancers. In: National Guideline Clearinghouse (NGC) [Web site]. Rockville (MD): Agency for Healthcare Research and Quality (AHRQ); [cited 2013 June 25]. Available: http://www.guideline.gov.

621. National Guideline Clearinghouse (NGC). Guideline summary: General principles of care. In: Management of early breast cancer. In: National Guideline Clearinghouse (NGC) [Web site]. Rockville (MD): Agency for Healthcare Research and Quality (AHRQ); [cited 2013 June 25]. Available: http://www.guideline.gov.

622. National Guideline Clearinghouse (NGC). Guideline summary: Breast cancer screening clinical practice guideline. In: National Guideline Clearinghouse (NGC) [Web site]. Rockville (MD): Agency for Healthcare Research and Quality (AHRQ); [cited 2013 June 25]. Available: http://www.guideline.gov.

623. Nggada HA, Yawe KD, Abdulazeez J, et al. Breast cancer burden in Maiduguri, North eastern Nigeria. Breast J. 2008 May-Jun;14(3):284-6. PMID: 18476884.

624. Niemann TH, Lucas JG, Marsh WL, Jr. To freeze or not to freeze. A comparison of methods for the handling of breast biopsies with no palpable abnormality. Am J Clin Pathol. 1996 Aug;106(2):225-8. PMID: 8712178.

625. Nishikawa RM, Pesce LL. Estimating sensitivity and specificity for technology assessment based on observer studies. Acad Radiol. 2013 Jul;20(7):825-30. PMID: 23660073.

626. Ocal K, Dag A, Turkmenoglu O, et al. Radioguided occult lesion localization versus wire-guided localization for non-palpable breast lesions: randomized controlled trial. Clinics (Sao Paulo). 2011;66(6):1003-7. PMID: 21808866.

627. O'Hanlon DM, Colbert ST, Keane PW, et al. Preemptive bupivacaine offers no advantages to postoperative wound infiltration in analgesia for outpatient breast biopsy. Am J Surg. 2000 Jul;180(1):29-32. PMID: 11036135.

628. Ohi Y, Umekita Y, Rai Y, et al. Mucocele-like lesions of the breast: a long-term follow-up study. Diagn Pathol. 2011;6:29. PMID: 21466711.

629. Ohlsson-Wilhelm BM, Wang G. Circulating killer cells in women undergoing needle-directed excisional breast biopsy. Eur J Histochem. 1994;38 Suppl 1:77-82. PMID: 8547715.

630. Ohtake E, Asaga T, Inaba M. Sentinel lymphoscintigraphy in patients with breast cancer undergoing excisional biopsy. Ann Nucl Med. 2005 Dec;19(8):671-5. PMID: 16444992.

631. Omranipour R, Alipour S, Hadji M, et al. Accuracy of estrogen and progesterone receptor assessment in core needle biopsy specimens of breast cancer. Iran Red Crescent Med J. 2013 Jun;15(6):515-8. PMID: 24349751.

632. Opie H, Estes NC, Jewell WR, et al. Breast biopsy for nonpalpable lesions: a worthwhile endeavor? Am Surg. 1993 Aug;59(8):490-3; discussion 3-4. PMID: 8393310.

633. Orel SG, Kay N, Reynolds C, et al. BI-RADS categorization as a predictor of malignancy. Radiology. 1999 Jun;211(3):845-50. PMID: 10352614.

634. Orel SG, Schnall MD, Powell CM, et al. Staging of suspected breast cancer: effect of MR imaging and MR-guided biopsy. Radiology. 1995 Jul;196(1):115-22. PMID: 7784554.

635. Osako T, Iwase T, Akiyama F. Reply: Isolated tumour cells and micrometastases in intraductal breast cancer: a simple mechanical question in some cases. Br J Cancer. 2013 May 14;108(9):1921. PMID: 23538389.

636. Owings DV, Hann L, Schnitt SJ. How thoroughly should needle localization breast biopsies be sampled for microscopic examination? A prospective mammographic/pathologic correlative study. Am J Surg Pathol. 1990 Jun;14(6):578-83. PMID: 2337206.

637. Ozumba BC, Nzegwu MA, Anyikam A, et al. Breast disease in children and adolescents in eastern Nigeria--a five-year study. J Pediatr Adolesc Gynecol. 2009 Jun;22(3):169-72. PMID: 19539203.

638. Palmedo H, Schomburg A, Grunwald F, et al. Technetium-99m-MIBI scintimammography for suspicious breast lesions. J Nucl Med. 1996 Apr;37(4):626-30. PMID: 8691253.

639. Palmer ML, Tsangaris TN. Breast biopsy in women 30 years old or less. Am J Surg. 1993 Jun;165(6):708-12. PMID: 8506971.

640. Palmieri FM, DePeri ER, Mincey BA, et al. Comprehensive diagnostic program for medically underserved women with abnormal breast screening evaluations in an urban population. Mayo Clin Proc. 2009 Apr;84(4):317-22. PMID: 19339648.

641. Parlakgumus A, Karakoc D, Ozenc A. Nine years' experience of needle localized breast biopsy in a university hospital: results and evaluation of the role of the surgeon in decision making. Acta Chir Belg. 2008 Sep-Oct;108(5):548-51. PMID: 19051464.

642. Patchefsky AS, Potok J, Hoch WS, et al. Increased detection of occult breast carcinoma after more thorough histologic examination of breast biopsies. Am J Clin Pathol. 1973 Dec;60(6):799-804. PMID: 4357121.

643. Paterson ML, Nathanson SD, Havstad S. Hematomas following excisional breast biopsies for invasive breast carcinoma: the influence of deep suture approximation of breast parenchyma. Am Surg. 1994 Nov;60(11):845-8. PMID: 7978679.

644. Pathmanathan P, Gavaghan DJ, Whiteley JP, et al. Predicting tumor location by modeling the deformation of the breast. IEEE Trans Biomed Eng. 2008 Oct;55(10):2471-80. PMID: 18838373.

645. Patton ML, Haith LR, Jr., Goldman WT. An improved technique for needle localized biopsy of occult lesions of the breast. Surg Gynecol Obstet. 1993 Jan;176(1):25-9. PMID: 8381241.

646. Pegolo E, Puppin C, Gerometta A, et al. One-step nucleic acid amplification (OSNA) for intraoperative evaluation of sentinel lymph node status in breast cancer: a comparative study between CK19 protein expression and CK19 mRNA level in primary tumors and lymph node metastasis. Virchows Arch. 2013 Jul;463(1):7-15. PMID: 23779101.

647. Perdue P, Page D, Nellestein M, et al. Early detection of breast carcinoma: a comparison of palpable and nonpalpable lesions. Surgery. 1992 Jun;111(6):656-9. PMID: 1595061.

648. Perdue PW, Galbo C, Ghosh BC. Stratification of palpable and nonpalpable breast cancer by method of detection and age. Ann Surg Oncol. 1995 Nov;2(6):512-5. PMID: 8591081.

649. Perfetto F, Fiorentino F, Urbano F, et al. Adjunctive diagnostic value of MRI in the breast radial scar. Radiol Med. 2009 Aug;114(5):757-70. PMID: 19484584.

650. Petit JY, Veronesi U, Rey P, et al. Nipple-sparing mastectomy: risk of nipple-areolar recurrences in a series of 579 cases. Breast Cancer Res Treat. 2009 Mar;114(1):97-101. PMID: 18360773.

651. Petrik DW, McCready DR, Goel V, et al. The rate of breast-conserving surgery for early breast cancer is not influenced by the surgical strategy of excisional biopsy followed by the definitive procedure. Breast J. 2001 May-Jun;7(3):158-65. PMID: 11469928.

652. Platt R, Zucker JR, Zaleznik DF, et al. Perioperative antibiotic prophylaxis and wound infection following breast surgery. J Antimicrob Chemother. 1993 Feb;31 Suppl B:43-8. PMID: 8449845.

653. Popiela TJ, Kibil W, Herman-Sucharska I, et al. The use of magnetic resonance mammography in women at increased risk for developing breast cancer. Wideochir Inne Tech Malo Inwazyjne. 2013 Mar;8(1):55-62. PMID: 23630555.

654. Purnell CA, Arnold RM. Retrospective analysis of communication with patients undergoing radiological breast biopsy. J Support Oncol. 2010 Nov-Dec;8(6):259-63. PMID: 21265393.

655. Qi CJ, Ning YL, Zhu YL, et al. In vitro chemosensitivity in breast cancer using ATP-tumor chemosensitivity assay. Arch Pharm Res. 2009 Dec;32(12):1737-42. PMID: 20162402.

656. Raghavan K, Shah AK, Cosgrove JM. Intraoperative breast problem--focused sonography a valuable tool in the training of surgical residents. J Surg Educ. 2008 Sep-Oct;65(5):350-3. PMID: 18809164.

657. Raju U. Mammographic Localization Biopsy for Ductal Carcinoma In Situ: A Simple Mapping Technique for Sampling and Size Estimation. Breast J. 2000 Nov;6(6):379-87. PMID: 11348396.

658. Ramsey-Stewart G, Lauer CS. Use of a specimen-evaluation device for the diagnosis of impalpable breast lesions detected by mammography. Med J Aust. 1992 Feb 17;156(4):244-6. PMID: 1310796.

659. Rao R, Lilley L, Andrews V, et al. Axillary staging by percutaneous biopsy: sensitivity of fine-needle aspiration versus core needle biopsy. Ann Surg Oncol. 2009 May;16(5):1170-5. PMID: 19263171.

660. Rappaport W, Thompson S, Wong R, et al. Complications associated with needle localization biopsy of the breast. Surg Gynecol Obstet. 1991 Apr;172(4):303-6. PMID: 2006456.

661. Raptopoulos V, Baum JK, Hochman M, et al. High resolution CT mammography of surgical biopsy specimens. J Comput Assist Tomogr. 1996 Mar-Apr;20(2):179-84. PMID: 8606220.

662. Reeves MJ, Osuch JR, Pathak DR. Development of a clinical decision rule for triage of women with palpable breast masses. J Clin Epidemiol. 2003 Jul;56(7):636-45. PMID: 12921932.

663. Reid SE, Jr., Scanlon EF, Bernstein JR, et al. An alternative approach to nonpalpable breast biopsies. J Surg Oncol. 1990 Jun;44(2):93-6. PMID: 2162454.

664. Rey JE, Gardner SM, Cushing RD. Determinants of surgical site infection after breast biopsy. Am J Infect Control. 2005 Mar;33(2):126-9. PMID: 15761414.

665. Reynolds HE, Jackson VP, Musick BS. Preoperative needle localization in the breast: utility of local anesthesia. Radiology. 1993 May;187(2):503-5. PMID: 8475298.

666. Ricci MD, Calvano Filho CM, Oliveira Filho HR, et al. Analysis of the concordance rates between core needle biopsy and surgical excision in patients with breast cancer. Rev Assoc Med Bras. 2012 Sep-Oct;58(5):532-6. PMID: 23090222.

667. Rickard MT, Lee W, Read JW, et al. Breast cancer diagnosis by screening mammography: early results of the Central Sydney Area Health Service Breast X-ray Programme. Med J Aust. 1991 Jan 21;154(2):126-31. PMID: 1986190.

668. Rikabi A, Hussain S. Diagnostic usefulness of tru-cut biopsy in the diagnosis of breast lesions. Oman Med J. 2013 Mar;28(2):125-7. PMID: 23599882.

669. Rimm DL, Stastny JF, Rimm EB, et al. Comparison of the costs of fine-needle aspiration and open surgical biopsy as methods for obtaining a pathologic diagnosis. Cancer. 1997 Feb 25;81(1):51-6. PMID: 9100542.

670. Roses DF, Mitnick J, Harris MN, et al. The risk of carcinoma in wire localization biopsies for mammographically detected clustered microcalcifications. Surgery. 1991 Nov;110(5):877-86. PMID: 1658957.

671. Rosner D, Lane WW, Penetrante R. Ductal carcinoma in situ with microinvasion. A curable entity using surgery alone without need for adjuvant therapy. Cancer. 1991 Mar 15;67(6):1498-503. PMID: 1848153.

672. Rubin P, O'Hanlon D, Browell D, et al. Tumour bed biopsy detects the presence of multifocal disease in patients undergoing breast conservation therapy for primary breast carcinoma. Eur J Surg Oncol. 1996 Feb;22(1):23-6. PMID: 8846861.

673. Ruckhaberle E, Karn T, Denkert C, et al. Predictive value of sphingosine kinase 1 expression in neoadjuvant treatment of breast cancer. J Cancer Res Clin Oncol. 2013 Oct;139(10):1681-9. PMID: 23955546.

674. Saarela AO, Kiviniemi HO, Rissanen TJ, et al. Cosmetic results after wire-guided biopsy of benign breast lesions. J Am Coll Surg. 1998 Dec;187(6):610-5. PMID: 9849734.

675. Sadeghi R, Forghani MN, Memar B, et al. Comparison of pre-operative lymphoscintigraphy with inter-operative gamma probe and dye technique regarding the number of detected sentinel lymph nodes. Hell J Nucl Med. 2009 Jan-Apr;12(1):30-2. PMID: 19330179.

676. Sailors DM, Crabtree JD, Land RL, et al. Needle localization for nonpalpable breast lesions. Am Surg. 1994 Mar;60(3):186-9. PMID: 8116978.

677. Sakakibara E, Kimachi S, Hashimoto K, et al. An aspiration material preparation system: application of a new liquid-based cytology technique for fine-needle aspiration of the breast. Acta Cytol. 2011;55(1):92-9. PMID: 21135528.

678. Sanders LM, Lacz NL, Lara J. 16 year experience with aspiration of noncomplex breast cysts: cytology results with focus on positive cases. Breast J. 2012 Sep;18(5):443-52. PMID: 22845618.

679. Sangoi A, Vose J, Atmodjo D, et al. A randomized controlled trial of the PEAK PlasmaBlade in open breast biopsy compared to scalpel and traditional electrosurgery. 2010. p. S186.

680. . A randomized controlled trial of the PEAK PlasmaBlade in open breast biopsy compared to scalpel and traditional electrosurgery. Ann Surg Oncol; 2010. SPRINGER 233 SPRING ST, NEW YORK, NY 10013 USA; 17.

681. Sari AA, Mobinizadeh M, Azadbakht M. A systematic review of the effects of diffuse optical imaging in breast diseases. Iran. J. Cancer Prev. 2013;6(1):44-51.

682. Sauer G, Schneiderhan-Marra N, Kazmaier C, et al. Prediction of nodal involvement in breast cancer based on multiparametric protein analyses from preoperative core needle biopsies of the primary lesion. Clin Cancer Res. 2008 Jun 1;14(11):3345-53. PMID: 18519762.

683. Saunders G, Lakra Y, Libcke J. Comparison of needle aspiration cytologic diagnosis with excisional biopsy tissue diagnosis of palpable tumors of the breast in a community hospital. Surg Gynecol Obstet. 1991 Jun;172(6):437-40. PMID: 1852078.

684. Saura C, Tseng L-M, Chan S, et al. Neoadjuvant Doxorubicin/Cyclophosphamide Followed by Ixabepilone or Paclitaxel in Early Stage Breast Cancer and Evaluation of βIII-Tubulin Expression as a Predictive Marker. Oncologist. 2013;18(7).

685. Scaperrotta G, Ferranti C, Costa C, et al. Role of sonoelastography in non-palpable breast lesions. Eur Radiol. 2008 Nov;18(11):2381-9. PMID: 18523780.

686. Scheiden R, Sand J, Tanous AM, et al. Accuracy of frozen section diagnoses of breast lesions after introduction of a national programme in mammographic screening. Histopathology. 2001 Jul;39(1):74-84. PMID: 11454047.

687. Schnur JB, Montgomery GH, Hallquist MN, et al. Anticipatory psychological distress in women scheduled for diagnostic and curative breast cancer surgery. Int J Behav Med. 2008 Jan-Mar;15(1):21-8. PMID: 18444017.

688. Schwab FD, Burger H, Isenschmid M, et al. Suspicious axillary lymph nodes in patients with unremarkable imaging of the breast. Eur J Obstet Gynecol Reprod Biol. 2010 May;150(1):88-91. PMID: 20189710.

689. Seah DS, Scott SM, Najita J, et al. Attitudes of patients with metastatic breast cancer toward research biopsies. Ann Oncol. 2013 Jul;24(7):1853-9. PMID: 23493137.

690. Seltzer MH. Preoperative prediction of open breast biopsy results. Cancer. 1997 May 1;79(9):1822-7. PMID: 9129002.

691. Sewell RF, Brenchley PE. Coupling of mono- and polyamino ligands to solid phases by nucleophilic attack on coupling groups that may be spontaneously hydrolysed. J Chromatogr. 1990 Jan 26;525(1):246-8. PMID: 2338446.

692. Shaheen E, Van Ongeval C, Zanca F, et al. The simulation of 3D microcalcification clusters in 2D digital mammography and breast tomosynthesis. Med Phys. 2011 Dec;38(12):6659-71. PMID: 22149848.

693. Shaikh A, Fatima S, Shaikh SM. Diagnostic value of needle-localization biopsy in the management of non-palpable breast lesions. Rawal Medical Journal. 2013;38(1):59-60.

694. Sharma H, Alekseychuk A, Leskovsky P, et al. Determining similarity in histological images using graph-theoretic description and matching methods for content-based image retrieval in medical diagnostics. Diagn Pathol. 2012;7:134. PMID: 23035717.

695. Sheikh HE, Abdulaziz NY. Intraoperative ultrasound localization of nonpalpable breast cancers: A valuable aid during breast-conserving surgery. The Egyptian Journal of Radiology and Nuclear Medicine. 2013;44(2):411-5.

696. Shigekawa T, Ijichi N, Ikeda K, et al. FOXP1, an estrogen-inducible transcription factor, modulates cell proliferation in breast cancer cells and 5-year recurrence-free survival of patients with tamoxifen-treated breast cancer. Horm Cancer. 2011 Oct;2(5):286-97. PMID: 21901488.

697. Shimauchi A, Jansen SA, Abe H, et al. Breast cancers not detected at MRI: review of false-negative lesions. AJR Am J Roentgenol. 2010 Jun;194(6):1674-9. PMID: 20489112.

698. Shin HJ, Kim HH, Ko MS, et al. BI-RADS descriptors for mammographically detected microcalcifications verified by histopathology after needle-localized open breast biopsy. AJR Am J Roentgenol. 2010 Dec;195(6):1466-71. PMID: 21098211.

699. Shroff JH, Lloyd LR, Schroder DM. Open breast biopsy. A critical analysis. Am Surg. 1991 Aug;57(8):481-5. PMID: 1928989.

700. Singhal H, Potter C, Osborne MP. No effect of timing of biopsy in the menstrual cycle on incidence of bone marrow micrometastasis in patients with breast cancer. Ann Surg Oncol. 1997 Sep;4(6):503-5. PMID: 9309341.

701. Skliris GP, Rowan BG, Al-Dhaheri M, et al. Immunohistochemical validation of multiple phospho-specific epitopes for estrogen receptor alpha (ERalpha) in tissue microarrays of ERalpha positive human breast carcinomas. Breast Cancer Res Treat. 2009 Dec;118(3):443-53. PMID: 19104930.

702. Skotnicki P, Łuczyńska E, Herman K, et al. USG-guided excision biopsy in case of ambiguous breast USG images. Polish Journal of Radiology. 2007;72(3):29-31.

703. Skripenova S, Layfield LJ. Initial margin status for invasive ductal carcinoma of the breast and subsequent identification of carcinoma in reexcision specimens. Arch Pathol Lab Med. 2010 Jan;134(1):109-14. PMID: 20073613.

704. Smith M, Zhai X, Harter R, et al. A novel MR-guided interventional device for 3D circumferential access to breast tissue. Med Phys. 2008 Aug;35(8):3779-86. PMID: 18777937.

705. Snell MJ, Ostrow LB, DuBois JJ, et al. Needle-localized biopsy of occult breast lesions: an update. Mil Med. 1992 Feb;157(2):61-4. PMID: 1318524.

706. Soluri A, Scopinaro F, De Vincentis G, et al. 99MTC [13LEU] bombesin and a new gamma camera, the imaging probe, are able to guide mammotome breast biopsy. Anticancer Res. 2003 May-Jun;23(3A):2139-42. PMID: 12894588.

707. Son BK, Bong JG, Park SH, et al. Ductal carcinoma in situ and sentinel lymph node biopsy. J Breast Cancer. 2011 Dec;14(4):301-7. PMID: 22323917.

708. SONUÇ MLSB-R, İÇİN K, DEĞERLERİ PÖ. POSITIVE PREDICTIVE VALUES OF THE SONOGRAPHIC BI-RADS FINAL ASSESSMENT CATEGORIES FOR BREAST LESIONS.

709. Stein MA, Karlan MS. Calcifications in breast biopsy specimens: discrepancies in radiologic-pathologic identification. Radiology. 1991 Apr;179(1):111-4. PMID: 2006260.

710. Stein T, Cosimo E, Yu X, et al. Loss of reelin expression in breast cancer is epigenetically controlled and associated with poor prognosis. Am J Pathol. 2010 Nov;177(5):2323-33. PMID: 20847288.

711. Steinberg JL, Trudeau ME, Ryder DE, et al. Combined fine-needle aspiration, physical examination and mammography in the diagnosis of palpable breast masses: their relation to outcome for women with primary breast cancer. Can J Surg. 1996 Aug;39(4):302-11. PMID: 8697321.

712. Steri V, Farnedi A, Montinari E, et al. Fast track biopsy method: a rapid approach to preoperative diagnoses. Pathologica. 2010 Apr;102(2):41-5. PMID: 23596755.

713. Tafra L, Guenther JM, Giuliano AE. Planned segmentectomy. A necessity for breast carcinoma. Arch Surg. 1993 Sep;128(9):1014-8; discussion 8-20. PMID: 8396387.

714. Takagi K, Ishida T, Miki Y, et al. Intratumoral concentration of estrogens and clinicopathological changes in ductal carcinoma in situ following aromatase inhibitor letrozole treatment. Br J Cancer. 2013 Jul 9;109(1):100-8. PMID: 23756858.

715. Takhellambam YS, Lourembam SS, Sapam OS, et al. Comparison of Ultrasonography and Fine Needle Aspiration Cytology in the Diagnosis of Malignant Breast Lesions. 2013.

716. Tanaka K, Komoike Y, Egawa C, et al. Indeterminate calcification and clustered cystic lesions are strongly predictive of the presence of mucocele-like tumor of the breast: a report of six cases. Breast Cancer. 2009;16(1):77-82. PMID: 18478314.

717. Tang J, Wang X, Wu YP, et al. Significance of methylene blue dye for localization biopsy of nonpalpable breast lesions. Ai Zheng. 2009 Jan;28(1):79-81. PMID: 19448424.

718. Tang J, Xie XM, Wang X, et al. Radiocolloid in combination with methylene dye localization, rather than wire localization, is a preferred procedure for excisional biopsy of nonpalpable breast lesions. Ann Surg Oncol. 2011 Jan;18(1):109-13. PMID: 20680696.

719. Tartter PI, Kaplan J, Bleiweiss I, et al. Lumpectomy margins, reexcision, and local recurrence of breast cancer. Am J Surg. 2000 Feb;179(2):81-5. PMID: 10773138.

720. Taxin A, Tartter PI, Zappetti D. Breast cancer diagnosis by fine needle aspiration and excisional biopsy. Recurrence and survival. Acta Cytol. 1997 Mar-Apr;41(2):302-6. PMID: 9100758.

721. Taylor L, Basro S, Apffelstaedt JP, et al. Time for a re-evaluation of mammography in the young? Results of an audit of mammography in women younger than 40 in a resource restricted environment. Breast Cancer Res Treat. 2011 Aug;129(1):99-106. PMID: 21698411.

722. Tez S, Dener C, Koktener A, et al. The value of fine needle aspiration and cytologic examination of impalpable complicated breast cysts. Bratisl Lek Listy. 2008;109(9):387-90. PMID: 19040143.

723. Tezuka K, Onoda N, Takashima T, et al. Clinical significance of intra-tumoral sinusoidal structures showing lympho-endothelial immunoreactivity in breast cancer. Oncol Rep. 2008 Jul;20(1):25-32. PMID: 18575714.

724. Thomas PA, Vazquez MF, Waisman J. Comparison of fine-needle aspiration and frozen section of palpable mammary lesions. Mod Pathol. 1990 Sep;3(5):570-4. PMID: 2235982.

725. Thomassin-Naggara I, Trop I, Chopier J, et al. Nonmasslike enhancement at breast MR imaging: the added value of mammography and US for lesion categorization. Radiology. 2011 Oct;261(1):69-79. PMID: 21771958.

726. Thompson WR, Bowen JR, Dorman BA, et al. Mammographic localization and biopsy of nonpalpable breast lesions. A 5-year study. Arch Surg. 1991 Jun;126(6):730-3; discussion 3-4. PMID: 1645516.

727. Thurley P, Evans A, Hamilton L, et al. Patient satisfaction and efficacy of vacuum-assisted excision biopsy of fibroadenomas. Clin Radiol. 2009 Apr;64(4):381-5. PMID: 19264182.

728. Tisi P, Langham-Brown J, Jackson A, et al. Localization biopsy for impalpable breast lesions in a district general hospital. Eur J Surg Oncol. 1994 Apr;20(2):115-7. PMID: 8181574.

729. Torres-Tabanera M, Alonso-Bartolome P, Vega-Bolivar A, et al. Percutaneous microductectomy with a directional vacuum-assisted system guided by ultrasonography for the treatment of breast discharge: experience in 63 cases. Acta Radiol. 2008 Apr;49(3):271-6. PMID: 18365813.

730. Troxel DB. Medicolegal aspects of error in pathology. Arch Pathol Lab Med. 2006 May;130(5):617-9. PMID: 16683874.

731. Tsai YM, Hsu HM, Chen CJ, et al. Association of estrogen receptor, progesterone receptor and HER2 following neoadjuvant systemic treatment in breast cancer patients undergoing surgery. Ir J Med Sci. 2014 Mar;183(1):71-5. PMID: 23757214.

732. Ueno E, Aiyoshi Y, Imamura A, et al. Ultrasonically guided biopsy of nonpalpable lesions of the breast by the spot method. Surg Gynecol Obstet. 1990 Feb;170(2):153-5. PMID: 2405524.

733. Uhercik M, Kybic J, Liebgott H, et al. Model fitting using RANSAC for surgical tool localization in 3-D ultrasound images. IEEE Trans Biomed Eng. 2010 Aug;57(8):1907-16. PMID: 20483680.

734. van Breest Smallenburg V, Duijm LE, Voogd AC, et al. Lower sensitivity of screening mammography after previous benign breast surgery. Int J Cancer. 2012 Jan 1;130(1):122-8. PMID: 21328339.

735. van Vlymen JM, Sa Rego MM, White PF. Benzodiazepine premedication: can it improve outcome in patients undergoing breast biopsy procedures? Anesthesiology. 1999 Mar;90(3):740-7. PMID: 10078675.

736. Venter A, Rosca E, Mutiu G, et al. The value of ultrasounds exam correlated with frozen section diagnosis in the breast tumors. Rom J Morphol Embryol. 2010;51(4):745-50. PMID: 21103636.

737. Verkooijen HM, Peeters PH, Pijnappel RM, et al. Diagnostic accuracy of needle-localized open breast biopsy for impalpable breast disease. Br J Surg. 2000 Mar;87(3):344-7. PMID: 10718805.

738. Volynskaya Z, Haka AS, Bechtel KL, et al. Diagnosing breast cancer using diffuse reflectance spectroscopy and intrinsic fluorescence spectroscopy. J Biomed Opt. 2008 Mar-Apr;13(2):024012. PMID: 18465975.

739. Wachter DL, Fasching PA, Haeberle L, et al. Prognostic molecular markers and neoadjuvant therapy response in anthracycline-treated breast cancer patients. Arch Gynecol Obstet. 2013 Feb;287(2):337-44. PMID: 22955249.

740. Wahner-Roedler DL, Hruska CB, O'Connor MK, et al. Molecular breast imaging for women presenting with a history of non-reproducible bloody nipple discharge and negative findings on routine imaging studies: A pilot study. J. Surg. Radiol. 2011;2(1):92-9.

741. Wakefield SE, Powis SJ. Benign breast surgery: is there a need for outpatient follow-up? Ann R Coll Surg Engl. 1995 Nov;77(6):457-9. PMID: 8540668.

742. Wang HY, Jiang YX, Zhu QL, et al. Differentiation of benign and malignant breast lesions: a comparison between automatically generated breast volume scans and handheld ultrasound examinations. Eur J Radiol. 2012 Nov;81(11):3190-200. PMID: 22386134.

743. Wang J, Chang KJ, Chen CY, et al. Evaluation of the diagnostic performance of infrared imaging of the breast: a preliminary study. Biomed Eng Online. 2010;9:3. PMID: 20055999.

744. Wang J, Xu B, Yuan P, et al. TOP2A amplification in breast cancer is a predictive marker of anthracycline-based neoadjuvant chemotherapy efficacy. Breast Cancer Res Treat. 2012 Sep;135(2):531-7. PMID: 22864769.

745. Wang T, Wang K, Yao Q, et al. Prospective study on combination of electrical impedance scanning and ultrasound in estimating risk of development of breast cancer in young women. Cancer Invest. 2010 Mar;28(3):295-303. PMID: 19857040.

746. Wang X, Lederman D, Tan J, et al. Computerized detection of breast tissue asymmetry depicted on bilateral mammograms: a preliminary study of breast risk stratification. Acad Radiol. 2010 Oct;17(10):1234-41. PMID: 20619697.

747. Wang ZL, Liu G, Li JL, et al. Sonographically guided percutaneous excision of clinically benign breast masses. J Clin Ultrasound. 2011 Jan;39(1):1-5. PMID: 20957735.

748. Warren HW, Griffith CD, McLean L, et al. Should breast biopsy cavities be drained? Ann R Coll Surg Engl. 1994 Jan;76(1):39-41. PMID: 8117018.

749. Weaver M. Breast cancer in nonpalpable lesions: can mammographic parenchymal pattern improve the predictive value of biopsy? Am Surg. 1992 Nov;58(11):692-4. PMID: 1485702.

750. Weise LM, Bruder M, Eibach S, et al. Efficacy and safety of local versus general anesthesia in stereotactic biopsies: a matched-pairs cohort study. J Neurosurg Anesthesiol. 2013 Apr;25(2):148-53. PMID: 23103527.

751. Weyant M, Carroccio A, Tartter PI, et al. Determinants of success with spot localization biopsy of the breast. J Am Coll Surg. 1995 Dec;181(6):521-4. PMID: 7582226.

752. Wiksell H, Schassburger KU, Janicijevic M, et al. Prevention of tumour cell dissemination in diagnostic needle procedures. Br J Cancer. 2010 Nov 23;103(11):1706-9. PMID: 21045831.

753. Wilkinson J, Appleton CM, Margenthaler JA. Utility of breast MRI for evaluation of residual disease following excisional biopsy. J Surg Res. 2011 Oct;170(2):233-9. PMID: 21550064.

754. Wilson R, Kavia S. Comparison of large-core vacuum-assisted breast biopsy and excision systems. Recent Results Cancer Res. 2009;173:23-41. PMID: 19763447.

755. Wiratkapun C, Bunyapaiboonsri W, Wibulpolprasert B, et al. Biopsy rate and positive predictive value for breast cancer in BI-RADS category 4 breast lesions. J Med Assoc Thai. 2010 Jul;93(7):830-7. PMID: 20649064.

756. Woodward S, Daly CP, Patterson SK, et al. Ensuring excision of intraductal lesions: marker placement at time of ductography. Acad Radiol. 2010 Nov;17(11):1444-8. PMID: 20650666.

757. Wulfkuhle JD, Berg D, Wolff C, et al. Molecular analysis of HER2 signaling in human breast cancer by functional protein pathway activation mapping. Clin Cancer Res. 2012 Dec 1;18(23):6426-35. PMID: 23045247.

758. Xiong J, Yu D, Wei N, et al. An estrogen receptor alpha suppressor, microRNA-22, is downregulated in estrogen receptor alpha-positive human breast cancer cell lines and clinical samples. FEBS J. 2010 Apr;277(7):1684-94. PMID: 20180843.

759. Yang JH, Lee WS, Kim SW, et al. Effect of core-needle biopsy vs fine-needle aspiration on pathologic measurement of tumor size in breast cancer. Arch Surg. 2005 Feb;140(2):125-8. PMID: 15723992.

760. Yang WT, Whitman GJ, Johnson MM, et al. Needle localization for excisional biopsy of breast lesions: comparison of effect of use of full-field digital versus screen-film mammographic guidance on procedure time. Radiology. 2004 Apr;231(1):277-81. PMID: 15068954.

761. Yararbas U, Argon AM, Yeniay L, et al. Problematic aspects of sentinel lymph node biopsy and its relation to previous excisional biopsy in breast cancer. Clin Nucl Med. 2009 Dec;34(12):854-8. PMID: 20139816.

762. Yom CK, Han W, Kim SW, et al. Clinical significance of annexin A1 expression in breast cancer. J Breast Cancer. 2011 Dec;14(4):262-8. PMID: 22323911.

763. Yom CK, Moon BI, Choe KJ, et al. Long-term results after excision of breast mass using a vacuum-assisted biopsy device. ANZ J Surg. 2009 Nov;79(11):794-8. PMID: 20078528.

764. Yoshinaga Y, Enomoto Y, Fujimitsu R, et al. Image and pathological changes after radiofrequency ablation of invasive breast cancer: a pilot study of nonsurgical therapy of early breast cancer. World J Surg. 2013 Feb;37(2):356-63. PMID: 23052813.

765. You SS, Jiang YX, Zhu QL, et al. US-guided diffused optical tomography: a promising functional imaging technique in breast lesions. Eur Radiol. 2010 Feb;20(2):309-17. PMID: 19707770.

766. Youk JH, Son EJ, Kim JA, et al. Scoring system based on BI-RADS lexicon to predict probability of malignancy in suspicious microcalcifications. Ann Surg Oncol. 2012 May;19(5):1491-8. PMID: 22173328.

767. Zhi W, Gu X, Qin J, et al. Solid breast lesions: clinical experience with US-guided diffuse optical tomography combined with conventional US. Radiology. 2012 Nov;265(2):371-8. PMID: 23012460.

768. Zhu Q, You S, Jiang Y, et al. Detecting angiogenesis in breast tumors: comparison of color Doppler flow imaging with ultrasound-guided diffuse optical tomography. Ultrasound Med Biol. 2011 Jun;37(6):862-9. PMID: 21531497.

769. Zografos GC, Zagouri F, Sergentanis TN, et al. Excisional breast biopsy under local anesthesia: stress-related neuroendocrine, metabolic and immune reactions during the procedure. In Vivo. 2009 Jul-Aug;23(4):649-52. PMID: 19567403.

770. National Guideline Clearinghouse (NGC). Guideline summary: ACR Appropriateness Criteria® palpable breast masses. In: National Guideline Clearinghouse (NGC) [Web site]. Rockville (MD): Agency for Healthcare Research and Quality (AHRQ); [cited 2013 June 25]. Available: http://www.guideline.gov.

771. Albarracin CT, Nguyen CV, Whitman GJ, et al. Identifying patients with atypical ductal hyperplasia diagnosed at core-needle biopsy who are at low risk of malignancy. Radiology. 2010 Dec;257(3):893-4; author reply 984. PMID: 21084420.

772. Amir E, Bedard PL, Ocana A, et al. Benefits and harms of detecting clinically occult breast cancer. J Natl Cancer Inst. 2012 Oct 17;104(20):1542-7. PMID: 22988040.

773. Bond M, Pavey T, Welch K, et al. Psychological consequences of false-positive screening mammograms in the UK. Evid Based Med. 2013 Apr;18(2):54-61. PMID: 22859786.

774. Bowman K, Munoz A, Mahvi DM, et al. Lobular neoplasia diagnosed at core biopsy does not mandate surgical excision. J Surg Res. 2007 Oct;142(2):275-80. PMID: 17662303.

775. Brant W. Percutaneous core biopsy of the breast. West J Med. 1996 Jul-Aug;165(1-2):52-3. PMID: 8855685.

776. Carkaci S, Santiago L, Adrada BE, et al. Screening for breast cancer with sonography. Semin Roentgenol. 2011 Oct;46(4):285-91. PMID: 22035671.

777. Cohen Y, Gekhtman D, Strano S. Mammography-sonography concordance. AJR Am J Roentgenol. 2011 Sep;197(3):765; author reply 6. PMID: 21862823.

778. Cooney CS, Khouri NF, Tsangaris TN. The role of breast MRI in the management of patients with breast disease. Adv Surg. 2008;42:299-312. PMID: 18953825.

779. Cusumano P, Polkowski WP, Liu H, et al. Percutaneous tissue acquisition: a treatment for breast cancer? Vacuum-assisted biopsy devices are not indicated for extended tissue removal. Eur J Cancer Prev. 2008 Aug;17(4):323-30. PMID: 18562956.

780. Damron TA. Vacuum-assisted biopsy is useful for breast tissue, but how useful is it for soft-tissue tumors in orthopaedics? Commentary on an article by Zarah Mohr, MD, et al.: "Vacuum-assisted minimally invasive biopsy of soft-tissue tumors". J Bone Joint Surg Am. 2012 Jan 18;94(2):e11. PMID: 22258008.

781. Dershaw DD. Stereotaxic breast biopsy. Semin Ultrasound CT MR. 1996 Oct;17(5):444-59. PMID: 8896110.

782. Eby PR, Lehman CD. Magnetic resonance imaging--guided breast interventions. Top Magn Reson Imaging. 2008 Jun;19(3):151-62. PMID: 18941395.

783. Giordano L, Giorgi D, Ventura L, et al. Time trends of process and impact indicators in Italian breast screening programmes (1999-2009). Epidemiol Prev. 2011 Sep-Dec;35(5-6 Suppl 5):28-38. PMID: 22166348.

784. Haid A, Knauer M, Dunzinger S, et al. Intra-operative sonography: a valuable aid during breast-conserving surgery for occult breast cancer. Ann Surg Oncol. 2007 Nov;14(11):3090-101. PMID: 17593330.

785. Hashimoto BE. New sonographic breast technologies. Semin Roentgenol. 2011 Oct;46(4):292-301. PMID: 22035672.

786. Kaiser WA, Pfleiderer SO, Baltzer PA. MRI-guided interventions of the breast. J Magn Reson Imaging. 2008 Feb;27(2):347-55. PMID: 18219688.

787. Karamouzis MV, Likaki-Karatza E, Ravazoula P, et al. Non-palpable breast carcinomas: correlation of mammographically detected malignant-appearing microcalcifications and molecular prognostic factors. Int J Cancer. 2002 Nov 1;102(1):86-90. PMID: 12353238.

788. Kettritz U. Modern concepts of ductal carcinoma in situ (DCIS) and its diagnosis through percutaneous biopsy. Eur Radiol. 2008 Feb;18(2):343-50. PMID: 17899107.

789. King V, Dershaw DD. Combining MRI with mammography: a more effective approach to breast cancer detection. Expert Rev Anticancer Ther. 2011 Aug;11(8):1155-8. PMID: 21916568.

790. Kluttig A, Trocchi P, Heinig A, et al. Reliability and validity of needle biopsy evaluation of breast-abnormalities using the B-categorization--design and objectives of the Diagnosis Optimisation Study (DIOS). BMC Cancer. 2007;7:100. PMID: 17570833.

791. Kontos M, Felekouras E, Fentiman IS. Radiofrequency ablation in the treatment of primary breast cancer: no surgical redundancies yet. Int J Clin Pract. 2008 May;62(5):816-20. PMID: 18412934.

792. Kopans DB. Review of stereotaxic large-core needle biopsy and surgical biopsy results in nonpalpable breast lesions. Radiology. 1993 Dec;189(3):665-6. PMID: 8234687.

793. Kopans DB. Caution on core. Radiology. 1994 Nov;193(2):325-6; discussion 6-8. PMID: 7972737.

794. Krupinski EA, Borders M, Fitzpatrick K. Processing stereotactic breast biopsy specimens: impact of specimen radiography system on workflow. Breast J. 2013 Jul-Aug;19(4):455-6. PMID: 23701431.

795. Marshall D, Laberge JM, Firetag B, et al. The changing face of percutaneous image-guided biopsy: molecular profiling and genomic analysis in current practice. J Vasc Interv Radiol. 2013 Aug;24(8):1094-103. PMID: 23806383.

796. Masood S. Reproducibility of breast biopsy. Eur J Radiol. 2012 Sep;81 Suppl 1:S95-6. PMID: 23083620.

797. Masood S, Vass L, Ibarra JA, Jr., et al. Breast pathology guideline implementation in low- and middle-income countries. Cancer. 2008 Oct 15;113(8 Suppl):2297-304. PMID: 18837021.

798. Mattheis J. Breast-cancer screening. N Engl J Med. 2012 Jan 12;366(2):190-1; author reply 1-2. PMID: 22236238.

799. Molleran V. Postbiopsy management. Semin Roentgenol. 2011 Jan;46(1):40-50. PMID: 21134527.

800. Monticciolo DL. Postbiopsy confirmation of MR-detected lesions biopsied using ultrasound. AJR Am J Roentgenol. 2012 Jun;198(6):W618-20. PMID: 22623580.

801. Morris EA, Kuhl CK, Lehman CD. Ensuring high-quality breast MR imaging technique and interpretation. Radiology. 2013 Mar;266(3):996-7. PMID: 23431233.

802. National Guideline Clearinghouse (NGC). Guideline summary: Diagnosis of breast disease. In: National Guideline Clearinghouse (NGC) [Web site]. Rockville (MD): Agency for Healthcare Research and Quality (AHRQ); [cited 2013 June 25]. Available: http://www.guideline.gov.

803. National Guideline Clearinghouse (NGC). Guideline summary: Breast cancer. In: Suspected cancer in primary care: guidelines for investigation, referral and reducing ethnic disparities. In: National Guideline Clearinghouse (NGC) [Web site]. Rockville (MD): Agency for Healthcare Research and Quality (AHRQ); [cited 2013 June 25]. Available: http://www.guideline.gov.

804. National Guideline Clearinghouse (NGC). Guideline summary: ACR Appropriateness Criteria® nonpalpable mammographic findings (excluding calcifications). In: National Guideline Clearinghouse (NGC) [Web site]. Rockville (MD): Agency for Healthcare Research and Quality (AHRQ); [cited 2013 June 25]. Available: http://www.guideline.gov.

805. National Guideline Clearinghouse (NGC). Guideline summary: Gynaecological cancer. In: Suspected cancer in primary care: guidelines for investigation, referral and reducing ethnic disparities. In: National Guideline Clearinghouse (NGC) [Web site]. Rockville (MD): Agency for Healthcare Research and Quality (AHRQ); [cited 2013 June 25]. Available: http://www.guideline.gov.

806. National Guideline Clearinghouse (NGC). Guideline summary: ACR Appropriateness Criteria® breast microcalcifications - initial diagnostic workup In: National Guideline Clearinghouse (NGC) [Web site]. Rockville (MD): Agency for Healthcare Research and Quality (AHRQ); [cited 2013 June 25]. Available: http://www.guideline.gov.

807. National Guideline Clearinghouse (NGC). Guideline summary: Early and locally advanced breast cancer. Diagnosis and treatment. In: National Guideline Clearinghouse (NGC) [Web site]. Rockville (MD): Agency for Healthcare Research and Quality (AHRQ); [cited 2013 June 25]. Available: http://www.guideline.gov.

808. Nields MW. Cost-effectiveness of image-guided core needle biopsy versus surgery in diagnosing breast cancer. Acad Radiol. 1996 Apr;3 Suppl 1:S138-40. PMID: 8796544.
809. Orel S. Who should have breast magnetic resonance imaging evaluation? J Clin Oncol. 2008 Feb 10;26(5):703-11. PMID: 18258977.
810. Park JM, Yang L, Laroia A, et al. Missed and/or misinterpreted lesions in breast ultrasound: reasons and solutions. Can Assoc Radiol J. 2011 Feb;62(1):41-9. PMID: 20947291.
811. Sardanelli F, Giuseppetti GM, Canavese G, et al. Indications for breast magnetic resonance imaging. Consensus document "Attualita in senologia", Florence 2007. Radiol Med. 2008 Dec;113(8):1085-95. PMID: 18953635.
812. Schousboe JT, Kerlikowske K, Loh A, et al. Personalizing mammography by breast density and other risk factors for breast cancer: analysis of health benefits and cost-effectiveness. Ann Intern Med. 2011 Jul 5;155(1):10-20. PMID: 21727289.
813. Schulz-Wendtl R. The vacora biopsy system. Recent Results Cancer Res. 2009;173:97-103. PMID: 19763449.
814. Sedgwick EL. Ultrasound-guided breast biopsy. Ultrasound Cln. 2011;6(3):327-33.
815. Sung JS, Lee CH, Morris EA, et al. Patient follow-up after concordant histologically benign imaging-guided biopsy of MRI-detected lesions. AJR Am J Roentgenol. 2012 Jun;198(6):1464-9. PMID: 22623564.
816. Trop I, Labelle M, David J, et al. Second-look targeted studies after breast magnetic resonance imaging: practical tips to improve lesion identification. Curr Probl Diagn Radiol. 2010 Sep-Oct;39(5):200-11. PMID: 20674767.
817. Tsang YY, Yau KK, Tang CN. Vacuum-assisted excision for benign breast lesions. Surgical Practice. 2013;17(3):129-.
818. Tse GM, Tan PH, Cheung HS, et al. Intermediate to highly suspicious calcification in breast lesions: a radio-pathologic correlation. Breast Cancer Res Treat. 2008 Jul;110(1):1-7. PMID: 17674189.
819. Tse GM, Tan PH, Lui PC, et al. Spindle cell lesions of the breast--the pathologic differential diagnosis. Breast Cancer Res Treat. 2008 May;109(2):199-207. PMID: 17636400.
820. Uematsu T. Screening and diagnosis of breast cancer in augmented women. Breast Cancer. 2008;15(2):159-64. PMID: 18293060.
821. Verkooijen HM. Needle core biopsy for screen detected breast lesions: time to raise the bar? Eur J Cancer. 2008 Nov;44(17):2540-1. PMID: 18930652.
822. Vogel VG. Epidemiology, genetics, and risk evaluation of postmenopausal women at risk of breast cancer. Menopause. 2008 Jul-Aug;15(4 Suppl):782-9. PMID: 18596599.
823. Warner E. Breast Surveillance of Patients with BRCA1 and BRCA2 Mutations. Current Breast Cancer Reports. 2013;5(3):255-61.
824. Z. PaSaNaSaSaCaHaCaLaAaaRa. The effect of a hypnotic intervention on anxiety and psychological distress in the breast biopsy suite: A pilot study [conference abstract].
825. Zagouri F, Sergentanis TN, Zografos GC. Vacuum-assisted breast biopsy: A role also on palpable lesions? Med Hypotheses. 2008;70(1):198-9. PMID: 17582694.
826. . [Update on current care guidelines: breast cancer diagnostics and screening]. Duodecim. 2010;126(10):1183-5. PMID: 20597348.
827. Aksoy F, Gundes E, Vatansev C, et al. Surgical treatment of phyllodes tumors of the breast: A single center experience: Memenin fillodes tumorlerinde cerrahi tedavi: Tek merkez deneyimi. J. Breast Health. 2013;9(2):52-6.

828. and X.-J. and Hu and D.-T. and Wu and J. and Chang and C. and and Zeng and W. DaJ-HaPaW-JaJaZ-XaLaG-YaJaY-JaZ. The first round imaging screening of breast cancer in Shanghai community: Primary results in 8234 patients. Chin. J. Radiol. 2013.

829. Apesteguia L, Ovelar A, Dominguez-Cunchillos F, et al. [Radiofrequency ablation of breast carcinomas: preliminary results of a clinical trial]. Radiologia. 2009 Nov-Dec;51(6):591-600. PMID: 19913265.

830. Aulmann S. [Ductal and lobular preneoplasia: role in breast cancer development]. Pathologe. 2011 Nov;32 Suppl 2:316-20. PMID: 21915665.

831. Bak M, Konyar E, Schneider F, et al. The "gray zone" in fi ne-needle aspiration cytology of the organized mammography screening. Cytohistological correlation: A "szurke zona" az emlorak mammografias szervezett szureseben. Citologiai-hisztologiai tanulmany. Orvosi Hetil. 2011;152(8):292-5.

832. Barreto AS, Mendes MF, Thuler LC. [Evaluation of a strategy adopted to expand adherence to breast cancer screening in Brazilian Northeast]. Rev Bras Ginecol Obstet. 2012 Feb;34(2):86-91. PMID: 22437768.

833. Bellolio JE, Guzman GP, Orellana CJ, et al. [Diagnostic value of frozen section biopsy during surgery for breast lesions or neoplasms]. Rev Med Chil. 2009 Sep;137(9):1173-8. PMID: 20011957.

834. Bettencourt H, Amendoeira I. Are core-needle biopsies representative of breast carcinomas?: Serao as microbiopsias representativas nos carcinomas da mama? Arq. Med. 2012;26(4):145-8.

835. Bilkova A, Janik V, Bendova M, et al. Computed tomography laser mamography (CTLM) - New imaging method in mammadiagnostics: Computed tomography laser mammography (CTLM) - Nova vysetrovaci metoda v mamarni diagnostice. Ceska Radiol. 2009;63(1):69-75.

836. Bokun ZV, Bokun R, Tatomirovic Z. [Determination of infiltrative ductal breast carcinoma differentiation grade in biopsy imprints]. Vojnosanit Pregl. 2009 Jul;66(7):527-33. PMID: 19678576.

837. Bouchlaka A, Ben Abdallah M, Ben Aissa R, et al. [Results and evaluation of 3 years of a large scale mammography program in the Ariana area of Tunisia]. Tunis Med. 2009 Jul;87(7):438-42. PMID: 20063676.

838. Bouhafa T, Masbah O, Bekkouch I, et al. [Phyllodes tumors of the breast: analysis of 53 patients]. Cancer Radiother. 2009 Apr;13(2):85-91. PMID: 19119040.

839. Brouwer OR, Donker M, Woerdeman LA, et al. [Local recurrence after skin-sparing mastectomy]. Ned Tijdschr Geneeskd. 2012;156(31):A4692. PMID: 22853767.

840. Chaveron C, Bachelle F, Fauquet I, et al. [Clip migration after stereotactic macrobiopsy and presurgical localization: technical considerations and tricks]. J Radiol. 2009 Jan;90(1 Pt 1):31-6. PMID: 19182711.

841. Contreras-Melendez L, Piottante-Becker A, Contreras-Seitz M, et al. The Chilean experience of variability in the assessment of HER2 status using immunohistochemistry: Variabilidad en la determinacion del estado de HER2 por inmunohistoquimica en Chile. Revista Esp. Patol. 2013;46(1):33-9.

842. Daubner D, Friedrich K, Spieth S. [Lactating adenoma of the breast - differential diagnosis in pregnancy and during breast feeding]. Rofo. 2012 Oct;184(10):934-5. PMID: 22744327.

843. de Lara CT, Fournier M, Macgrogan G. Ganglions sentinelles et carcinome canalaire in situ. Oncologie. 2013;15(6):331-5.

844. de Souza E, de Souza LF, Batista Mda C, et al. [Breast biopsy performed by the helicoid biopsy technique: an experimental study]. Rev Bras Ginecol Obstet. 2010 Dec;32(12):597-601. PMID: 21484028.

845. Ding Jianhui eaSCwwbcsrotfrotiaR-. Shanghai Community 8234 women with breast cancer screening results of the first round of the image analysis.

846. Dumay-Levesque T, Lemery S, Dauplat MM, et al. [Evaluation of stereotactic core biopsies of the breast with the 10-gauge Vacora(R) biopsy device: a review of 541 procedures]. J Radiol. 2011 Mar;92(3):226-35. PMID: 21501761.

847. Engvad B, Laenkholm AV, Schwartz W, et al. [Fine needle aspiration cytology of mammography screening]. Ugeskr Laeger. 2009 Aug 17;171(34):2379-82. PMID: 19732519.

848. Fischer T, Grigoryev M, Bossenz S, et al. [Sonographic detection of microcalcifications - potential of new method]. Ultraschall Med. 2012 Aug;33(4):357-65. PMID: 22322544.

849. Fischer U, Schwethelm L, Baum FT, et al. [Effort, accuracy and histology of MR-guided vacuum biopsy of suspicious breast lesions--retrospective evaluation after 389 interventions]. Rofo. 2009 Aug;181(8):774-81. PMID: 19582655.

850. Fouche CJ, Tabareau F, Michenet P, et al. [Specimen radiography assessment of surgical margins status in subclinical breast carcinoma: a diagnostic study]. J Gynecol Obstet Biol Reprod (Paris). 2011 Jun;40(4):314-22. PMID: 21349659.

851. Frankel PP, Esteves VF, Thuler LC, et al. [Diagnostic accuracy of the fine needle aspiration cytology and core needle biopsy as a diagnostic method for breast lesions]. Rev Bras Ginecol Obstet. 2011 Mar;33(3):139-43. PMID: 21829998.

852. Frikha M, Yaiche O, Elloumi F, et al. [Results of a pilot study for breast cancer screening by mammography in Sfax region, Tunisia]. J Gynecol Obstet Biol Reprod (Paris). 2013 May;42(3):252-61. PMID: 23478043.

853. G. TDLaCaFaMaaMa. Sentinel lymph nodes and ductal carcinoma in situ: Ganglions sentinelles et carcinome canalaire in situ. Oncologie.

854. Gomi N, Iwase T, Akiyama F. [VAB (vacuum-assisted breast biopsy system)]. Nihon Rinsho. 2012 Sep;70 Suppl 7:302-5. PMID: 23350410.

855. Gong J, Yao Y, Tang J, et al. Impact of preoperative chemotherapy on expression of hormone receptor and drug-resistant related proteins in breast cancer tissue. Chin. J. Clin. Oncol. 2012;39(23):1896-8.

856. Hahn M, Fischbach E, Fehm T, et al. [Are breast biopsies adequately funded? A process cost & revenue analysis]. Rofo. 2011 Apr;183(4):347-57. PMID: 21113867.

857. He YJ, Li JF, Wang TF, et al. [Diagnostic value and health economic evaluation of ultrasound-combined fine-needle aspiration cytology in primary breast cancer]. Zhonghua Yi Xue Za Zhi. 2012 Dec 11;92(46):3288-90. PMID: 23328516.

858. Heineke A, Bendel M, Tronnier M, et al. [Grouped papules on the left chest wall]. J Dtsch Dermatol Ges. 2010 Sep;8(9):715-7. PMID: 20821831.

859. Horak M, Barta J, Andryskova H, et al. Breast biopsy guided by magnetic resonance - First experiences: Biopsie prsu se zamerenim cile na magneticke rezonanci - Prvni zkusenosti. Ceska Radiol. 2009;63(1):56-60.

860. Jiang H, Fu J, Zhang F, et al. Value of steel wire implantation with prone table stereotactic digital mammography in the detection of microcalcification of the breast. Chin. J. Clin. Oncol. 2010;37(1):1-4.

861. Jing Z, Yu-xin J, Qing-li Z, et al. Impact of lesion size on the detection rate of non-palpable breast malignant lesions. Zhongguo Yi Xue Ke Xue Yuan Xue Bao. 2011 Apr;33(2):136-41. PMID: 21529439.

862. Kanayev SV, Novikov SN, Semiglazov VF, et al. The role of scintimammography and ultrasound in diagnosis of early (less than 10 mm) breast cancer. Vopr. Onkol. 2011;57(5):622-6.

863. Khlifi A, Ziadi S, Trimeche M, et al. Clinicopathological study of breast lobular carcinoma in Central Tunisia: A report of 74 cases: Etude clinicopathologique des carcinomes lobulaires du sein dans le Centre tunisien: a propos de 74 cas. J. Afr. Cancer. 2011;3(3):155-62.

864. Kosa C, Garami Z, Dinya T, et al. [Predictive factors of invasion with initial diagnosis of ductal carcinoma in situ based on core biopsy]. Magy Seb. 2012 Aug;65(4):218-21. PMID: 22940391.

865. Kuipers IM, Oostenbroek RJ, Storm RK, et al. [Suppose a mammary carcinoma is absent from the surgical specimen]. Ned Tijdschr Geneeskd. 2009;153:A3. PMID: 19900338.

866. L. ZaL-YaZaR-ZaZaC-WaLaJaaWa. Quantitative dynamic contrast enhanced MR in the prediction of response in breast cancer patients undergoing neoadjuvant chemotherapy. Chin. J. Radiol.

867. Langhans L, Vejborg TS, Vejborg I, et al. [Marking of non-palpable changes in breast tissue]. Ugeskr Laeger. 2012 Aug 20;174(34):1891-4. PMID: 22909568.

868. Li TY, Yu ZY, Wang LX, et al. Value of ultrasound-guided Mammotome rotation system in diagnosis and treatment of breast lesions. Chin. J. Cancer Prev. Treat. 2010;17(24):2060-1.

869. Li Y, Tong XS, Mu WM, et al. [Evaluation of the value of ultrasound-guided core needle biopsy in the diagnosis of breast lesions]. Zhonghua Zhong Liu Za Zhi. 2010 Jun;32(6):470-1. PMID: 20819494.

870. Liu M, Chen W, Li XR, et al. [Study on diagnostic accuracy of ultrasound-guided core needle breast biopsy]. Zhonghua Bing Li Xue Za Zhi. 2010 Nov;39(11):739-42. PMID: 21215163.

871. Lobato Miguélez J, Moreno Domingo J, Martinez Urruzola J, et al. Riesgo de invasión en carcinoma in situ de mama diagnosticado por biopsia percutánea: estudio retrospectivo. Clínica e Investigación en Ginecología y Obstetricia. 2013.

872. Ma WY, Zhang P, Zhang BL, et al. [Phase II clinical trial of neoadjuvant therapy with carboplatin plus paclitaxel for locally advanced triple-negative breast cancer]. Zhonghua Zhong Liu Za Zhi. 2012 Oct;34(10):770-4. PMID: 23291072.

873. Manych M. MR-detected lesions of the breast - When should a specific sonography follow?: MR-Lsionen der Brust - Wann Sollte Eine Gezielte Sonografie Folgen? RoFo Fortschr. Geb. Rontgenstr. Bildgebenden Verfahren. 2010;182(4):305.

874. MAO F, PAN B, SUN Q, et al. Diagnosis and treatment of neuroendocrine breast cancer: A retrospective analysis of ten cases and review of the literature. TUMOR. 2013;33(2):171-6.

875. Martins EC, Soares A, Guimaraes CM, et al. [Ultrasound guided core biopsy for breast lesions using 16G needle]. Rev Col Bras Cir. 2009 Aug;36(4):312-5. PMID: 20076920.

876. Mercier-Vogel L, Couson F, Kohlik M, et al. [Impact of breast MRI and PET-CT in breast cancer staging]. Rev Med Suisse. 2010 May 26;6(250):1076-8, 80. PMID: 20564867.

877. Mohajeri G, Khezreh H, Kushki AM, et al. Evaluation of fine needle aspiration versus core needle biopsy for breast cancer detection. J. Isfahan Med. Sch. 2012;30(174).

878. Monter SEP, Gómez ACA, Chávez VG, et al. Abordaje quirúrgico de nódulos mamarios durante el embarazo•. Ginecol Obstet Mex. 2009;77(4):191-8.

879. Neira P, Aguirre B, Taub T, et al. [Breast MRI--histologic correlation for ductal carcinoma in situ]. Radiologia. 2009 Jul-Aug;51(4):396-402. PMID: 19406443.

880. Nicolas F, Voltzenlogel MC, Lavoue V, et al. [Pleomorphic lobular intraepithelial neoplasia: clinical, histological and prognostic study of nine cases]. J Gynecol Obstet Biol Reprod (Paris). 2013 Apr;42(2):130-6. PMID: 23265671.

881. Obermann EC, Eppenberger-Castori S, Tapia C. [Assessment of proliferation: core biopsy or resection specimen? Discrepancies in breast cancer with low and high proliferation]. Pathologe. 2012 May;33(3):245-50. PMID: 22576598.

882. Ouldamer L, Body G, Arbion F, et al. [Mucocele-like lesions of the breast: management after diagnosis on ultrasound guided core biopsy or stereotactic vacuum-assisted biopsy]. Gynecol Obstet Fertil. 2010 Jul-Aug;38(7-8):455-9. PMID: 20605510.

883. Peres A, Becette V, Guinebretiere JM, et al. [The lesions of flat epithelial atypia diagnosed on breast biopsy]. Gynecol Obstet Fertil. 2011 Oct;39(10):579-85. PMID: 21924938.

884. Perez Monter SE, Arteaga Gomez AC, Gorbea Chavez V, et al. [Surgical approach of breast nodules during pregnancy]. Ginecol Obstet Mex. 2009 Apr;77(4):189-96. PMID: 19496511.

885. Perlet C, Schneider P, Amaya B, et al. MR-Guided vacuum biopsy of 206 contrast-enhancing breast lesions. Rofo. 2002 Jan;174(1):88-95. PMID: 11793291.

886. Plaza Loma S, Rodriguez de Diego Y, Gonzalez Blanco I, et al. Stereotactic vacuum-assisted breast biopsy. Correlation with surgical excisional biopsy: Biopsia mamaria asistida por vacio y guiada por estereotaxia. Correlacion con la biopsia quirurgica. Prog. Obstet. Ginecol. 2012;55(2):66-70.

887. Prutki M, Stern-Padovan R, Jakic-Razumovic J, et al. [Ultrasound guided breast biopsy--a retrospective study and literature review]. Lijec Vjesn. 2012 Sep-Oct;134(9-10):270-5. PMID: 23297511.

888. Qin NS, Wang XY, Wu CX, et al. Correlation of tumor vessel morphologic features with clinical and pathological characteristics of breast cancer on dynamic contrast enhanced MRI. Chin. J. Med. Imaging Technol. 2009;25(2):244-7.

889. Ren AH, Zhang XP, Li J, et al. Dynamic contrast-enhanced breast MRI for patients with BI-RADS 3-5 microcalcifications detected by digital mammography. Chin. J. Med. Imaging Technol. 2009;25(1):89-92.

890. Ricart Selma V, Camps Herrero J, Martinez Rubio C, et al. [Diabetic mastopathy: clinical presentation, imaging and histologic findings, and treatment]. Radiologia. 2011 Jul-Aug;53(4):349-54. PMID: 21530989.

891. Ruvalcaba Limon E, Espejo Fonseca R, Bautista Pina V, et al. [Radiological control intraoperatory of a surgical piece in non palpable breast lesions]. Ginecol Obstet Mex. 2009 Sep;77(9):407-18. PMID: 19899430.

892. Salem A, Debabria H, Mehiri S, et al. [Retrospective results of ultrasonographically-guided biopsy the breast cancer screening program of the Ariana area of Tunisia]. Tunis Med. 2009 Jul;87(7):463-70. PMID: 20063681.

893. Schulz-Wendtland R, Adamietz B, Meier-Meitinger M, et al. Ultrasound-guided core cut biopsy: 15 years' follow-up: Sonografisch gezielte Stanzbiopsie: 15 Jahre Follow-up. Geburtshilfe Frauenheilkd. 2010;70(6):478-82.

894. Semiglazov VV, Semiglazov VF, Ermchenkova AM. [Minimal breast carcinomas]. Vopr Onkol. 2011;57(6):702-6. PMID: 22416384.

895. Shi SH, Deng YC, Li XJ. Ultrasound-guided mammotome biopsy in diagnosis and management of single intraductal breast papilloma. J. Pract. Oncol. 2012;27(4):390-2.
896. Siegmann KC, Moron HU, Baur A, et al. [Diagnostic value of a breast MRI score for the prediction of malignancy of breast lesions detected solely with MRI]. Rofo. 2009 Jun;181(6):556-63. PMID: 19452398.
897. Stoblen F, Landt S, Koninger A, et al. [Detection of microcalcifications by high-resolution B-mode sonography in patients with BI-RADS 4a lesions]. Gynakol Geburtshilfliche Rundsch. 2009;49(4):292-8. PMID: 20530944.
898. Su KL, Xu HB, Hu ZJ, et al. [Vacuum-assisted biopsy and wire localization for the diagnosis of non-palpable breast lesions]. Zhonghua Zhong Liu Za Zhi. 2010 Jun;32(6):472-5. PMID: 20819495.
899. Traore B, Eric Douanla D, Diallo Y, et al. Problems in the management of breast cancers diagnosed post-surgery in the unit of surgical oncology, teaching hospital Donka, Conakry (Guinea): Problematique de la prise en charge des cancers du sein de << diagnostic postoperatoire >> a l'unite de chirurgie oncologique, CHU de Donka, Conakry (Guinee). J. Afr. Cancer. 2010;2(3):140-5.
900. Uehara M. [Breast surgery and biopsy in anticoagulated patients]. Nihon Rinsho. 2012 Sep;70 Suppl 7:706-9. PMID: 23350490.
901. Uhara M, Matsuda K, Shimojyo Y, et al. [Comparison of two HER-2 FISH kits on formalin-fixed paraffin-embedded tissues: signal detection and simple procedure]. Rinsho Byori. 2010 Jan;58(1):25-9. PMID: 20169940.
902. Utzschneider S, Weber P, Fottner A, et al. [Prognosis-adapted surgical management of bone metastases]. Orthopade. 2009 Apr;38(4):308, 10-12, 14-5. PMID: 19296081.
903. Wang Q, Zhu CX, Zhang AQ, et al. Clinical and pathological analysis of breast cancer with false-negative mammogram. Chin. J. Cancer Prev. Treat. 2009;16(2):138-40.
904. X.-J. LaJ-CaFaX-LaZaW-MaaZa. Analysis of 278 breast biopsy cases guided by mammography. Cancer Res. Clin.
905. Xu J, Wang Q, Xia J, et al. Primary efficacy of physical examination combined with ultragraphy and complemented with mammography for breast cancer screening in 280 thousand Chinese women. European Journal of Cancer. 2013;49:S322-S3.
906. Xu Juan, et al. Complement the X-ray and ultrasonic examination mammography for breast cancer screening mode preliminary application evaluation. Chinese Journal of Cancer. 2013.
907. Yan L, Qiang S, Wei-Xuan Z. Role of fine needle aspiration cytology in surgical treatment of breast cancer. Zhongguo Yi Xue Ke Xue Yuan Xue Bao. 2011 Feb;33(1):80-2. PMID: 21375944.
908. Ye JM, Xu L, Wang DM, et al. [Prospective study on the role of MRI and B ultrasonography in evaluating the tumor response to neoadjuvant chemotherapy in breast cancer]. Zhonghua Wai Ke Za Zhi. 2009 Mar 1;47(5):349-52. PMID: 19595011.
909. Yin CF, Zhao HJ, Gao WR. Diagnostic value of three-dimensional stereotactic localization for nonpalpable breast lesions. Chin. J. Med. Imaging Technol. 2010;26(8):1492-4.
910. Yin HF, Wang YH, Qin XQ, et al. [Effect of neoadjuvant chemotherapy on histologic grade and expression of biological markers in breast cancer]. Zhonghua Zhong Liu Za Zhi. 2009 Nov;31(11):858-62. PMID: 20137353.
911. Zhang Y, Tang Y, Bai L, et al. Clinical significance of ultrasound and needle biopsy in diagnosis of breast cancer with liver metastasis. Chin. J. Cancer Prev. Treat. 2010;17(2):142-4.

912. Zhao HJ, Yin CF, Zhao AL. Comparison of two-dimensional and three-dimensional X-ray guided wire localization breast biopsy. Chin. J. Intervent. Imaging Ther. 2011;8(4):307-9.

913. Zhao JH, Ding J, Xu SB, et al. Comparison of diagnosis value between 18F-FDG PET/CT and MRI in breast cancer. J. Jilin Univ. Med. Ed. 2011;37(4):746-9.

914. Zhou YJ, Ying M, He YJ, et al. [Analysis of associations between molecular subtypes and responses to neoadjuvant chemotherapy in primary breast cancer patients]. Zhonghua Yi Xue Za Zhi. 2013 Jun 11;93(22):1711-5. PMID: 24124677.

915. Abbas H, Imran S, Waris NA, et al. Importance of physical examination in early detection of lump in breast in women of different age groups. J Ayub Med Coll Abbottabad. 2010 Apr-Jun;22(2):79-82. PMID: 21702273.

916. Abdel-Hadi M, Abdel-Hamid GF, Abdel-Razek N, et al. Should fine-needle aspiration cytology be the first choice diagnostic modality for assessment of all nonpalpable breast lesions? The experience of a breast cancer screening center in Alexandria, Egypt. Diagn Cytopathol. 2010 Dec;38(12):880-9. PMID: 20049973.

917. Adamietz BR, Kahmann L, Fasching PA, et al. Differentiation between phyllodes tumor and fibroadenoma using real-time elastography. Ultraschall Med. 2011 Dec;32 Suppl 2:E75-9. PMID: 22194044.

918. Adibelli ZH, Ergenc R, Oztekin O, et al. Observer Variability of the Breast Imaging Reporting and Data System (BI-RADS) Lexicon for Mammography. Breast Care (Basel). 2010 Mar;5(1):11-6. PMID: 22619635.

919. Adler DD, Riba MB, Eggly S. Breaking bad news in the breast imaging setting. Acad Radiol. 2009 Feb;16(2):130-5. PMID: 19124097.

920. Aellig A, Maillard M, Phavorin A, et al. The energy metabolism of the leukocyte. VIII. The determination of the concentration of the coenzymes NAD, NADH, NADP and NADPH in polymorphonuclear leukocytes at rest and after incubation by enzymatic cycling. Enzyme. 1977;22(3):196-206. PMID: 16746.

921. Al-Attar MA, Michell MJ, Ralleigh G, et al. The impact of image guided needle biopsy on the outcome of mammographically detected indeterminate microcalcification. Breast. 2006 Oct;15(5):635-9. PMID: 16488148.

922. Albert US, Duda V, Hadji P, et al. Imprint cytology of core needle biopsy specimens of breast lesions. A rapid approach to detecting malignancies, with comparison of cytologic and histopathologic analyses of 173 cases. Acta Cytol. 2000 Jan-Feb;44(1):57-62. PMID: 10667161.

923. Al-Hallaq HA, Mell LK, Bradley JA, et al. Magnetic resonance imaging identifies multifocal and multicentric disease in breast cancer patients who are eligible for partial breast irradiation. Cancer. 2008 Nov 1;113(9):2408-14. PMID: 18823018.

924. Al-Harethee WA, Kalles V, Papapanagiotou I, et al. Thermal damage of the specimen during breast biopsy with the use of the Breast Lesion Excision System: does it affect diagnosis? Breast Cancer. 2013 Mar 16PMID: 23504263.

925. Alimoglu E, Bayraktar SD, Bozkurt S, et al. Follow-up versus tissue diagnosis in BI-RADS category 3 solid breast lesions at US: a cost-consequence analysis. Diagn Interv Radiol. 2012 Jan-Feb;18(1):3-10. PMID: 21997885.

926. Al-Rikabi A, Husain S. Increasing prevalence of breast cancer among Saudi patients attending a tertiary referral hospital: a retrospective epidemiologic study. Croat Med J. 2012 Jun;53(3):239-43. PMID: 22661137.

927. Al-Sobhi SS, Helvie MA, Pass HA, et al. Extent of lumpectomy for breast cancer after diagnosis by stereotactic core versus wire localization biopsy. Ann Surg Oncol. 1999;6(4):330-5.

928. Anania G, Bazzocchi M, di Loreto C, et al. Percutaneous large core needle biopsy versus surgical biopsy in the diagnosis of breast lesions. Int Surg. 1997 Jan-Mar;82(1):52-5. PMID: 9189803.

929. Andersen SB, Vejborg I, von Euler-Chelpin M. Participation behaviour following a false positive test in the Copenhagen mammography screening programme. Acta Oncol. 2008;47(4):550-5. PMID: 18465321.

930. Andreu FJ, Sentis M, Castaner E, et al. The impact of stereotactic large-core needle biopsy in the treatment of patients with nonpalpable breast lesions: a study of diagnostic accuracy in 510 consecutive cases. Eur Radiol. 1998;8(8):1468-74. PMID: 9853239.

931. Arentz C, Baxter K, Boneti C, et al. Ten-year experience with hematoma-directed ultrasound-guided (HUG) breast lumpectomy. Ann Surg Oncol. 2010 Oct;17 Suppl 3:378-83. PMID: 20853061.

932. Ariyarathenam AV, Currie R, Cooper MJ, et al. Impact of age extension to include 47-49 year old women on the workload of the surgical department of a single Breast Cancer Screening Unit--The first non-randomized experience in UK. Int J Surg. 2013;11(7):535-7. PMID: 23684821.

933. Arleo EK, Dashevsky BZ, Reichman M, et al. Screening mammography for women in their 40s: a retrospective study of the potential impact of the U.S. Preventive Service Task Force's 2009 breast cancer screening recommendations. AJR Am J Roentgenol. 2013 Dec;201(6):1401-6. PMID: 24261383.

934. Arora N, Martins D, Ruggerio D, et al. Effectiveness of a noninvasive digital infrared thermal imaging system in the detection of breast cancer. Am J Surg. 2008 Oct;196(4):523-6. PMID: 18809055.

935. Arrangoiz R, Garand S, Slomski C, et al. What is the diagnostic accuracy of hypocellular fine needle aspiration of the breast in the context of an otherwise negative triple screen. Int. J. Oncol. 2009;6(1).

936. Ashbeck EL, Rosenberg RD, Stauber PM, et al. Benign breast biopsy diagnosis and subsequent risk of breast cancer. Cancer Epidemiol Biomarkers Prev. 2007 Mar;16(3):467-72. PMID: 17337650.

937. Aslam HM, Saleem S, Shaikh HA, et al. Clinico- pathological profile of patients with breast diseases. Diagn Pathol. 2013;8:77. PMID: 23659667.

938. Awad FM. Role of supersonic shear wave imaging quantitative elastography (SSI) in differentiating benign and malignant solid breast masses. The Egyptian Journal of Radiology and Nuclear Medicine. 2013;44(3):681-5.

939. Ballesio L, Maggi C, Savelli S, et al. Role of breast magnetic resonance imaging (MRI) in patients with unilateral nipple discharge: preliminary study. Radiol Med. 2008 Mar;113(2):249-64. PMID: 18386126.

940. Ballo MS, Sneige N. Can core needle biopsy replace fine-needle aspiration cytology in the diagnosis of palpable breast carcinoma. A comparative study of 124 women. Cancer. 1996 Aug 15;78(4):773-7. PMID: 8756371.

941. Baltzer PA, Yang F, Dietzel M, et al. Sensitivity and specificity of unilateral edema on T2w-TSE sequences in MR-Mammography considering 974 histologically verified lesions. Breast J. 2010 May-Jun;16(3):233-9. PMID: 20565468.

942. Barman I, Dingari NC, Saha A, et al. Application of Raman spectroscopy to identify microcalcifications and underlying breast lesions at stereotactic core needle biopsy. Cancer Res. 2013 Jun 1;73(11):3206-15. PMID: 23729641.

943. Barr RG. Real-time ultrasound elasticity of the breast: initial clinical results. Ultrasound Q. 2010 Jun;26(2):61-6. PMID: 20498561.

944. Barr RG, Lackey AE. The utility of the" bull's-eye" artifact on breast elasticity imaging in reducing breast lesion biopsy rate. Ultrasound Q. 2011;27(3):151-5.

945. Barra Ade A, Gobbi H, de LRCA, et al. A comparision of aspiration cytology and core needle biopsy according to tumor size of suspicious breast lesions. Diagn Cytopathol. 2008 Jan;36(1):26-31. PMID: 18064684.

946. Battaglia TA, Howard MB, Kavanah M, et al. The addition of internists to a breast health program. Breast J. 2012 Jan-Feb;18(1):58-64. PMID: 22098389.

947. Beattie A. Detecting breast cancer in a general practice - Like finding needles in a haystack? Aust Fam Physician. 2009 Dec;38(12):1003-6. PMID: 20369155.

948. Beckmann KR, Farshid G, Roder DM, et al. Impact of hormone replacement therapy use on mammographic screening outcomes. Cancer Causes Control. 2013 Jul;24(7):1417-26. PMID: 23649232.

949. Bent CK, Bassett LW, D'Orsi CJ, et al. The positive predictive value of BI-RADS microcalcification descriptors and final assessment categories. AJR Am J Roentgenol. 2010 May;194(5):1378-83. PMID: 20410428.

950. Berg WA, Jaeger B, Campassi C, et al. Predictive value of specimen radiography for core needle biopsy of noncalcified breast masses. AJR Am J Roentgenol. 1998 Dec;171(6):1671-8. PMID: 9843311.

951. Berna JD, Nieves FJ, Romero T, et al. A multimodality approach to the diagnosis of breast hamartomas with atypical mammographic appearance. Breast J. 2001 Jan-Feb;7(1):2-7. PMID: 11348408.

952. Berna-Serna JD, Torres-Ales C, Berna-Mestre JD, et al. Role of Galactography in the Early Diagnosis of Breast Cancer. Breast Care. 2013;8(2):122-6.

953. Berube M, Curpen B, Ugolini P, et al. Level of suspicion of a mammographic lesion: use of features defined by BI-RADS lexicon and correlation with large-core breast biopsy. Can Assoc Radiol J. 1998 Aug;49(4):223-8. PMID: 9709675.

954. Bianchi S, Caini S, Renne G, et al. Positive predictive value for malignancy on surgical excision of breast lesions of uncertain malignant potential (B3) diagnosed by stereotactic vacuum-assisted needle core biopsy (VANCB): a large multi-institutional study in Italy. Breast. 2011 Jun;20(3):264-70. PMID: 21208804.

955. Bleznak AD, Magaram D. Surgical biopsy techniques for mammographically detected abnormalities. The Breast Journal. 1998;4(6):426-9.

956. Boba M, Koltun U, Bobek-Billewicz B, et al. False-negative results of breast core needle biopsies - retrospective analysis of 988 biopsies. Pol J Radiol. 2011 Jan;76(1):25-9. PMID: 22802813.

957. Bodai BI, Boyd B, Brown L, et al. Total cost comparison of 2 biopsy methods for nonpalpable breast lesions. Am J Manag Care. 2001 May;7(5):527-38. PMID: 11388132.

958. Bonifacino A, Petrocelli V, Pisani T, et al. Accuracy rates of US-guided vacuum-assisted breast biopsy. Anticancer Res. 2005 May-Jun;25(3c):2465-70. PMID: 16080477.

959. Bowers GJ, Getz JB, Roettger RH, et al. Nonpalpable breast lesions: association of mammographic abnormalities with diagnosis after needle-directed biopsy. South Med J. 1993 Jul;86(7):748-52. PMID: 8391719.

960. Brem RF, Floerke AC, Rapelyea JA, et al. Breast-specific gamma imaging as an adjunct imaging modality for the diagnosis of breast cancer. Radiology. 2008 Jun;247(3):651-7. PMID: 18487533.

961. Brenner RJ, Sickles EA. Surveillance mammography and stereotactic core breast biopsy for probably benign lesions: a cost comparison analysis. Acad Radiol. 1997 Jun;4(6):419-25. PMID: 9189199.

962. Breslin TM, Caughran J, Pettinga J, et al. Improving breast cancer care through a regional quality collaborative. Surgery. 2011 Oct;150(4):635-42. PMID: 22000174.

963. Britton P, McCann J. Needle biopsy in the NHS breast screening programme 1996/97: how much and how accurate? The Breast. 1999;8(1):5-11.

964. Brown ML, Houn F, Sickles EA, et al. Screening mammography in community practice: positive predictive value of abnormal findings and yield of follow-up diagnostic procedures. AJR Am J Roentgenol. 1995 Dec;165(6):1373-7. PMID: 7484568.

965. Buijs-van der Woude T, Verkooijen HM, Pijnappel RM, et al. Cost comparison between stereotactic large-core-needle biopsy versus surgical excision biopsy in The Netherlands. Eur J Cancer. 2001 Sep;37(14):1736-45. PMID: 11549426.

966. Bulte JP, Polman L, Schlooz-Vries M, et al. One-day core needle biopsy in a breast clinic: 4 years experience. Breast Cancer Res Treat. 2013 Jan;137(2):609-16. PMID: 23239152.

967. Bundred SM, Zhou J, Whiteside S, et al. Impact of full-field digital mammography on pre-operative diagnosis and surgical treatment of mammographic microcalcification. Breast Cancer Res Treat. 2014 Jan;143(2):359-66. PMID: 24318468.

968. Burbank F. Stereotactic breast biopsy: comparison of 14- and 11-gauge Mammotome probe performance and complication rates. Am Surg. 1997 Nov;63(11):988-95. PMID: 9358788.

969. Burbank F, Forcier N. Tissue marking clip for stereotactic breast biopsy: initial placement accuracy, long-term stability, and usefulness as a guide for wire localization. Radiology. 1997 Nov;205(2):407-15. PMID: 9356621.

970. Burbank F, Parker SH, Fogarty TJ. Stereotactic breast biopsy: improved tissue harvesting with the Mammotome. Am Surg. 1996 Sep;62(9):738-44. PMID: 8751765.

971. Burnside ES, Rubin DL, Fine JP, et al. Bayesian network to predict breast cancer risk of mammographic microcalcifications and reduce number of benign biopsy results: initial experience. Radiology. 2006 Sep;240(3):666-73. PMID: 16926323.

972. Caines JS, Schaller GH, Iles SE, et al. Ten years of breast screening in the Nova Scotia Breast Screening Program, 1991-2001. experience: use of an adaptable stereotactic device in the diagnosis of screening-detected abnormalities. Can Assoc Radiol J. 2005 Apr;56(2):82-93. PMID: 15957275.

973. Calhoun K, Giuliano A, Brenner RJ. Intraoperative loss of core biopsy clips: clinical implications. AJR Am J Roentgenol. 2008 Mar;190(3):W196-200. PMID: 18287412.

974. Candelaria R, Fornage BD. Second-look US examination of MR-detected breast lesions. J Clin Ultrasound. 2011 Mar-Apr;39(3):115-21. PMID: 21387324.

975. Cangiarella J, Gross J, Symmans WF, et al. The incidence of positive margins with breast conserving therapy following mammotome biopsy for microcalcification. J Surg Oncol. 2000 Aug;74(4):263-6. PMID: 10962457.

976. Cangiarella J, Mercado CL, Symmans WF, et al. Stereotaxic aspiration biopsy in the evaluation of mammographically detected clustered microcalcification. Cancer. 1998 Aug 25;84(4):226-30. PMID: 9723597.

977. Cangiarella JF, Waisman J, Weg N, et al. The Use of Stereotaxic Core Biopsy and Stereotaxic Aspiration Biopsy as Diagnostic Tools in the Evaluation of Mammary Calcification. Breast J. 2000 Nov;6(6):366-72. PMID: 11348394.

978. Carbonaro LA, Verardi N, Di Leo G, et al. Handling a high relaxivity contrast material for dynamic breast MR imaging using higher thresholds for the initial enhancement. Invest Radiol. 2010 Mar;45(3):114-20. PMID: 20065856.

979. Carney PA, Parikh J, Sickles EA, et al. Diagnostic mammography: identifying minimally acceptable interpretive performance criteria. Radiology. 2013 May;267(2):359-67. PMID: 23297329.

980. Carty NJ, Ravichandran D, Carter C, et al. Randomized comparison of fine-needle aspiration cytology and Biopty-Cut needle biopsy after unsatisfactory initial cytology of discrete breast lesions. Br J Surg. 1994 Sep;81(9):1313-4. PMID: 7953396.

981. Chan KKK, Lui CY, Chu T, et al. Stratifying risk for malignancy using microcalcification descriptors from the breast imaging reporting and data system 4th edition: Experience in a single centre in Hong Kong. J. HK Coll. Radiol. 2009;11(4):149-53.

982. Chang JM, Moon WK, Cho N, et al. Breast mass evaluation: factors influencing the quality of US elastography. Radiology. 2011 Apr;259(1):59-64. PMID: 21330569.

983. Chang JM, Moon WK, Cho N, et al. Breast cancers initially detected by hand-held ultrasound: detection performance of radiologists using automated breast ultrasound data. Acta Radiol. 2011 Feb 1;52(1):8-14. PMID: 21498319.

984. Chang JM, Moon WK, Cho N, et al. Radiologists' performance in the detection of benign and malignant masses with 3D automated breast ultrasound (ABUS). Eur J Radiol. 2011 Apr;78(1):99-103. PMID: 21330080.

985. Chang JM, Moon WK, Cho N, et al. Clinical application of shear wave elastography (SWE) in the diagnosis of benign and malignant breast diseases. Breast Cancer Res Treat. 2011 Aug;129(1):89-97. PMID: 21681447.

986. Chare MJ, Flowers CI, O'Brien CJ, et al. Image-guided core biopsy in patients with breast disease. Br J Surg. 1996 Oct;83(10):1415-6. PMID: 8944459.

987. Chasteen ND, White LK, Campbell RF. Metal site conformational states of vanadyl(IV) human serotransferrin complexes. Biochemistry. 1977 Feb 8;16(3):363-5. PMID: 13814.

988. Cheng J, Qiu S, Raju U, et al. Benign breast disease heterogeneity: association with histopathology, age, and ethnicity. Breast Cancer Res Treat. 2008 Sep;111(2):289-96. PMID: 17917807.

989. Cheng YC, Wu NY, Ko JS, et al. Breast cancers detected by breast MRI screening and ultrasound in asymptomatic Asian women: 8 years of experience in Taiwan. Oncology. 2012;82(2):98-107. PMID: 22328009.

990. Cheung KL, Wong AW, Parker H, et al. Pathological features of primary breast cancer in the elderly based on needle core biopsies--a large series from a single centre. Crit Rev Oncol Hematol. 2008 Sep;67(3):263-7. PMID: 18524618.

991. Cheung YC, Wan YL, Chen SC, et al. Sonographic evaluation of mammographically detected microcalcifications without a mass prior to stereotactic core needle biopsy. J Clin Ultrasound. 2002 Jul-Aug;30(6):323-31. PMID: 12116093.

992. Chlebowski RT, Anderson G, Pettinger M, et al. Estrogen plus progestin and breast cancer detection by means of mammography and breast biopsy. Arch Intern Med. 2008 Feb 25;168(4):370-7; quiz 45. PMID: 18299491.

993. Cho N, Moon WK. Digital mammography-guided skin marking for sonographically guided biopsy of suspicious microcalcifications. AJR Am J Roentgenol. 2009 Mar;192(3):W132-6. PMID: 19234241.

994. Cho N, Moon WK, Cha JH, et al. Ultrasound-guided vacuum-assisted biopsy of microcalcifications detected at screening mammography. Acta Radiol. 2009 Jul;50(6):602-9. PMID: 19449232.

995. Cho N, Moon WK, Cha JH, et al. Sonographically guided core biopsy of the breast: comparison of 14-gauge automated gun and 11-gauge directional vacuum-assisted biopsy methods. Korean J Radiol. 2005 Apr-Jun;6(2):102-9. PMID: 15968149.

996. Cho N, Moon WK, Chang JM, et al. Aliasing artifact depicted on ultrasound (US)-elastography for breast cystic lesions mimicking solid masses. Acta Radiol. 2011 Feb 1;52(1):3-7. PMID: 21498318.

997. Chu TY, Lui CY, Hung WK, et al. Localisation of occult breast lesion: a comparative analysis of hookwire and radioguided procedures. Hong Kong Med J. 2010 Oct;16(5):367-72. PMID: 20890001.

998. Chuo CB, Corder AP. Core biopsy vs fine needle aspiration cytology in a symptomatic breast clinic. Eur J Surg Oncol. 2003 May;29(4):374-8. PMID: 12711292.

999. Ciatto S, Del Turco MR, Marrazzo A, et al. Time trends of benign/malignant breast biopsy ratios a multicenter Italian study. Tumori. 1996 Jul-Aug;82(4):325-8. PMID: 8890964.

1000. Clarke D, Sudhakaran N, Gateley CA. Replace fine needle aspiration cytology with automated core biopsy in the triple assessment of breast cancer. Ann R Coll Surg Engl. 2001 Mar;83(2):110-2. PMID: 11320918.

1001. Clarke-Pearson EM, Jacobson AF, Boolbol SK, et al. Quality assurance initiative at one institution for minimally invasive breast biopsy as the initial diagnostic technique. J Am Coll Surg. 2009 Jan;208(1):75-8. PMID: 19228506.

1002. Clifford EJ, De Vol EB, Pockaj BA, et al. Early results from a novel quality outcomes program: the American Society Of Breast Surgeons' Mastery of Breast Surgery. Ann Surg Oncol. 2010 Oct;17 Suppl 3:233-41. PMID: 20853039.

1003. Coldman AJ, Phillips N. False-positive screening mammograms and biopsies among women participating in a Canadian provincial breast screening program. Can J Public Health. 2012 Nov-Dec;103(6):e420-4. PMID: 23618020.

1004. Cole EB, Toledano AY, Lundqvist M, et al. Comparison of radiologist performance with photon-counting full-field digital mammography to conventional full-field digital mammography. Acad Radiol. 2012 Aug;19(8):916-22. PMID: 22537503.

1005. Corn CC. Review of 125 SiteSelect stereotactic large-core breast biopsy procedures. Breast J. 2003 May-Jun;9(3):147-52. PMID: 12752621.

1006. Cornea V, Jaffer S, Bleiweiss IJ, et al. Adequate histologic sampling of breast magnetic resonance imaging-guided core needle biopsy. Arch Pathol Lab Med. 2009 Dec;133(12):1961-4. PMID: 19961252.

1007. Corsetti V, Houssami N, Ferrari A, et al. Breast screening with ultrasound in women with mammography-negative dense breasts: evidence on incremental cancer detection and false positives, and associated cost. Eur J Cancer. 2008 Mar;44(4):539-44. PMID: 18267357.

1008. Crotch-Harvey M, Loughran C. Combined stereotactic wide-core needle biopsy and fine-needle aspiration cytology in the assessment of impalpable mammographic abnormalities detected in a breast-screening programme. The Breast. 1996;5(1):48-9.

1009. Crowe JP, Jr., Rim A, Patrick R, et al. A prospective review of the decline of excisional breast biopsy. Am J Surg. 2002 Oct;184(4):353-5. PMID: 12383901.

1010. Crump SR, Shipp MP, McCray GG, et al. Abnormal mammogram follow-up: do community lay health advocates make a difference? Health Promot Pract. 2008 Apr;9(2):140-8. PMID: 18340089.

1011. Cui Y, Page DL, Lane DS, et al. Menstrual and reproductive history, postmenopausal hormone use, and risk of benign proliferative epithelial disorders of the breast: a cohort study. Breast Cancer Res Treat. 2009 Mar;114(1):113-20. PMID: 18360772.

1012. Dahlstrom JE, Sutton S, Jain S. Histological precision of stereotactic core biopsy in diagnosis of malignant and premalignant breast lesions. Histopathology. 1996 Jun;28(6):537-41. PMID: 8803597.

1013. Dahlstrom JE, Sutton S, Jain S. Histologic-radiologic correlation of mammographically detected microcalcification in stereotactic core biopsies. Am J Surg Pathol. 1998 Feb;22(2):256-9. PMID: 9500229.

1014. Daly CP, Bailey JE, Klein KA, et al. Complicated breast cysts on sonography: is aspiration necessary to exclude malignancy? Acad Radiol. 2008 May;15(5):610-7. PMID: 18423318.

1015. Damascelli B, Frigerio LF, Lanocita R, et al. Stereotactic excisional breast biopsy performed by interventional radiologists using the advanced breast biopsy instrumentation system. Br J Radiol. 1998 Oct;71(850):1003-11. PMID: 10211058.

1016. Damascelli B, Frigerio LF, Patelli G, et al. Stereotactic breast biopsy: en bloc excision of microcalcifications with a large-bore cannula device. AJR Am J Roentgenol. 1999 Oct;173(4):895-900. PMID: 10511143.

1017. D'Angelo PC, Galliano DE, Rosemurgy AS. Stereotactic excisional breast biopsies utilizing the advanced breast biopsy instrumentation system. Am J Surg. 1997 Sep;174(3):297-302. PMID: 9324141.

1018. Demir F, Donmez YC, Ozsaker E, et al. Patients' lived experiences of excisional breast biopsy: a phenomenological study. J Clin Nurs. 2008 Mar;17(6):744-51. PMID: 18279277.

1019. Dennison G, Anand R, Makar SH, et al. A prospective study of the use of fine-needle aspiration cytology and core biopsy in the diagnosis of breast cancer. Breast J. 2003 Nov-Dec;9(6):491-3. PMID: 14616944.

1020. Denton ER, Ryan S, Beaconfield T, et al. Image-guided breast biopsy: analysis of pain and discomfort related to technique. Breast. 1999 Oct;8(5):257-60. PMID: 14965740.

1021. Dershaw DD, Morris EA, Liberman L, et al. Nondiagnostic stereotaxic core breast biopsy: results of rebiopsy. Radiology. 1996 Feb;198(2):323-5. PMID: 8596825.

1022. Destounis S, Arieno A, Morgan R, et al. Clinical experience with elasticity imaging in a community-based breast center. J Ultrasound Med. 2013 Feb;32(2):297-302. PMID: 23341386.

1023. Destounis S, Skolny MN, Morgan R, et al. Rates of pathological underestimation for 9 and 12 gauge breast needle core biopsies at surgical excision. Breast Cancer. 2011 Jan;18(1):42-50. PMID: 20204553.

1024. Deurloo EE, Gilhuijs KG, Kool LJS, et al. Displacement of breast tissue and needle deviations during stereotactic procedures. Invest Radiol. 2001;36(6):347-53.

1025. Deutscher SL, Dickerson M, Gui G, et al. Carbohydrate antigens in nipple aspirate fluid predict the presence of atypia and cancer in women requiring diagnostic breast biopsy. BMC Cancer. 2010;10:519. PMID: 20920311.

1026. Devia A, Murray KA, Nelson EW. Stereotactic core needle biopsy and the workup of mammographic breast lesions. Arch Surg. 1997 May;132(5):512-5; discussion 5-7. PMID: 9161394.

1027. Dietzel M, Baltzer PA, Vag T, et al. The necrosis sign in magnetic resonance-mammography: diagnostic accuracy in 1,084 histologically verified breast lesions. Breast J. 2010 Nov-Dec;16(6):603-8. PMID: 21070437.

1028. Dillon MF, Maguire AA, McDermott EW, et al. Needle core biopsy characteristics identify patients at risk of compromised margins in breast conservation surgery. Mod Pathol. 2008 Jan;21(1):39-45. PMID: 17948023.

1029. Dittus K, Geller B, Weaver DL, et al. Impact of mammography screening interval on breast cancer diagnosis by menopausal status and BMI. J Gen Intern Med. 2013 Nov;28(11):1454-62. PMID: 23760741.

1030. Docktor BJ, MacGregor JH, Burrowes PW. Ultrasonographic findings 6 months after 11-gauge vacuum-assisted large-core breast biopsy. Can Assoc Radiol J. 2004 Jun;55(3):151-6. PMID: 15237775.

1031. Donaldson LA, Cliff A, Gardiner L, et al. Surgeon-controlled ultrasound-guided core biopsies in the breast--a prospective study and a new use for surgeons in the clinic. Eur J Surg Oncol. 2003 Mar;29(2):139-42. PMID: 12633556.

1032. Doridot V, Meunier M, El Khoury C, et al. Stereotactic radioguided surgery by siteSelect for subclinical mammographic lesions. Ann Surg Oncol. 2005 Feb;12(2):181-8. PMID: 15827800.

1033. D'Orsi CJ, Getty DJ, Pickett RM, et al. Stereoscopic digital mammography: improved specificity and reduced rate of recall in a prospective clinical trial. Radiology. 2013 Jan;266(1):81-8. PMID: 23150865.

1034. Dowlatshahi K, Yaremko ML, Kluskens LF, et al. Nonpalpable breast lesions: findings of stereotaxic needle-core biopsy and fine-needle aspiration cytology. Radiology. 1991 Dec;181(3):745-50. PMID: 1947091.

1035. Doyle AJ, King AR, Miller MV, et al. Implementation of image-guided large-core needle biopsy of the breast on a limited budget. Australas Radiol. 1998 Aug;42(3):199-203. PMID: 9727241.

1036. Doyle JM, O'Doherty A, Coffey L, et al. Can the radiologist accurately predict the adequacy of sampling when performing ultrasound-guided core biopsy of BI-RADS category 4 and 5 lesions detected on screening mammography? Clin Radiol. 2005 Sep;60(9):999-1005. PMID: 16124982.

1037. Duijm LE, Groenewoud JH, de Koning HJ, et al. Delayed diagnosis of breast cancer in women recalled for suspicious screening mammography. Eur J Cancer. 2009 Mar;45(5):774-81. PMID: 19046632.

1038. Duijm LE, Groenewoud JH, Fracheboud J, et al. Utilization and cost of diagnostic imaging and biopsies following positive screening mammography in the southern breast cancer screening region of the Netherlands, 2000-2005. Eur Radiol. 2008 Nov;18(11):2390-7. PMID: 18491102.

1039. Duijm LE, Louwman MW, Groenewoud JH, et al. Inter-observer variability in mammography screening and effect of type and number of readers on screening outcome. Br J Cancer. 2009 Mar 24;100(6):901-7. PMID: 19259088.

1040. Dunning K, Liedtke E, Toedter L, et al. Outpatient surgery centers draw cases away from hospitals, impact resident training volume. J Surg Educ. 2008 Nov-Dec;65(6):460-4. PMID: 19059178.

1041. E. FaBDaCaCJaFaKaGaTaaMaS. Core needle biopsy: A useful adjunct to fine-needle aspiration in select patients with palpable breast lesions. Cancer.

1042. El Khouli RH, Macura KJ, Barker PB, et al. MRI-guided vacuum-assisted breast biopsy: a phantom and patient evaluation of targeting accuracy. J Magn Reson Imaging. 2009 Aug;30(2):424-9. PMID: 19629977.

1043. El Khoury M, Mesurolle B, Omeroglu A, et al. Values of pathological analysis of lost tissue fragments in the vacuum canister during a vacuum-assisted stereotactic biopsy of the breast. Br J Radiol. 2013 May;86(1025):20120270. PMID: 23520227.

1044. Elkum NB, Myles JD, Kumar P. Analyzing biological rhythms in clinical trials. Contemp Clin Trials. 2008 Sep;29(5):720-6. PMID: 18571991.

1045. El-Sayed ME, Rakha EA, Reed J, et al. Audit of performance of needle core biopsy diagnoses of screen detected breast lesions. Eur J Cancer. 2008 Nov;44(17):2580-6. PMID: 18632261.

1046. Elter M, Schulz-Wendtland R, Wittenberg T. The prediction of breast cancer biopsy outcomes using two CAD approaches that both emphasize an intelligible decision process. Med Phys. 2007 Nov;34(11):4164-72. PMID: 18072480.

1047. Ertas G, Gulcur HO, Tunaci M, et al. A preliminary study on computerized lesion localization in MR mammography using 3D nMITR maps, multilayer cellular neural networks, and fuzzy c-partitioning. Med Phys. 2008 Jan;35(1):195-205. PMID: 18293575.

1048. Eser M, Kaptanoglu L, Kement M, et al. A Challenging entity in the differential diagnosis of breast cancer: A retrospective analysis of 17 cases with granulomatous lobular mastitis: Meme kanserinin ayirici tanisinda zor bir durum: Granulomatoz lobuler mastitli 17 olgunun retrospektif analizi. J. Breast Health. 2013;9(2):69-75.

1049. Evans A, Whelehan P, Thomson K, et al. Differentiating benign from malignant solid breast masses: value of shear wave elastography according to lesion stiffness combined with greyscale ultrasound according to BI-RADS classification. Br J Cancer. 2012 Jul 10;107(2):224-9. PMID: 22691969.

1050. Evans A, Whelehan P, Thomson K, et al. Quantitative shear wave ultrasound elastography: initial experience in solid breast masses. Breast Cancer Res. 2010;12(6):R104. PMID: 21122101.

1051. Evans LA. Feasibility of family member presence in the OR during breast biopsy procedures. AORN J. 2008 Oct;88(4):568-86. PMID: 18928960.

1052. Fahy BN, Bold RJ, Schneider PD, et al. Cost-benefit analysis of biopsy methods for suspicious mammographic lesions; discussion 994-5. Arch Surg. 2001 Sep;136(9):990-4. PMID: 11529819.

1053. Fajardo LL. Cost-effectiveness of stereotaxic breast core needle biopsy. Acad Radiol. 1996 Apr;3 Suppl 1:S21-3. PMID: 8796501.

1054. Fajardo LL, Bird RE, Herman CR, et al. Placement of endovascular embolization microcoils to localize the site of breast lesions removed at stereotactic core biopsy. Radiology. 1998 Jan;206(1):275-8. PMID: 9423683.

1055. Farshid G, Pieterse S. Core imprint cytology of screen-detected breast lesions is predictive of the histologic results. Cancer. 2006 Jun 25;108(3):150-6. PMID: 16634070.

1056. Farshid G, Rush G. The use of fine-needle aspiration cytology and core biopsy in the assessment of highly suspicious mammographic microcalcifications: analysis of outcome for 182 lesions detected in the setting of a population-based breast cancer screening program. Cancer. 2003 Dec 25;99(6):357-64. PMID: 14681944.

1057. Faulkner K, McCormack S, Bennison K. A retrospective analysis of digital stereotaxis in breast screening. Br J Radiol. 2007 Jul;80(955):563-8. PMID: 17621605.

1058. Feeley L, Kiernan D, Mooney T, et al. Digital mammography in a screening programme and its implications for pathology: a comparative study. J Clin Pathol. 2011 Mar;64(3):215-9. PMID: 21177749.

1059. Fenton JJ, Xing G, Elmore JG, et al. Short-term outcomes of screening mammography using computer-aided detection: a population-based study of medicare enrollees. Ann Intern Med. 2013 Apr 16;158(8):580-7. PMID: 23588746.

1060. Feoli F, Paesmans M, Van Eeckhout P. Fine needle aspiration cytology of the breast: impact of experience on accuracy, using standardized cytologic criteria. Acta Cytol. 2008 Mar-Apr;52(2):145-51. PMID: 18499986.

1061. Ferguson J, Chamberlain P, Cramer HM, et al. ER, PR, and Her2 immunocytochemistry on cell-transferred cytologic smears of primary and metastatic breast carcinomas: a comparison study with formalin-fixed cell blocks and surgical biopsies. Diagn Cytopathol. 2013 Jul;41(7):575-81. PMID: 22807465.

1062. Ferzli GS, Hurwitz JB, Puza T, et al. Advanced breast cancer biopsy instrumentation: a critique. J Am Coll Surg. 1997 Aug;185(2):145-51. PMID: 9249081.

1063. Ferzli GS, Puza T, Vanvorst-Bilotti S, et al. Breast Biopsies with ABBI(R): Experience with 183 Attempted Biopsies. Breast J. 1999 Jan;5(1):26-8. PMID: 11348252.

1064. Fiaschetti V, Salimbeni C, Gaspari E, et al. The role of second-look ultrasound of BIRADS-3 mammary lesions detected by breast MR imaging. Eur J Radiol. 2012 Nov;81(11):3178-84. PMID: 22417393.

1065. Fine RE, Boyd BA. Stereotactic breast biopsy: a practical approach. Am Surg. 1996 Feb;62(2):96-102. PMID: 8554199.

1066. Fine RE, Boyd BA, Whitworth PW, et al. Percutaneous removal of benign breast masses using a vacuum-assisted hand-held device with ultrasound guidance. Am J Surg. 2002 Oct;184(4):332-6. PMID: 12383895.

1067. Fine RE, Israel PZ, Walker LC, et al. A prospective study of the removal rate of imaged breast lesions by an 11-gauge vacuum-assisted biopsy probe system. Am J Surg. 2001 Oct;182(4):335-40. PMID: 11720666.

1068. Fitzpatrick P, Fleming P, O'Neill S, et al. False-positive mammographic screening: factors influencing re-attendance over a decade of screening. J Med Screen. 2011;18(1):30-3. PMID: 21536814.

1069. Fleury EF, Rinaldi JF, Piato S, et al. Appearance of breast masses on sonoelastography with special focus on the diagnosis of fibroadenomas. Eur Radiol. 2009 Jun;19(6):1337-46. PMID: 19159934.

1070. Fornasa F, Pinali L, Gasparini A, et al. Diffusion-weighted magnetic resonance imaging in focal breast lesions: analysis of 78 cases with pathological correlation. Radiol Med. 2011 Mar;116(2):264-75. PMID: 21076884.

1071. Fournier LS, Vanel D, Athanasiou A, et al. Dynamic optical breast imaging: a novel technique to detect and characterize tumor vessels. Eur J Radiol. 2009 Jan;69(1):43-9. PMID: 18829193.

1072. Frayne J, Sterrett GF, Harvey J, et al. Stereotactic 14 gauge core-biopsy of the breast: results from 101 patients. Aust N Z J Surg. 1996 Sep;66(9):585-91. PMID: 8859155.

1073. Freeman S. One-stop clinic can diagnose suspect lesions in a day. Oncol. Rep. 2010(SEPTEMBER-OCTOBER):14+5.

1074. Friedlander LC, Roth SO, Gavenonis SC. Results of MR imaging screening for breast cancer in high-risk patients with lobular carcinoma in situ. Radiology. 2011 Nov;261(2):421-7. PMID: 21900618.

1075. Fu CY, Hsu HH, Yu JC, et al. Influence of age on PPV of sonographic BI-RADS categories 3, 4, and 5. Ultraschall Med. 2011 Jan;32 Suppl 1:S8-13. PMID: 20603785.

1076. Gajdos C, Levy M, Herman Z, et al. Complete removal of nonpalpable breast malignancies with a stereotactic percutaneous vacuum-assisted biopsy instrument. J Am Coll Surg. 1999 Sep;189(3):237-40. PMID: 10472922.

1077. Gala I, Fisher P, Hermann GA. Usefulness of Telfa pads in the histologic assessment of stereotactic-guided breast biopsy specimens. Mod Pathol. 1999 May;12(5):553-7. PMID: 10349996.

1078. Gallagher R, Schafer G, Redick M, et al. Microcalcifications of the breast: a mammographic-histologic correlation study using a newly designed Path/Rad Tissue Tray. Ann Diagn Pathol. 2012 Jun;16(3):196-201. PMID: 22225905.

1079. Gan FY, Wettlaufer JR, Lundell AL. Breast imaging in a military setting: a comparison with civilian breast imaging. Mil Med. 2004 May;169(5):361-7. PMID: 15186000.

1080. Geller BM, Oppenheimer RG, Mickey RM, et al. Patient perceptions of breast biopsy procedures for screen-detected lesions. Am J Obstet Gynecol. 2004 Apr;190(4):1063-9. PMID: 15118643.

1081. Gentry CL, Henry CA. Stereotactic Percutaneous Breast Biopsy: A Comparative Analysis Between Surgeon and Radiologist. Breast J. 1999 Mar;5(2):101-4. PMID: 11348267.

1082. Ghosh K, Melton LJ, 3rd, Suman VJ, et al. Breast biopsy utilization: a population-based study. Arch Intern Med. 2005 Jul 25;165(14):1593-8. PMID: 16043676.

1083. Giordano L, Giorgi D, Piccini P, et al. Time trends of process and impact indicators in Italian breast screening programmes: 1998-2007. Epidemiol Prev. 2009 May-Jun;33(3 Suppl 2):29-39. PMID: 19776485.

1084. Giordano L, Giorgi D, Piccini P, et al. Time trends of process and impact indicators in Italian breast screening programmes--1996-2005. Epidemiol Prev. 2008 Mar-Apr;32(2 Suppl 1):23-36. PMID: 18770993.

1085. Giordano L, Giorgi D, Ventura L, et al. Time trends of process and impact indicators in Italian breast screening programmes: 1998-2008. Epidemiol Prev. 2010 Sep-Dec;34(5-6 Suppl 4):27-34. PMID: 21220835.

1086. Girardi V, Tonegutti M, Ciatto S, et al. Breast ultrasound in 22,131 asymptomatic women with negative mammography. Breast. 2013 Oct;22(5):806-9. PMID: 23558244.

1087. Gittleman MA. Single-step ultrasound localization of breast lesions and lumpectomy procedure. Am J Surg. 2003 Oct;186(4):386-90. PMID: 14553856.

1088. Goldman LE, Walker R, Hubbard R, et al. Timeliness of abnormal screening and diagnostic mammography follow-up at facilities serving vulnerable women. Med Care. 2013 Apr;51(4):307-14. PMID: 23358386.

1089. Goldman LE, Walker R, Miglioretti DL, et al. Facility characteristics do not explain higher false-positive rates in diagnostic mammography at facilities serving vulnerable women. Med Care. 2012 Mar;50(3):210-6. PMID: 22186768.

1090. Golub RM, Bennett CL, Stinson T, et al. Cost minimization study of image-guided core biopsy versus surgical excisional biopsy for women with abnormal mammograms. Journal of clinical oncology. 2004;22(12):2430-7.

1091. Goodman KA, Birdwell RL, Ikeda DM. Compliance with recommended follow-up after percutaneous breast core biopsy. AJR Am J Roentgenol. 1998 Jan;170(1):89-92. PMID: 9423606.

1092. Gray RE, Benson GW, Lustig DD. Stereotactic breast biopsy: experience in a community setting. J Miss State Med Assoc. 1999 Jan;40(1):3-7. PMID: 9919043.

1093. Grimes MM, Karageorge LS, Hogge JP. Does exhaustive search for microcalcifications improve diagnostic yield in stereotactic core needle breast biopsies? Mod Pathol. 2001 Apr;14(4):350-3. PMID: 11301352.

1094. Groenewoud JH, Pijnappel RM, van den Akker-Van Marle ME, et al. Cost-effectiveness of stereotactic large-core needle biopsy for nonpalpable breast lesions compared to open-breast biopsy. Br J Cancer. 2004 Jan 26;90(2):383-92. PMID: 14735181.

1095. Gruber S, Debski BK, Pinker K, et al. Three-dimensional proton MR spectroscopic imaging at 3 T for the differentiation of benign and malignant breast lesions. Radiology. 2011 Dec;261(3):752-61. PMID: 21998046.

1096. Gufler H, Wagner S, Franke FE. The interior structure of breast microcalcifications assessed with micro computed tomography. Acta Radiol. 2011 Jul 1;52(6):592-6. PMID: 21498282.

1097. Gumus H, Gumus M, Devalia H, et al. Causes of failure in removing calcium in microcalcification-only lesions using 11-gauge stereotactic vacuum-assisted breast biopsy. Diagn Interv Radiol. 2012 Jul-Aug;18(4):354-9. PMID: 22477646.

1098. Gumus H, Gumus M, Mills P, et al. Clinically palpable breast abnormalities with normal imaging: is clinically guided biopsy still required? Clin Radiol. 2012 May;67(5):437-40. PMID: 22119297.

1099. Gumus H, Mills P, Fish D, et al. Breast microcalcification: diagnostic value of calcified and non-calcified cores on specimen radiographs. Breast J. 2013 Mar-Apr;19(2):156-61. PMID: 23294155.

1100. Gur D, Wallace LP, Klym AH, et al. Trends in recall, biopsy, and positive biopsy rates for screening mammography in an academic practice. Radiology. 2005 May;235(2):396-401. PMID: 15770039.

1101. Gurel K, Karabay O, Gurel S, et al. Does prebiopsy, nonsterile ultrasonography gel affect biopsy-site asepsis? Cardiovasc Intervent Radiol. 2008 Jan-Feb;31(1):131-4. PMID: 17978849.

1102. Gutwein LG, Ang DN, Liu H, et al. Utilization of minimally invasive breast biopsy for the evaluation of suspicious breast lesions. Am J Surg. 2011 Aug;202(2):127-32. PMID: 21295284.

1103. Gweon HM, Youk JH, Son EJ, et al. Visually assessed colour overlay features in shear-wave elastography for breast masses: quantification and diagnostic performance. Eur Radiol. 2013 Mar;23(3):658-63. PMID: 22976918.

1104. Haj M, Kniaz D, Eitan A, et al. Three years of experience with advanced breast biopsy instrumentation (ABBI). Breast J. 2002 Sep-Oct;8(5):275-80. PMID: 12199754.

1105. Hamilton LJ, Cornford EJ, Maxwell AJ. A survey of current UK practice regarding the biopsy of clinically and radiologically benign breast masses in young women. Clin Radiol. 2011 Aug;66(8):738-41. PMID: 21513922.

1106. Hann LE, Liberman L, Dershaw DD, et al. Mammography immediately after stereotaxic breast biopsy: is it necessary? AJR Am J Roentgenol. 1995 Jul;165(1):59-62. PMID: 7785633.

1107. Hanna WC, Demyttenaere SV, Ferri LE, et al. The use of stereotactic excisional biopsy in the management of invasive breast cancer. World J Surg. 2005 Nov;29(11):1490-4; discussion 5-6. PMID: 16240063.

1108. Harlow SP, Krag DN, Ames SE, et al. Intraoperative ultrasound localization to guide surgical excision of nonpalpable breast carcinoma. J Am Coll Surg. 1999 Sep;189(3):241-6. PMID: 10472923.

1109. Harman SM, Gucciardo F, Heward CB, et al. Discrimination of breast cancer by anti-malignin antibody serum test in women undergoing biopsy. Cancer Epidemiol Biomarkers Prev. 2005 Oct;14(10):2310-5. PMID: 16214910.

1110. Harvey JA, Nicholson BT, Lorusso AP, et al. Short-term follow-up of palpable breast lesions with benign imaging features: evaluation of 375 lesions in 320 women. AJR Am J Roentgenol. 2009 Dec;193(6):1723-30. PMID: 19933671.

1111. Hassan HHM, Mahmoud Zahran MH, El-Prince Hassan H, et al. Diffusion magnetic resonance imaging of breast lesions: Initial experience at Alexandria University. Alexandria Journal of Medicine. 2013;49(3):265-72.

1112. Hatada T, Ishii H, Ichii S, et al. Diagnostic value of ultrasound-guided fine-needle aspiration biopsy, core-needle biopsy, and evaluation of combined use in the diagnosis of breast lesions. J Am Coll Surg. 2000 Mar;190(3):299-303. PMID: 10703854.

1113. Hayes BD, Brodie C, O'Doherty A, et al. High-grade histologic features of DCIS are associated with R5 rather than R3 calcifications in breast screening mammography. Breast J. 2013 May-Jun;19(3):319-24. PMID: 23600490.

1114. Hemmer JM, Kelder JC, van Heesewijk HP. Stereotactic large-core needle breast biopsy: analysis of pain and discomfort related to the biopsy procedure. Eur Radiol. 2008 Feb;18(2):351-4. PMID: 17909818.

1115. Henderson LM, Hubbard RA, Onega TL, et al. Assessing health care use and cost consequences of a new screening modality: the case of digital mammography. Med Care. 2012 Dec;50(12):1045-52. PMID: 22922432.

1116. Heywang-Koebrunner S, Bock K, Heindel W, et al. Mammography Screening–as of 2013. Geburtshilfe und Frauenheilkunde. 2013;73(10):1007-16.

1117. Hille H, Vetter M, Hackeloer BJ. The accuracy of BI-RADS classification of breast ultrasound as a first-line imaging method. Ultraschall Med. 2012 Apr;33(2):160-3. PMID: 21877320.

1118. Hillhouse RA, Norvill KA, Buchanan SW, et al. Analysis of malignancy detected by needle-localized breast biopsy. J Am Osteopath Assoc. 1996 Jul;96(7):398-400. PMID: 8758871.

1119. Hillner BE, Bear HD, Fajardo LL. Estimating the cost-effectiveness of stereotaxic biopsy for nonpalpable breast abnormalities: a decision analysis model. Acad Radiol. 1996 Apr;3(4):351-60. PMID: 8796686.

1120. Hoffmann J. Analysis of surgical and diagnostic quality at a specialist breast unit. The Breast. 2006;15(4):490-7.

1121. Hofvind S, Ponti A, Patnick J, et al. False-positive results in mammographic screening for breast cancer in Europe: a literature review and survey of service screening programmes. J Med Screen. 2012;19 Suppl 1:57-66. PMID: 22972811.

1122. Holloway CM, Gagliardi AR. Percutaneous needle biopsy for breast diagnosis: how do surgeons decide? Ann Surg Oncol. 2009 Jun;16(6):1629-36. PMID: 19357925.

1123. Holloway CM, Saskin R, Paszat L. Geographic variation and physician specialization in the use of percutaneous biopsy for breast cancer diagnosis. Can J Surg. 2008 Dec;51(6):453-63. PMID: 19057734.

1124. Homesh NA, Issa MA, El-Sofiani HA. The diagnostic accuracy of fine needle aspiration cytology versus core needle biopsy for palpable breast lump(s). Saudi Med J. 2005 Jan;26(1):42-6. PMID: 15756351.

1125. Hooley RJ, Greenberg KL, Stackhouse RM, et al. Screening US in patients with mammographically dense breasts: initial experience with Connecticut Public Act 09-41. Radiology. 2012 Oct;265(1):59-69. PMID: 22723501.

1126. Hoorntje LE, Peeters PH, Mali WP, et al. Is stereotactic large-core needle biopsy beneficial prior to surgical treatment in BI-RADS 5 lesions? Breast Cancer Res Treat. 2004 Jul;86(2):165-70. PMID: 15319568.

1127. Hrung JM, Langlotz CP, Orel SG, et al. Cost-effectiveness of MR imaging and core-needle biopsy in the preoperative work-up of suspicious breast lesions. Radiology. 1999 Oct;213(1):39-49. PMID: 10540638.

1128. Hsu HH, Yu JC, Lee HS, et al. Complex cystic lesions of the breast on ultrasonography: feature analysis and BI-RADS assessment. Eur J Radiol. 2011 Jul;79(1):73-9. PMID: 20116191.

1129. Hubbard RA, Kerlikowske K, Flowers CI, et al. Cumulative Probability of False-Positive Recall or Biopsy Recommendation After 10 Years of Screening MammographyA Cohort Study. Ann Intern Med. 2011;155(8):481-92.

1130. Hubbard RA, Zhu W, Horblyuk R, et al. Diagnostic imaging and biopsy pathways following abnormal screen-film and digital screening mammography. Breast Cancer Res Treat. 2013 Apr;138(3):879-87. PMID: 23471650.

1131. Hubbard RA, Zhu W, Onega TL, et al. Effects of digital mammography uptake on downstream breast-related care among older women. Med Care. 2012 Dec;50(12):1053-9. PMID: 23132199.

1132. Hung WK, Lam HS, Lau Y, et al. Diagnostic accuracy of vacuum-assisted biopsy device for image-detected breast lesions. ANZ J Surg. 2001 Aug;71(8):457-60. PMID: 11504288.

1133. Hunter TB, Roberts CC, Hunt KR, et al. Occurrence of fibroadenomas in postmenopausal women referred for breast biopsy. J Am Geriatr Soc. 1996 Jan;44(1):61-4. PMID: 8537592.

1134. Ibrahim AE, Bateman AC, Theaker JM, et al. The role and histological classification of needle core biopsy in comparison with fine needle aspiration cytology in the preoperative assessment of impalpable breast lesions. J Clin Pathol. 2001 Feb;54(2):121-5. PMID: 11215280.

1135. Idowu MO, Hardy LB, Souers RJ, et al. Pathologic diagnostic correlation with breast imaging findings: a College of American Pathologists Q-Probes study of 48 institutions. Arch Pathol Lab Med. 2012 Jan;136(1):53-60. PMID: 22208488.

1136. Ikeda K, Ogawa Y, Takii M, et al. A role for elastography in the diagnosis of breast lesions by measuring the maximum fat lesion ratio (max-FLR) by tissue Doppler imaging. Breast Cancer. 2012 Jan;19(1):71-6. PMID: 21567172.

1137. Insausti LP, Alberro JA, Regueira FM, et al. An experience with the Advanced Breast Biopsy Instrumentation (ABBI) system in the management of non-palpable breast lesions. Eur Radiol. 2002 Jul;12(7):1703-10. PMID: 12111061.

1138. Iwatani T, Matsuda A, Kawabata H, et al. Predictive factors for psychological distress related to diagnosis of breast cancer. Psychooncology. 2013 Mar;22(3):523-9. PMID: 23577351.

1139. Jackman RJ, Marzoni FA, Jr. Needle-localized breast biopsy: why do we fail? Radiology. 1997 Sep;204(3):677-84. PMID: 9280243.

1140. Jackman RJ, Marzoni FA, Jr. Stereotactic histologic biopsy with patients prone: technical feasibility in 98% of mammographically detected lesions. AJR Am J Roentgenol. 2003 Mar;180(3):785-94. PMID: 12591697.

1141. Jackman RJ, Rodriguez-Soto J. Breast microcalcifications: retrieval failure at prone stereotactic core and vacuum breast biopsy--frequency, causes, and outcome. Radiology. 2006 Apr;239(1):61-70. PMID: 16567483.

1142. Jacobs IA, Chevinsky AH, Diehl W, et al. Advanced breast biopsy instrumentation (ABBI) and management of nonpalpable breast abnormalities: a community hospital experience. Breast. 2001 Oct;10(5):421-6. PMID: 14965618.

1143. Jacobs TW, Silverman JF, Schroeder B, et al. Accuracy of touch imprint cytology of image-directed breast core needle biopsies. Acta Cytol. 1999 Mar-Apr;43(2):169-74. PMID: 10097705.

1144. Jaffer S, Bleiweiss IJ, Nagi C. Incidental intraductal papillomas (<2 mm) of the breast diagnosed on needle core biopsy do not need to be excised. Breast J. 2013 Mar-Apr;19(2):130-3. PMID: 23336823.

1145. Jan WA, Zada N, Samieulla, et al. Comparison of FNAC and core biopsy for evaluating breast lumps. Med Forum Mon. 2002;13(12):26-8.

1146. Jara-Lazaro AR, Tan PH. Comparing digital and optical microscopy diagnoses of breast and prostate core biopsies. Pathology. 2012 Jan;44(1):46-8. PMID: 22157691.

1147. Jensen A, Rank F, Dyreborg U, et al. Performance of combined clinical mammography and needle biopsy: a nationwide study from Denmark. APMIS. 2006 Dec;114(12):884-92. PMID: 17207089.

1148. Johnson KS, Baker JA, Lee SS, et al. Cancelation of MRI guided breast biopsies for suspicious breast lesions identified at 3.0 T MRI: reasons, rates, and outcomes. Acad Radiol. 2013 May;20(5):569-75. PMID: 23473719.

1149. Jones L, Lott MF, Calder CJ, et al. Imprint cytology from ultrasound-guided core biopsies: accurate and immediate diagnosis in a one-stop breast clinic. Clin Radiol. 2004 Oct;59(10):903-8. PMID: 15451349.

1150. Jung HJ, Hahn SY, Choi HY, et al. Breast sonographic elastography using an advanced breast tissue-specific imaging preset: initial clinical results. J Ultrasound Med. 2012 Feb;31(2):273-80. PMID: 22298871.

1151. Kaiser CG, Reich C, Wasser K, et al. Economic aspects of MR-mammography in dense breasts. Eur J Radiol. 2012 Sep;81 Suppl 1:S69-71. PMID: 23083609.

1152. Kaplan SS, Collado-Mesa F, Ekens J, et al. Palpable solid breast masses with probably benign sonographic features: can biopsy be avoided? Breast J. 2013 Mar-Apr;19(2):212-4. PMID: 23316805.

1153. Kasahara Y, Kawai M, Tsuji I, et al. Harms of screening mammography for breast cancer in Japanese women. Breast Cancer. 2013 Oct;20(4):310-5. PMID: 22282164.

1154. Kass R, Henry-Tillman RS, Nurko J, et al. Touch preparation of breast core needle specimens is a new method for same-day diagnosis. Am J Surg. 2003 Dec;186(6):737-41; discussion 42. PMID: 14672788.

1155. Kass R, Kumar G, Klimberg VS, et al. Clip migration in stereotactic biopsy. Am J Surg. 2002 Oct;184(4):325-31. PMID: 12383894.

1156. Kaufman HJ, Witherspoon LE, Gwin JL, Jr., et al. Stereotactic breast biopsy: a study of first core samples. Am Surg. 2001 Jun;67(6):572-5; discussion 5-6. PMID: 11409806.

1157. Kawasaki T, Mochizuki K, Yamauchi H, et al. High prevalence of neuroendocrine carcinoma in breast lesions detected by the clinical symptom of bloody nipple discharge. Breast. 2012 Oct;21(5):652-6. PMID: 22397895.

1158. Kaye MD, Vicinanza-Adami CA, Sullivan ML. Mammographic findings after stereotaxic biopsy of the breast performed with large-core needles. Radiology. 1994 Jul;192(1):149-51. PMID: 8208927.

1159. Kelaher M, Cawson J, Miller J, et al. Use of breast cancer screening and treatment services by Australian women aged 25-44 years following Kylie Minogue's breast cancer diagnosis. Int J Epidemiol. 2008 Dec;37(6):1326-32. PMID: 18515324.

1160. Kelley WE, Bailey R, Bertelsen C, et al. Stereotactic automated surgical biopsy using the ABBI biopsy device: a multicenter study. The Breast Journal. 1998;4(5):302-6.

1161. Kennedy G, Markert M, Alexander JR, et al. Predictive value of BI-RADS classification for breast imaging in women under age 50. Breast Cancer Res Treat. 2011 Dec;130(3):819-23. PMID: 21748292.

1162. Kessler R, Sutcliffe JB, Bell L, et al. Negative predictive value of breast-specific gamma imaging in low suspicion breast lesions: a potential means for reducing benign biopsies. Breast J. 2011 May-Jun;17(3):319-21. PMID: 21492299.

1163. Khanna AK, Singh MR, Khanna S, et al. Fine needle aspiration cytology, imprint cytology and tru-cut needle biopsy in breast lumps: a comparative evaluation. J Indian Med Assoc. 1991 Jul;89(7):192-5. PMID: 1940411.

1164. Kiaer HW, Laenkholm AV, Nielsen BB, et al. Classical pathological variables recorded in the Danish Breast Cancer Cooperative Group's register 1978-2006. Acta Oncol. 2008;47(4):778-83. PMID: 18465348.

1165. Kibil W, Hodorowicz-Zaniewska D, Popiela TJ, et al. Mammotome biopsy in diagnosing and treatment of intraductal papilloma of the breast. Polish Journal of Surgery. 2013;85(4):210-5.

1166. Kim BS. Usefulness of breast-specific gamma imaging as an adjunct modality in breast cancer patients with dense breast: a comparative study with MRI. Ann Nucl Med. 2012 Feb;26(2):131-7. PMID: 22006539.

1167. Kim C, Yoon C, Park JH, et al. Evaluation of ultrasound synthetic aperture imaging using bidirectional pixel-based focusing: preliminary phantom and in vivo breast study. IEEE Trans Biomed Eng. 2013 Oct;60(10):2716-24. PMID: 23686939.

1168. Kim MJ, Kim JY, Youn JH, et al. US-guided diffuse optical tomography for breast lesions: the reliability of clinical experience. Eur Radiol. 2011 Jul;21(7):1353-63. PMID: 21274716.

1169. Kim SJ, Chang JM, Cho N, et al. Outcome of breast lesions detected at screening ultrasonography. Eur J Radiol. 2012 Nov;81(11):3229-33. PMID: 22591758.

1170. Kim WH, Chang JM, Moon WK, et al. Intraductal mass on breast ultrasound: final outcomes and predictors of malignancy. AJR Am J Roentgenol. 2013 Apr;200(4):932-7. PMID: 23521472.

1171. Kim YW, Kim SK, Youn HJ, et al. The clinical utility of automated breast volume scanner: a pilot study of 139 cases. J Breast Cancer. 2013 Sep;16(3):329-34. PMID: 24155763.

1172. Klein RL, Mook JA, Euhus DM, et al. Evaluation of a hydrogel based breast biopsy marker (HydroMARK(R)) as an alternative to wire and radioactive seed localization for non-palpable breast lesions. J Surg Oncol. 2012 May;105(6):591-4. PMID: 22095610.

1173. Klevesath MB, Godwin RJ, Bannon R, et al. Touch imprint cytology of core needle biopsy specimens: a useful method for immediate reporting of symptomatic breast lesions. Eur J Surg Oncol. 2005 Jun;31(5):490-4. PMID: 15922884.

1174. Ko ES, Choi HY, Kim RB, et al. Application of sonoelastography: comparison of performance between mass and non-mass lesion. Eur J Radiol. 2012 Apr;81(4):731-6. PMID: 21306848.

1175. Kontos M, Wilson R, Fentiman I. Digital infrared thermal imaging (DITI) of breast lesions: sensitivity and specificity of detection of primary breast cancers. Clin Radiol. 2011 Jun;66(6):536-9. PMID: 21377664.

1176. Kooistra B, Wauters C, Strobbe L. Indeterminate breast fine-needle aspiration: repeat aspiration or core needle biopsy? Ann Surg Oncol. 2009 Feb;16(2):281-4. PMID: 19050965.

1177. Koskela A, Berg M, Sudah M, et al. Learning curve for add-on stereotactic core needle breast biopsy. Acta Radiol. 2006 Jun;47(5):454-60. PMID: 16796305.

1178. Kotsianos-Hermle D, Hiltawsky KM, Wirth S, et al. Analysis of 107 breast lesions with automated 3D ultrasound and comparison with mammography and manual ultrasound. Eur J Radiol. 2009 Jul;71(1):109-15. PMID: 18468829.

1179. Krainick-Strobel U, Flugel B, Hahn M, et al. Complete resection of benign breast lesions with an ultrasound-guided vacuum biopsy system with a median follow-up of 13 months: Komplettresektion benigner Mammabefunde mittels ultraschallgefuhrter grosslumiger Vakuumbiopsie: Medianes Follow-up von 13 Monaten. Tumor Diagn. Ther. 2010;31(6):338-42.

1180. Kruger BM, Burrowes P, MacGregor JH. Accuracy of marker clip placement after mammotome breast biopsy. Can Assoc Radiol J. 2002 Jun;53(3):137-40. PMID: 12101533.

1181. Kuhl CK, Morakkabati N, Leutner CC, et al. MR imaging--guided large-core (14-gauge) needle biopsy of small lesions visible at breast MR imaging alone. Radiology. 2001 Jul;220(1):31-9. PMID: 11425969.

1182. Kumm TR, Szabunio MM. Elastography for the characterization of breast lesions: initial clinical experience. Cancer Control. 2010 Jul;17(3):156-61. PMID: 20664512.

1183. Kuo YL, Chang TW. Can concurrent core biopsy and fine needle aspiration biopsy improve the false negative rate of sonographically detectable breast lesions? BMC Cancer. 2010;10:371. PMID: 20637074.

1184. Lacquement MA, Mitchell D, Hollingsworth AB. Positive predictive value of the Breast Imaging Reporting and Data System. J Am Coll Surg. 1999 Jul;189(1):34-40. PMID: 10401738.

1185. Lamm RL, Jackman RJ. Mammographic abnormalities caused by percutaneous stereotactic biopsy of histologically benign lesions evident on follow-up mammograms. AJR Am J Roentgenol. 2000 Mar;174(3):753-6. PMID: 10701620.

1186. Lang EV, Berbaum KS, Lutgendorf SK. Large-core breast biopsy: abnormal salivary cortisol profiles associated with uncertainty of diagnosis. Radiology. 2009 Mar;250(3):631-7. PMID: 19244038.

1187. Lannin DR, Ponn T, Andrejeva L, et al. Should all breast cancers be diagnosed by needle biopsy? Am J Surg. 2006 Oct;192(4):450-4. PMID: 16978947.

1188. LaRaja RD, Saber AA, Sickles A. Early experience in the use of the Advanced Breast Biopsy Instrumentation: a report of one hundred twenty-seven patients. Surgery. 1999 Apr;125(4):380-4. PMID: 10216528.

1189. Larrieux G, Cupp JA, Liao J, et al. Effect of introducing hematoma ultrasound-guided lumpectomy in a surgical practice. J Am Coll Surg. 2012 Aug;215(2):237-43. PMID: 22632911.

1190. Larson BT, Erdman AG, Tsekos NV, et al. Design of an MRI-compatible robotic stereotactic device for minimally invasive interventions in the breast. J Biomech Eng. 2004 Aug;126(4):458-65. PMID: 15543863.

1191. Laudico A, Redaniel MT, Mirasol-Lumague MR, et al. Epidemiology and clinicopathology of breast cancer in metro Manila and Rizal Province, Philippines. Asian Pac J Cancer Prev. 2009 Jan-Mar;10(1):167-72. PMID: 19469648.

1192. Layfield LJ, Factor RE, Jarboe EA. Clinician compliance with laboratory regulations requiring submission of relevant clinical data: A one year retrospective analysis. Pathol Res Pract. 2012 Nov 15;208(11):668-71. PMID: 22999368.

1193. LeCarpentier GL, Roubidoux MA, Fowlkes JB, et al. Suspicious breast lesions: assessment of 3D Doppler US indexes for classification in a test population and fourfold cross-validation scheme. Radiology. 2008 Nov;249(2):463-70. PMID: 18936310.

1194. Leconte I, Abraham C, Galant C, et al. Fibroadenoma: can fine needle aspiration biopsy avoid short term follow-up? Diagn Interv Imaging. 2012 Oct;93(10):750-6. PMID: 22999986.

1195. Lee A, Chang J, Lim W, et al. Effectiveness of breast-specific gamma imaging (BSGI) for breast cancer in Korea: a comparative study. Breast J. 2012 Sep;18(5):453-8. PMID: 22897514.

1196. Lee AH, Villena Salinas NM, Hodi Z, et al. The value of examination of multiple levels of mammary needle core biopsy specimens taken for investigation of lesions other than calcification. J Clin Pathol. 2012 Dec;65(12):1097-9. PMID: 22918889.

1197. Lee CI, Wells CJ, Bassett LW. Cost minimization analysis of ultrasound-guided diagnostic evaluation of probably benign breast lesions. Breast J. 2013 Jan-Feb;19(1):41-8. PMID: 23186174.

1198. Lee EJ, Jung HK, Ko KH, et al. Diagnostic performances of shear wave elastography: which parameter to use in differential diagnosis of solid breast masses? Eur Radiol. 2013 Jul;23(7):1803-11. PMID: 23423637.

1199. Lee HJ, Kim EK, Kim MJ, et al. Observer variability of Breast Imaging Reporting and Data System (BI-RADS) for breast ultrasound. Eur J Radiol. 2008 Feb;65(2):293-8. PMID: 17531417.

1200. Lee JH, Fulp W, Wells KJ, et al. Patient navigation and time to diagnostic resolution: results for a cluster randomized trial evaluating the efficacy of patient navigation among patients with breast cancer screening abnormalities, Tampa, FL. PLoS One. 2013;8(9):e74542. PMID: 24066145.

1201. Lee SH, Chang JM, Kim WH, et al. Differentiation of benign from malignant solid breast masses: comparison of two-dimensional and three-dimensional shear-wave elastography. Eur Radiol. 2013 Apr;23(4):1015-26. PMID: 23085867.

1202. Lefkowitz RJ. Identification of adenylate cyclase-coupled beta-adrenergic receptors with radiolabeled beta-adrenergic antagonists. Biochem Pharmacol. 1975 Sep 15;24(18):1651-8. PMID: 11.

1203. Lehman CD, Shook JE. Position of clip placement after vacuum-assisted breast biopsy: is a unilateral two-view postbiopsy mammogram necessary? Breast J. 2003 Jul-Aug;9(4):272-6. PMID: 12846859.

1204. Leifland K, Lagerstedt U, Svane G. Comparison of stereotactic fine needle aspiration cytology and core needle biopsy in 522 non-palpable breast lesions. Acta Radiol. 2003 Jul;44(4):387-91. PMID: 12846688.

1205. Leifland K, Lundquist H, Lagerstedt U, et al. Comparison of preoperative simultaneous stereotactic fine needle aspiration biopsy and stereotactic core needle biopsy in ductal carcinoma in situ of the breast. Acta Radiol. 2003 Mar;44(2):213-7. PMID: 12694110.

1206. Leong LC, Sim LS, Lee YS, et al. A prospective study to compare the diagnostic performance of breast elastography versus conventional breast ultrasound. Clin Radiol. 2010 Nov;65(11):887-94. PMID: 20933643.

1207. Leucht W, Leucht D, Kiesel L. Sonographic demonstration and evaluation of microcalcifications in the breast. Breast disease. 1992;5(2):105-23.

1208. Levin DC, Parker L, Schwartz GF, et al. Percutaneous needle vs surgical breast biopsy: previous allegations of overuse of surgery are in error. J Am Coll Radiol. 2012 Feb;9(2):137-40. PMID: 22305700.

1209. Li M, Song Y, Cho N, et al. An HR-MAS MR metabolomics study on breast tissues obtained with core needle biopsy. PLoS One. 2011;6(10):e25563. PMID: 22028780.

1210. Liao MN, Chen PL, Chen MF, et al. Effect of supportive care on the anxiety of women with suspected breast cancer. J Adv Nurs. 2010 Jan;66(1):49-59. PMID: 19968726.

1211. Liao MN, Chen PL, Chen MF, et al. Supportive care for Taiwanese women with suspected breast cancer during the diagnostic period: effect on healthcare and support needs. Oncol Nurs Forum. 2009 Sep;36(5):585-92. PMID: 19726399.

1212. Liberman L, Benton CL, Dershaw DD, et al. Learning curve for stereotactic breast biopsy: how many cases are enough? AJR Am J Roentgenol. 2001 Mar;176(3):721-7. PMID: 11222213.

1213. Liberman L, Dershaw DD, Morris EA, et al. Clip placement after stereotactic vacuum-assisted breast biopsy. Radiology. 1997 Nov;205(2):417-22. PMID: 9356622.

1214. Liberman L, Dershaw DD, Rosen PP, et al. Stereotaxic 14-gauge breast biopsy: how many core biopsy specimens are needed? Radiology. 1994 Sep;192(3):793-5. PMID: 8058949.

1215. Liberman L, Dershaw DD, Rosen PP, et al. Percutaneous removal of malignant mammographic lesions at stereotactic vacuum-assisted biopsy. Radiology. 1998 Mar;206(3):711-5. PMID: 9494489.

1216. Liberman L, Dershaw DD, Rosen PP, et al. Core needle biopsy of synchronous ipsilateral breast lesions: impact on treatment. AJR Am J Roentgenol. 1996 Jun;166(6):1429-32. PMID: 8633457.

1217. Liberman L, Evans WP, 3rd, Dershaw DD, et al. Radiography of microcalcifications in stereotaxic mammary core biopsy specimens. Radiology. 1994 Jan;190(1):223-5. PMID: 8259409.

1218. Liberman L, Goodstine SL, Dershaw DD, et al. One operation after percutaneous diagnosis of nonpalpable breast cancer: frequency and associated factors. AJR Am J Roentgenol. 2002 Mar;178(3):673-9. PMID: 11856696.

1219. Liberman L, Hann LE, Dershaw DD, et al. Mammographic findings after stereotactic 14-gauge vacuum biopsy. Radiology. 1997 May;203(2):343-7. PMID: 9114086.

1220. Liberman L, Smolkin JH, Dershaw DD, et al. Calcification retrieval at stereotactic, 11-gauge, directional, vacuum-assisted breast biopsy. Radiology. 1998 Jul;208(1):251-60. PMID: 9646821.

1221. Lieske B, Ravichandran D, Wright D. Role of fine-needle aspiration cytology and core biopsy in the preoperative diagnosis of screen-detected breast carcinoma. Br J Cancer. 2006 Jul 3;95(1):62-6. PMID: 16755293.

1222. Lieu D. Cytopathologist-performed ultrasound-guided fine-needle aspiration and core-needle biopsy: a prospective study of 500 consecutive cases. Diagn Cytopathol. 2008 May;36(5):317-24. PMID: 18418854.

1223. Lifrange E, Dondelinger RF, Foidart JM, et al. Percutaneous stereotactic en bloc excision of nonpalpable breast carcinoma: a step in the direction of supraconservative surgery. Breast. 2002 Dec;11(6):501-8. PMID: 14965717.

1224. Lifrange E, Dondelinger RF, Fridman V, et al. En bloc excision of nonpalpable breast lesions using the advanced breast biopsy instrumentation system: an alternative to needle guided surgery? Eur Radiol. 2001;11(5):796-801. PMID: 11372610.

1225. Lifrange E, Kridelka F, Colin C. Stereotaxic needle-core biopsy and fine-needle aspiration biopsy in the diagnosis of nonpalpable breast lesions: controversies and future prospects. Eur J Radiol. 1997 Jan;24(1):39-47. PMID: 9056148.

1226. Linda A, Zuiani C, Londero V, et al. Outcome of initially only magnetic resonance mammography-detected findings with and without correlate at second-look sonography: distribution according to patient history of breast cancer and lesion size. Breast. 2008 Feb;17(1):51-7. PMID: 17709249.

1227. Lindfors KK, O'Connor J, Acredolo CR, et al. Short-interval follow-up mammography versus immediate core biopsy of benign breast lesions: assessment of patient stress. AJR Am J Roentgenol. 1998 Jul;171(1):55-8. PMID: 9648763.

1228. Lister D, Evans AJ, Burrell HC, et al. The accuracy of breast ultrasound in the evaluation of clinically benign discrete, symptomatic breast lumps. Clin Radiol. 1998 Jul;53(7):490-2. PMID: 9714387.

1229. Liu X, Inciardi M, Bradley JP, et al. Microcalcifications of the breast: size matters! A mammographic-histologic correlation study. Pathologica. 2007 Feb;99(1):5-10. PMID: 17566305.

1230. Lo GG, Ai V, Chan JK, et al. Diffusion-weighted magnetic resonance imaging of breast lesions: first experiences at 3 T. J Comput Assist Tomogr. 2009 Jan-Feb;33(1):63-9. PMID: 19188787.

1231. Logan-Young W, Dawson AE, Wilbur DC, et al. The cost-effectiveness of fine-needle aspiration cytology and 14-gauge core needle biopsy compared with open surgical biopsy in the diagnosis of breast carcinoma. Cancer. 1998 May 15;82(10):1867-73. PMID: 9587118.

1232. Lovrics PJ, Gordon M, Cornacchi SD, et al. Practice patterns and perceptions of margin status for breast conserving surgery for breast carcinoma: National Survey of Canadian General Surgeons. Breast. 2012 Dec;21(6):730-4. PMID: 22901975.

1233. Lyon D, Walter J, Munro CL, et al. Challenges in interpreting cytokine biomarkers in biobehavioral research: a breast cancer exemplar. Biol Res Nurs. 2011 Jan;13(1):25-31. PMID: 21199813.

1234. Mack LA, Dabbs K, Temple WJ. Synoptic operative record for point of care outcomes: a leap forward in knowledge translation. Eur J Surg Oncol. 2010 Sep;36 Suppl 1:S44-9. PMID: 20609548.

1235. Madabhushi A, Agner S, Basavanhally A, et al. Computer-aided prognosis: predicting patient and disease outcome via quantitative fusion of multi-scale, multi-modal data. Comput Med Imaging Graph. 2011 Oct-Dec;35(7-8):506-14. PMID: 21333490.

1236. Mahoney MC. Initial clinical experience with a new MRI vacuum-assisted breast biopsy device. J Magn Reson Imaging. 2008 Oct;28(4):900-5. PMID: 18821610.

1237. Mainiero MB, Koelliker SL, Lazarus E, et al. Ultrasound-guided large-core needle biopsy of the breast. JOURNAL OF WOMENS IMAGING. 2002;4(2):52-7.

1238. Majek O, Danes J, Skovajsova M, et al. Breast cancer screening in the Czech Republic: time trends in performance indicators during the first seven years of the organised programme. BMC Public Health. 2011;11:288. PMID: 21554747.

1239. Manfrin E, Mariotto R, Remo A, et al. Is there still a role for fine-needle aspiration cytology in breast cancer screening? Experience of the Verona Mammographic Breast Cancer Screening Program with real-time integrated radiopathologic activity (1999-2004). Cancer. 2008 Apr 25;114(2):74-82. PMID: 18306357.

1240. Mann RM. The effectiveness of MR imaging in the assessment of invasive lobular carcinoma of the breast. Magn Reson Imaging Clin N Am. 2010 May;18(2):259-76, ix. PMID: 20494311.

1241. Mansour SM, Omar OS. Elastography ultrasound and questionable breast lesions: does it count? Eur J Radiol. 2012 Nov;81(11):3234-44. PMID: 22591761.

1242. March DE, Walker MT, Bur M, et al. Touch-preparation cytologic examination of breast core biopsy specimens: accuracy in predicting benign or malignant core histologic results. Acad Radiol. 1999 Jun;6(6):333-8. PMID: 10376063.

1243. Margolin FR, Kaufman L, Denny SR, et al. Metallic marker placement after stereotactic core biopsy of breast calcifications: comparison of two clips and deployment techniques. AJR Am J Roentgenol. 2003 Dec;181(6):1685-90. PMID: 14627597.

1244. Margolin FR, Kaufman L, Jacobs RP, et al. Stereotactic core breast biopsy of malignant calcifications: diagnostic yield of cores with and cores without calcifications on specimen radiographs. Radiology. 2004 Oct;233(1):251-4. PMID: 15333764.

1245. Marti WR, Zuber M, Oertli D, et al. Advanced breast biopsy instrumentation for the evaluation of impalpable lesions: a reliable diagnostic tool with little therapeutic potential. European Journal of Surgery. 2001;167(1):15-8.

1246. Masood S, Antley CM, Mooney EE, et al. A Comparison of Accuracy Rates Between Open Biopsy, Cutting-Needle Biopsy, and Fine-Needle Aspiration Biopsy of the Breast: A 3-Year Experience. The Breast Journal. 1998;4(1):3-8.

1247. Masood S, Feng D, Tutuncuoglu O, et al. Diagnostic value of imprint cytology during image-guided core biopsy in improving breast health care. Ann Clin Lab Sci. 2011 Fall;41(1):8-13. PMID: 21325248.

1248. Masroor I. Effectiveness of assigning BI-RADS category-3 to breast lesion with respect to follow-up. J Coll Physicians Surg Pak. 2008 Apr;18(4):209-12. PMID: 18474152.

1249. Matthews BD, Williams GB. Initial experience with the advanced breast biopsy instrumentation system. Am J Surg. 1999 Feb;177(2):97-101. PMID: 10204548.

1250. Mazouni C, Sneige N, Rouzier R, et al. A nomogram to predict for malignant diagnosis of BI-RADS Category 4 breast lesions. J Surg Oncol. 2010 Sep 1;102(3):220-4. PMID: 20740578.

1251. Mazzini RC, Elias S, Nazario AC, et al. Prevalence of c-myc expression in breast lesions associated with microcalcifications detected by routine mammography. Sao Paulo Med J. 2009 May;127(2):66-70. PMID: 19597680.

1252. McKee MD, Cropp MD, Hyland A, et al. Provider case volume and outcome in the evaluation and treatment of patients with mammogram-detected breast carcinoma. Cancer. 2002 Aug 15;95(4):704-12. PMID: 12209712.

1253. Meloni GB, Dessole S, Becchere MP, et al. Ultrasound-guided mammotome vacuum biopsy for the diagnosis of impalpable breast lesions. Ultrasound Obstet Gynecol. 2001 Nov;18(5):520-4. PMID: 11844176.

1254. Melotti MK, Berg WA. Core needle breast biopsy in patients undergoing anticoagulation therapy: preliminary results. AJR Am J Roentgenol. 2000 Jan;174(1):245-9. PMID: 10628487.

1255. Mendez A, Cabanillas F, Echenique M, et al. Mammographic features and correlation with biopsy findings using 11-gauge stereotactic vacuum-assisted breast biopsy (SVABB). Ann Oncol. 2004 Mar;15(3):450-4. PMID: 14998847.

1256. Menes TS, Kerlikowske K, Jaffer S, et al. Rates of atypical ductal hyperplasia have declined with less use of postmenopausal hormone treatment: findings from the Breast Cancer Surveillance Consortium. Cancer Epidemiol Biomarkers Prev. 2009 Nov;18(11):2822-8. PMID: 19900937.

1257. Mercado CL, Guth AA, Toth HK, et al. Sonographically guided marker placement for confirmation of removal of mammographically occult lesions after localization. AJR Am J Roentgenol. 2008 Oct;191(4):1216-9. PMID: 18806168.

1258. Mesurolle B, Bining HJ, El Khoury M, et al. Contribution of tissue harmonic imaging and frequency compound imaging in interventional breast sonography. J Ultrasound Med. 2006 Jul;25(7):845-55. PMID: 16798895.

1259. Meyer JE, Smith DN, DiPiro PJ, et al. Stereotactic breast biopsy of clustered microcalcifications with a directional, vacuum-assisted device. Radiology. 1997 Aug;204(2):575-6. PMID: 9240556.

1260. Milenkovic J, Hertl K, Kosir A, et al. Characterization of spatiotemporal changes for the classification of dynamic contrast-enhanced magnetic-resonance breast lesions. Artif Intell Med. 2013 Jun;58(2):101-14. PMID: 23548472.

1261. Moon HJ, Kim EK, Kwak JY, et al. Interval growth of probably benign breast lesions on follow-up ultrasound: how can these be managed? Eur Radiol. 2011 May;21(5):908-18. PMID: 21113596.

1262. Moon HJ, Kim MJ, Kwak JY, et al. Probably benign breast lesions on ultrasonography: a retrospective review of ultrasonographic features and clinical factors affecting the BI-RADS categorization. Acta Radiol. 2010 May;51(4):375-82. PMID: 20350247.

1263. Moon HJ, Kim MJ, Kwak JY, et al. Malignant lesions initially categorized as probably benign breast lesions: retrospective review of ultrasonographic, clinical and pathologic characteristics. Ultrasound Med Biol. 2010 Apr;36(4):551-9. PMID: 20350681.

1264. Moon JH, Kim HH, Shin HJ, et al. Supplemental use of optical diffusion breast imaging for differentiation between benign and malignant breast lesions. AJR Am J Roentgenol. 2011 Sep;197(3):732-9. PMID: 21862818.

1265. Moon WK, Huang CS, Shen WC, et al. Analysis of elastographic and B-mode features at sonoelastography for breast tumor classification. Ultrasound Med Biol. 2009 Nov;35(11):1794-802. PMID: 19767139.

1266. Moore SG, Shenoy PJ, Fanucchi L, et al. Cost-effectiveness of MRI compared to mammography for breast cancer screening in a high risk population. BMC Health Serv Res. 2009;9:9. PMID: 19144138.

1267. Moritz JD, Luftner-Nagel S, Westerhof JP, et al. A comparison of conventional mammographic magnification, ultra high magnification and industrial magnification radiography in the radiographic detection of microcalcifications within core biopsies of the breast. Br J Radiol. 1997 Nov;70(839):1099-103. PMID: 9536898.

1268. Moritz JD, Mertens C, Westerhof JP, et al. Role of high magnification specimen radiography in surgical and core biopsies of the breast. Br J Radiol. 2000 Nov;73(875):1170-7. PMID: 11144794.

1269. Morrogh M, Morris EA, Liberman L, et al. MRI identifies otherwise occult disease in select patients with Paget disease of the nipple. J Am Coll Surg. 2008 Feb;206(2):316-21. PMID: 18222386.

1270. Morrogh M, Park A, Elkin EB, et al. Lessons learned from 416 cases of nipple discharge of the breast. Am J Surg. 2010 Jul;200(1):73-80. PMID: 20079481.

1271. Morrow M, Venta L, Stinson T, et al. Prospective comparison of stereotactic core biopsy and surgical excision as diagnostic procedures for breast cancer patients. Ann Surg. 2001 Apr;233(4):537-41. PMID: 11303136.

1272. Mouton JP, Apffelstaedt J, Baatjes K. Surgical mammography reporting in a limited resource environment. World J Surg. 2010 Nov;34(11):2530-6. PMID: 20577769.

1273. Moy L, Elias K, Patel V, et al. Is breast MRI helpful in the evaluation of inconclusive mammographic findings? AJR Am J Roentgenol. 2009 Oct;193(4):986-93. PMID: 19770320.

1274. Moy L, Noz ME, Maguire GQ, Jr., et al. Role of fusion of prone FDG-PET and magnetic resonance imaging of the breasts in the evaluation of breast cancer. Breast J. 2010 Jul-Aug;16(4):369-76. PMID: 20443788.

1275. Moyle P, Sonoda L, Britton P, et al. Incidental breast lesions detected on CT: what is their significance? Br J Radiol. 2010 Mar;83(987):233-40. PMID: 19546179.

1276. Mullen DJ, Eisen RN, Newman RD, et al. The use of carbon marking after stereotactic large-core-needle breast biopsy. Radiology. 2001 Jan;218(1):255-60. PMID: 11152811.

1277. Nakhleh RE, Grimm EE, Idowu MO, et al. Laboratory compliance with the American Society of Clinical Oncology/college of American Pathologists guidelines for human epidermal growth factor receptor 2 testing: a College of American Pathologists survey of 757 laboratories. Arch Pathol Lab Med. 2010 May;134(5):728-34. PMID: 20441503.

1278. National Guideline Clearinghouse (NGC). Guideline summary: Cancer in children and young people. In: Suspected cancer in primary care: guidelines for investigation, referral and reducing ethnic disparities. In: National Guideline Clearinghouse (NGC) [Web site]. Rockville (MD): Agency for Healthcare Research and Quality (AHRQ); [cited 2013 June 25]. Available: http://www.guideline.gov.

1279. Neary M, Lowery AJ, O'Conghaile A, et al. NCCP breast cancer referral guidelines--are breast cancer patients prioritised? Ir Med J. 2011 Feb;104(2):39-41. PMID: 21465872.

1280. Nederend J, Duijm LE, Louwman MW, et al. Impact of the transition from screen-film to digital screening mammography on interval cancer characteristics and treatment - a population based study from the Netherlands. Eur J Cancer. 2014 Jan;50(1):31-9. PMID: 24275518.

1281. Nederend J, Duijm LE, Louwman MW, et al. Impact of transition from analog screening mammography to digital screening mammography on screening outcome in The Netherlands: a population-based study. Ann Oncol. 2012 Dec;23(12):3098-103. PMID: 22745215.

1282. Ng AK, Garber JE, Diller LR, et al. Prospective study of the efficacy of breast magnetic resonance imaging and mammographic screening in survivors of Hodgkin lymphoma. J Clin Oncol. 2013 Jun 20;31(18):2282-8. PMID: 23610104.

1283. Ng CH, Lee KT, Taib NA, et al. Experience with hookwire localisation excision biopsy at a medical centre in Malaysia. Singapore Med J. 2010 Apr;51(4):306-10. PMID: 20505908.

1284. Ngotho J, Githaiga J, Kaisha W. Palpable discrete breast masses in young women: two of the components of the modified triple test may be adequate. S Afr J Surg. 2013 May;51(2):58-60. PMID: 23725894.

1285. Nguansangiam S, Jesdapatarakul S, Tangjitgamol S. Accuracy of fine needle aspiration cytology from breast masses in Thailand. Asian Pac J Cancer Prev. 2009 Oct-Dec;10(4):623-6. PMID: 19827882.

1286. Nizri E, Schneebaum S, Klausner JM, et al. Current management practice of breast borderline lesions--need for further research and guidelines. Am J Surg. 2012 Jun;203(6):721-5. PMID: 22153085.

1287. Noroozian M, Hadjiiski L, Rahnama-Moghadam S, et al. Digital breast tomosynthesis is comparable to mammographic spot views for mass characterization. Radiology. 2012 Jan;262(1):61-8. PMID: 21998048.

1288. Nurko J, Mancino AT, Whitacre E, et al. Surgical benefits conveyed by biopsy site marking system using ultrasound localization. Am J Surg. 2005 Oct;190(4):618-22. PMID: 16164935.

1289. O'Flynn EA, Currie RJ, Mohammed K, et al. Pre-operative factors indicating risk of multiple operations versus a single operation in women undergoing surgery for screen detected breast cancer. Breast. 2013 Feb;22(1):78-82. PMID: 22789490.

1290. Ogura A, Hayakawa K, Yoshida S, et al. Use of dynamic phase subtraction (DPS) map in dynamic contrast-enhanced MRI of the breast. J Comput Assist Tomogr. 2011 Nov-Dec;35(6):749-52. PMID: 22082548.

1291. Ohene-Yeboah M. Breast pain in Ghanaian women: clinical, ultrasonographic, mammographic and histological findings in 1612 consecutive patients. West Afr J Med. 2008 Jan;27(1):20-3. PMID: 18689298.

1292. Oikonomou V, Fotou M, Zagouri F, et al. Imprint cytology of vacuum-assisted breast biopsy specimens: a rapid diagnostic tool in non-palpable solid lesions. Cytopathology. 2008 Oct;19(5):311-5. PMID: 17953690.

1293. Okazaki H, Tsujimoto F, Maeda I, et al. Radiologic-pathological correlation of punctate hyperechoic foci by ultrasound in stereotactic vacuum-assisted breast biopsy samples. Jpn J Radiol. 2009 Dec;27(10):438-43. PMID: 20035416.

1294. Okines AF, Thompson LC, Cunningham D, et al. Effect of HER2 on prognosis and benefit from peri-operative chemotherapy in early oesophago-gastric adenocarcinoma in the MAGIC trial. Ann Oncol. 2013 May;24(5):1253-61. PMID: 23233651.

1295. Olaya W, Bae W, Wong J, et al. Are percutaneous biopsy rates a reasonable quality measure in breast cancer management? Ann Surg Oncol. 2010 Oct;17 Suppl 3:268-72. PMID: 20853045.

1296. O'Leary R, Hawkins K, Beazley JC, et al. Agreement between preoperative core needle biopsy and postoperative invasive breast cancer histopathology is not dependent on the amount of clinical material obtained. J Clin Pathol. 2004 Feb;57(2):193-5. PMID: 14747449.

1297. Oliveira TM, Brasileiro Sant'Anna TK, Mauad FM, et al. Breast imaging: is the sonographic descriptor of orientation valid for magnetic resonance imaging? J Magn Reson Imaging. 2012 Dec;36(6):1383-8. PMID: 22911937.

1298. Olsen ML, Morton MJ, Stan DL, et al. Is there a role for magnetic resonance imaging in diagnosing palpable breast masses when mammogram and ultrasound are negative? J Womens Health (Larchmt). 2012 Nov;21(11):1149-54. PMID: 23046046.

1299. O'Meara ES, Zhu W, Hubbard RA, et al. Mammographic screening interval in relation to tumor characteristics and false-positive risk by race/ethnicity and age. Cancer. 2013 Nov 15;119(22):3959-67. PMID: 24037812.

1300. Ooi GJ, Fox J, Siu K, et al. Fourier transform infrared imaging and small angle x-ray scattering as a combined biomolecular approach to diagnosis of breast cancer. Med Phys. 2008 May;35(5):2151-61. PMID: 18561690.

1301. Oster NV, Carney PA, Allison KH, et al. Development of a diagnostic test set to assess agreement in breast pathology: practical application of the Guidelines for Reporting Reliability and Agreement Studies (GRRAS). BMC Womens Health. 2013;13:3. PMID: 23379630.

1302. Ozulker T, Ozulker F, Ozpacaci T, et al. The efficacy of (99m)Tc-MIBI scintimammography in the evaluation of breast lesions and axillary involvement: a comparison with X-rays mammography, ultrasonography and magnetic resonance imaging. Hell J Nucl Med. 2010 May-Aug;13(2):144-9. PMID: 20808988.

1303. Pacheco JM, Gao F, Bumb C, et al. Racial differences in outcomes of triple-negative breast cancer. Breast Cancer Res Treat. 2013 Feb;138(1):281-9. PMID: 23400579.

1304. Pagni F, Bosisio FM, Salvioni D, et al. Application of the British National Health Service Breast Cancer Screening Programme classification in 226 breast core needle biopsies: correlation with resected specimens. Ann Diagn Pathol. 2012 Apr;16(2):112-8. PMID: 22056037.

1305. Park YM, Kim EK, Lee JH, et al. Palpable breast masses with probably benign morphology at sonography: can biopsy be deferred? Acta Radiol. 2008 Dec;49(10):1104-11. PMID: 18855166.

1306. Parker SJ, Wheaton M, Wallis MG, et al. Why should diagnostic benign breast biopsies weight less than twenty grams? Ann R Coll Surg Engl. 2001 Mar;83(2):113-6. PMID: 11320919.

1307. Partridge SC, DeMartini WB, Kurland BF, et al. Quantitative diffusion-weighted imaging as an adjunct to conventional breast MRI for improved positive predictive value. AJR Am J Roentgenol. 2009 Dec;193(6):1716-22. PMID: 19933670.

1308. Pegolo E, Pandolfi M, Di Loreto C. Implementation of a microwave-assisted tissue-processing system and an automated embedding system for breast needle core biopsy samples: morphology, immunohistochemistry, and FISH evaluation. Appl Immunohistochem Mol Morphol. 2013 Jul;21(4):362-70. PMID: 23060302.

1309. Pelletier M, Knauper B, Loiselle CG, et al. Moderators of psychological recovery from benign cancer screening results. Curr Oncol. 2012 Jun;19(3):e191-200. PMID: 22670109.

1310. Perelman VS, Colapinto ND, Lee S, et al. Experience with the advanced breast biopsy instrumentation system. Can J Surg. 2000 Dec;43(6):437-41. PMID: 11129832.

1311. Perez-Stable EJ, Afable-Munsuz A, Kaplan CP, et al. Factors influencing time to diagnosis after abnormal mammography in diverse women. J Womens Health (Larchmt). 2013 Feb;22(2):159-66. PMID: 23350859.

1312. Pezner RD, Lorant JA, Terz J, et al. Wound-healing complications following biopsy of the irradiated breast. Arch Surg. 1992 Mar;127(3):321-4. PMID: 1550480.

1313. Philpotts LE, Lee CH, Horvath LJ, et al. Canceled stereotactic core-needle biopsy of the breast: analysis of 89 cases. Radiology. 1997 Nov;205(2):423-8. PMID: 9356623.

1314. Philpotts LE, Shaheen NA, Carter D, et al. Comparison of rebiopsy rates after stereotactic core needle biopsy of the breast with 11-gauge vacuum suction probe versus 14-gauge needle and automatic gun. AJR Am J Roentgenol. 1999 Mar;172(3):683-7. PMID: 10063860.

1315. Pijnappel RM, van Dalen A, Borel Rinkes IH, et al. The diagnostic accuracy of core biopsy in palpable and non-palpable breast lesions. Eur J Radiol. 1997 Feb;24(2):120-3. PMID: 9097053.

1316. Pilgrim S, Ravichandran D. Fine needle aspiration cytology as an adjunct to core biopsy in the assessment of symptomatic breast carcinoma. The Breast. 2005;14(5):411-4.

1317. Piron CA, Causer P, Jong R, et al. A hybrid breast biopsy system combining ultrasound and MRI. IEEE Trans Med Imaging. 2003 Sep;22(9):1100-10. PMID: 12956265.

1318. Pocock B, Taback B, Klein L, et al. Preoperative needle biopsy as a potential quality measure in breast cancer surgery. Ann Surg Oncol. 2009 May;16(5):1108-11. PMID: 18953610.

1319. Pogacnik A, Strojan Flezar M, Rener M. Ultrasonographically and stereotactically guided fine-needle aspiration cytology of non-palpable breast lesions: cyto-histological correlation. Cytopathology. 2008 Oct;19(5):303-10. PMID: 17944953.

1320. Poole GH, Willsher PC, Pinder SE, et al. Diagnosis of breast cancer with core-biopsy and fine needle aspiration cytology. Aust N Z J Surg. 1996 Sep;66(9):592-4. PMID: 8859156.

1321. Portincasa G, Lucci E, Navarra GG, et al. Initial experience with breast biopsy utilizing the Advanced Breast Biopsy Instrumentation (ABBI). J Surg Oncol. 2000;74(3):201-3.

1322. Povoski SP, Jimenez RE. A comprehensive evaluation of the 8-gauge vacuum-assisted Mammotome® system for ultrasound-guided diagnostic biopsy and selective excision of breast lesions. World journal of surgical oncology. 2007;5(1):83.

1323. Prat X, Sittek H, Grosse A, et al. European quadricentric evaluation of a breast MR biopsy and localization device: technical improvements based on phase-I evaluation. Eur Radiol. 2002 Jul;12(7):1720-7. PMID: 12111063.

1324. Price J, Chen SW. Screening for breast cancer with MRI: recent experience from the Australian Capital Territory. J Med Imaging Radiat Oncol. 2009 Feb;53(1):69-80. PMID: 19453531.

1325. Prieto-Granada C, Setia N, Otis CN. Lymph node extramedullary hematopoiesis in breast cancer patients receiving neoadjuvant therapy: a potential diagnostic pitfall. Int J Surg Pathol. 2013 Jun;21(3):264-6. PMID: 23493877.

1326. Pritchard MG, Townend JN, Lester WA, et al. Management of patients taking antiplatelet or anticoagulant medication requiring invasive breast procedures: United Kingdom survey of radiologists' and surgeons' current practice. Clin Radiol. 2008 Mar;63(3):305-11. PMID: 18275871.

1327. Provatopoulou X, Gounaris A, Kalogera E, et al. Circulating levels of matrix metalloproteinase-9 (MMP-9), neutrophil gelatinase-associated lipocalin (NGAL) and their complex MMP-9/NGAL in breast cancer disease. BMC Cancer. 2009;9:390. PMID: 19889214.

1328. Pruthi S, Shmidt E, Sherman MM, et al. Promoting a breast cancer screening clinic for underserved women: a community collaboration. Ethn Dis. 2010 Autumn;20(4):463-6. PMID: 21305838.

1329. Psooy BJ, Schreuer D, Borgaonkar J, et al. Patient navigation: improving timeliness in the diagnosis of breast abnormalities. Can Assoc Radiol J. 2004 Jun;55(3):145-50. PMID: 15237774.

1330. Qazi DES, Mohayuddin N. Role of fine needle aspiration cytology and core biopsy in the diagnosis of breast lumps. J Postgrad med Inst. 2005;19(1):67-70.

1331. Qi J, Ye Z. CTLM as an adjunct to mammography in the diagnosis of patients with dense breast. Clin Imaging. 2013 Mar-Apr;37(2):289-94. PMID: 23465981.

1332. Qin W, Gui G, Zhang K, et al. Proteins and carbohydrates in nipple aspirate fluid predict the presence of atypia and cancer in women requiring diagnostic breast biopsy. BMC Cancer. 2012;12:52. PMID: 22296682.

1333. Qureshi NA, Beresford A, Sami S, et al. Imprint cytology of needle core-biopsy specimens of breast lesions: is it a useful adjunt to rapid assessment breast clinics? Breast. 2007 Feb;16(1):81-5. PMID: 16952454.

1334. Raj V, Sivashanmugam T, Gupta S, et al. Influence of imaging on touch imprint cytology of breast lesions. Cancer Epidemiol. 2010 Aug;34(4):457-60. PMID: 20537609.

1335. Rebner M, Chesbrough R, Gregory N. Initial experience with the advanced breast biopsy instrumentation device. AJR Am J Roentgenol. 1999 Jul;173(1):221-6. PMID: 10397130.

1336. Regini E, Bagnera S, Tota D, et al. Role of sonoelastography in characterising breast nodules. Preliminary experience with 120 lesions. Radiol Med. 2010 Jun;115(4):551-62. PMID: 20177990.

1337. Renshaw AA. Minimal (< or =0.1 cm) invasive carcinoma in breast core needle biopsies. Incidence, sampling, associated findings, and follow-up. Arch Pathol Lab Med. 2004 Sep;128(9):996-9. PMID: 15335264.

1338. Reynolds HE. Marker clip placement following directional, vacuum-assisted breast biopsy. Am Surg. 1999 Jan;65(1):59-60. PMID: 9915534.

1339. Rhodes DJ, Hruska CB, Phillips SW, et al. Dedicated dual-head gamma imaging for breast cancer screening in women with mammographically dense breasts. Radiology. 2011 Jan;258(1):106-18. PMID: 21045179.

1340. Riedl CC, Pfarl G, Memarsadeghi M, et al. Lesion miss rates and false-negative rates for 1115 consecutive cases of stereotactically guided needle-localized open breast biopsy with long-term follow-up. Radiology. 2005 Dec;237(3):847-53. PMID: 16237133.

1341. Robbins J, Jeffries D, Roubidoux M, et al. Accuracy of diagnostic mammography and breast ultrasound during pregnancy and lactation. AJR Am J Roentgenol. 2011 Mar;196(3):716-22. PMID: 21343518.

1342. Roe SM, Mathews JA, Burns RP, et al. Stereotactic and ultrasound core needle breast biopsy performed by surgeons. Am J Surg. 1997 Dec;174(6):699-703; discussion -4. PMID: 9409600.

1343. Roman M, Hubbard RA, Sebuodegard S, et al. The cumulative risk of false-positive results in the Norwegian Breast Cancer Screening Program: Updated results. Cancer. 2013 Nov 15;119(22):3952-8. PMID: 23963877.

1344. Romero C, Varela C, Munoz E, et al. Impact on breast cancer diagnosis in a multidisciplinary unit after the incorporation of mammography digitalization and computer-aided detection systems. AJR Am J Roentgenol. 2011 Dec;197(6):1492-7. PMID: 22109307.

1345. Rominger MB, Sax EV, Figiel JH, et al. Occurrence and Positive Predictive Value of Additional Nonmass Findings for Risk Stratification of Breast Microcalcifications in Mammography. Can Assoc Radiol J. 2013 Jan 5PMID: 23298860.

1346. Rose A, Collins JP, Neerhut P, et al. Carbon localisation of impalpable breast lesions. Breast. 2003 Aug;12(4):264-9. PMID: 14659311.

1347. Rosen EL, Baker JA, Soo MS. Accuracy of a collagen-plug biopsy site marking device deployed after stereotactic core needle breast biopsy. AJR Am J Roentgenol. 2003 Nov;181(5):1295-9. PMID: 14573422.

1348. Rosen EL, Vo TT. Metallic clip deployment during stereotactic breast biopsy: retrospective analysis. Radiology. 2001 Feb;218(2):510-6. PMID: 11161170.

1349. Rotten D, Levaillant JM, Leridon H, et al. Ultrasonographically guided fine needle aspiration cytology and core-needle biopsy in the diagnosis of breast tumors. Eur J Obstet Gynecol Reprod Biol. 1993 May;49(3):175-86. PMID: 8405632.

1350. Ruano R, Ramos M, Garcia-Talavera JR, et al. Staging the axilla with selective sentinel node biopsy in patients with previous excision of non-palpable and palpable breast cancer. Eur J Nucl Med Mol Imaging. 2008 Jul;35(7):1299-304. PMID: 18274744.

1351. Rubin E, Dempsey PJ, Pile NS, et al. Needle-localization biopsy of the breast: impact of a selective core needle biopsy program on yield. Radiology. 1995 Jun;195(3):627-31. PMID: 7753985.

1352. Rulli A, Lauro A, Bisacci C, et al. Non-palpable breast lesion-biopsy by ABBI® system. A diagnostic tool. CHIRURGIA-TORINO-. 2005;18(4):175.

1353. Saad Z, Vincent M, Bramwell V, et al. Timing of surgery influences survival in receptor-negative as well as receptor-positive breast cancer. Eur J Cancer. 1994;30A(9):1348-52. PMID: 7999424.

1354. Sadler GP, McGee S, Dallimore NS, et al. Role of fine-needle aspiration cytology and needle-core biopsy in the diagnosis of lobular carcinoma of the breast. Br J Surg. 1994 Sep;81(9):1315-7. PMID: 7953397.

1355. Saha A, Barman I, Dingari NC, et al. Precision of Raman spectroscopy measurements in detection of microcalcifications in breast needle biopsies. Anal Chem. 2012 Aug 7;84(15):6715-22. PMID: 22746329.

1356. Sahiner B, Chan HP, Hadjiiski LM, et al. Multi-modality CADx: ROC study of the effect on radiologists' accuracy in characterizing breast masses on mammograms and 3D ultrasound images. Acad Radiol. 2009 Jul;16(7):810-8. PMID: 19375953.

1357. Sakuma T, Mimura A, Tanigawa N, et al. Rapid on-site cytologic examination of 1500 breast lesions using the modified Shorr's stain. Breast Cancer. 2013 Jun 4PMID: 23733595.

1358. Sanchez Gomez S, Torres Tabanera M, Vega Bolivar A, et al. Impact of a CAD system in a screen-film mammography screening program: a prospective study. Eur J Radiol. 2011 Dec;80(3):e317-21. PMID: 20863639.

1359. Sanders MA, Roland L, Sahoo S. Clinical implications of subcategorizing BI-RADS 4 breast lesions associated with microcalcification: a radiology-pathology correlation study. Breast J. 2010 Jan-Feb;16(1):28-31. PMID: 19929890.

1360. Satchithananda K, Fernando RA, Ralleigh G, et al. An audit of pain/discomfort experienced during image-guided breast biopsy procedures. Breast J. 2005 Nov-Dec;11(6):398-402. PMID: 16297083.

1361. Sauter ER, Davis W, Qin W, et al. Identification of a beta-casein-like peptide in breast nipple aspirate fluid that is associated with breast cancer. Biomark Med. 2009 Oct;3(5):577-88. PMID: 20477526.

1362. Sauven P, Bishop H, Patnick J, et al. The National Health Service Breast Screening Programme and British Association of Surgical Oncology audit of quality assurance in breast screening 1996-2001. Br J Surg. 2003 Jan;90(1):82-7. PMID: 12520580.

1363. Sayed S, Moloo Z, Bird P, et al. Breast cancer diagnosis in a resource poor environment through a collaborative multidisciplinary approach: the Kenyan experience. J Clin Pathol. 2013 Apr;66(4):307-11. PMID: 23378268.

1364. Scaranelo AM, Crystal P, Bukhanov K, et al. Sensitivity of a direct computer-aided detection system in full-field digital mammography for detection of microcalcifications not associated with mass or architectural distortion. Can Assoc Radiol J. 2010 Jun;61(3):162-9. PMID: 20137883.

1365. Schabel MC, Morrell GR, Oh KY, et al. Pharmacokinetic mapping for lesion classification in dynamic breast MRI. J Magn Reson Imaging. 2010 Jun;31(6):1371-8. PMID: 20512889.

1366. Schaefer FK, Eden I, Schaefer PJ, et al. Factors associated with one step surgery in case of non-palpable breast cancer. Eur J Radiol. 2007 Dec;64(3):426-31. PMID: 17386990.

1367. Schaefer FK, Heer I, Schaefer PJ, et al. Breast ultrasound elastography--results of 193 breast lesions in a prospective study with histopathologic correlation. Eur J Radiol. 2011 Mar;77(3):450-6. PMID: 19773141.

1368. Schaub NP, Jones KJ, Nyalwidhe JO, et al. Serum proteomic biomarker discovery reflective of stage and obesity in breast cancer patients. J Am Coll Surg. 2009 May;208(5):970-8; discussion 8-80. PMID: 19476873.

1369. Schiffhauer LM, Boger JN, Bonfiglio TA, et al. Confocal microscopy of unfixed breast needle core biopsies: a comparison to fixed and stained sections. BMC Cancer. 2009;9:265. PMID: 19650910.

1370. Schiller DE, Le LW, Cho BC, et al. Factors associated with negative margins of lumpectomy specimen: potential use in selecting patients for intraoperative radiotherapy. Ann Surg Oncol. 2008 Mar;15(3):833-42. PMID: 18163174.

1371. Schneider J, Lucas R, Tejerina A. Predicting complete removal of impalpable breast carcinomas using stereotactic radiologically guided surgery. Br J Surg. 2005 May;92(5):563-4. PMID: 15739212.

1372. Schneider P, Piper S, Schmitz CH, et al. Fast 3D Near-infrared breast imaging using indocyanine green for detection and characterization of breast lesions. Rofo. 2011 Oct;183(10):956-63. PMID: 21972043.

1373. Schnur JB, Bovbjerg DH, David D, et al. Hypnosis decreases presurgical distress in excisional breast biopsy patients. Anesth Analg. 2008 Feb;106(2):440-4, table of contents. PMID: 18227298.

1374. Schonberg MA, Silliman RA, Marcantonio ER. Weighing the benefits and burdens of mammography screening among women age 80 years or older. J Clin Oncol. 2009 Apr 10;27(11):1774-80. PMID: 19255318.

1375. Schwartz JC, Rishi M, Christy CJ, et al. What do breast surgeons do? Am J Surg. 2009 Oct;198(4):544-6. PMID: 19800465.

1376. Schwartzberg BS, Goates JJ, Keeler SA, et al. Use of advanced breast biopsy instrumentation while performing stereotactic breast biopsies: review of 150 consecutive biopsies. J Am Coll Surg. 2000 Jul;191(1):9-15. PMID: 10898178.

1377. Seigneurin A, Exbrayat C, Labarere J, et al. Association of diagnostic work-up with subsequent attendance in a breast cancer screening program for false-positive cases. Breast Cancer Res Treat. 2011 May;127(1):221-8. PMID: 20809364.

1378. Seow JH, Metcalf C, Wylie E. Nipple discharge in a screening programme: imaging findings with pathological correlation. J Med Imaging Radiat Oncol. 2011 Dec;55(6):577-86. PMID: 22141605.

1379. Setz-Pels W, Duijm LE, Coebergh JW, et al. Re-attendance after false-positive screening mammography: a population-based study in the Netherlands. Br J Cancer. 2013 Oct 15;109(8):2044-50. PMID: 24052045.

1380. Setz-Pels W, Duijm LE, Louwman MW, et al. Characteristics and screening outcome of women referred twice at screening mammography. Eur Radiol. 2012 Dec;22(12):2624-32. PMID: 22696156.

1381. Shaaban MA, Aly AEAK. Real-time ultrasound elastography: Does it improve B-mode ultrasound characterization of solid breast lesions? Egypt. J. Radiol. Nucl. Med. 2012;43(2):301-9.

1382. Shabaik AS, Cox CE, Clark RA, et al. Imprint cytology of needle-localized breast lesions. Acta Cytol. 1993 Jan-Feb;37(1):10-5. PMID: 8434486.

1383. Shafqat G, Agha A, Masror I, et al. Dynamic contrast enhanced MRI breast for lesion detection and characterization with histopathological co relation: preliminary experience at tertiary care hospital. J Pak Med Assoc. 2011 Mar;61(3):252-5. PMID: 21465939.

1384. Shannon J, Douglas-Jones AG, Dallimore NS. Conversion to core biopsy in preoperative diagnosis of breast lesions: is it justified by results? J Clin Pathol. 2001 Oct;54(10):762-5. PMID: 11577122.

1385. Sharifi S, Peterson MK, Baum JK, et al. Assessment of pathologic prognostic factors in breast core needle biopsies. Mod Pathol. 1999 Oct;12(10):941-5. PMID: 10530557.

1386. Sheth D, Wesen CA, Schroder D, et al. The advanced breast biopsy instrumentation (ABBI) experience at a community hospital. Am Surg. 1999 Aug;65(8):726-9; discussion 9-30. PMID: 10432081.

1387. Shields MW, Smith RS, Bardwil MF, et al. Is needle-directed breast biopsy overused? West J Med. 1994 Mar;160(3):229-31. PMID: 8191754.

1388. Shin HJ, Sneige N, Staerkel GA. Utility of punch biopsy for lesions that are hard to aspirate by conventional fine-needle aspiration. Cancer. 1999 Jun 25;87(3):149-54. PMID: 10385446.

1389. Shin S, Schneider HB, Cole FJ, et al. Follow-Up Recommendations for Benign Breast Biopsies. Breast J. 2006;12(5):413-7.

1390. Shirley SE, Mitchell DI, Soares DP, et al. Clinicopathologic features of breast disease in Jamaica: findings of the Jamaican Breast Disease Study, 2000-2002. West Indian Med J. 2008 Mar;57(2):90-4. PMID: 19565948.

1391. Siegal E, Angelakis E, Morris P, et al. Breast molecular imaging: a retrospective review of one institutions experience with this modality and analysis of its potential role in breast imaging decision making. Breast J. 2012 Mar-Apr;18(2):111-7. PMID: 22300043.

1392. Simpson WL, Jr., Hermann G, Rausch DR, et al. Ultrasound detection of nonpalpable mammographically occult malignancy. Can Assoc Radiol J. 2008 Apr;59(2):70-6. PMID: 18533395.

1393. Skaane P, Gullien R, Bjorndal H, et al. Digital breast tomosynthesis (DBT): initial experience in a clinical setting. Acta Radiol. 2012 Jun 1;53(5):524-9. PMID: 22593120.

1394. Slanetz PJ, Giardino AA, McCarthy KA, et al. Previous breast biopsy for benign disease rarely complicates or alters interpretation on screening mammography. AJR Am J Roentgenol. 1998 Jun;170(6):1539-41. PMID: 9609170.

1395. Smathers RL. Advanced breast biopsy instrumentation device: percentages of lesion and surrounding tissue removed. AJR Am J Roentgenol. 2000 Sep;175(3):801-3. PMID: 10954470.

1396. Sneige N, Tulbah A. Accuracy of cytologic diagnoses made from touch imprints of image-guided needle biopsy specimens of nonpalpable breast abnormalities. Diagn Cytopathol. 2000 Jul;23(1):29-34. PMID: 10907929.

1397. Soares JS, Barman I, Dingari NC, et al. Diagnostic power of diffuse reflectance spectroscopy for targeted detection of breast lesions with microcalcifications. Proc Natl Acad Sci U S A. 2013 Jan 8;110(2):471-6. PMID: 23267090.

1398. Somerville P, Seifert PJ, Destounis SV, et al. Anticoagulation and bleeding risk after core needle biopsy. AJR Am J Roentgenol. 2008 Oct;191(4):1194-7. PMID: 18806164.

1399. Soo MS, Kliewer MA, Ghate S, et al. Stereotactic breast biopsy of noncalcified lesions: a cost-minimization analysis comparing 14-gauge multipass automated core biopsy to 14-and 11-gauge vacuum-assisted biopsy. Clin Imaging. 2005;29(1):26-33.

1400. Staren ED, O'Neill TP. Ultrasound-guided needle biopsy of the breast. Surgery. 1999 Oct;126(4):629-34; discussion 34-5. PMID: 10520908.

1401. Stojadinovic A, Nissan A, Shriver CD, et al. Electrical impedance scanning as a new breast cancer risk stratification tool for young women. J Surg Oncol. 2008;97(2):112-20.

1402. Stolier AJ, Rupley DG. The impact of image-directed core biopsy on the practice of breast surgery: a new algorithm for a changing technology. Am Surg. 1997 Sep;63(9):827-30. PMID: 9290531.

1403. Stomper PC, Budnick RM, Stewart CC. Breast stereotactic core biopsy washings: abundant cell samples from clinically occult lesions for flow cytometric DNA analysis. Invest Radiol. 1998 Jan;33(1):51-5. PMID: 9438510.

1404. Stomper PC, Cholewinski SP, Penetrante RB, et al. Atypical hyperplasia: frequency and mammographic and pathologic relationships in excisional biopsies guided with mammography and clinical examination. Radiology. 1993 Dec;189(3):667-71. PMID: 8234688.

1405. Su MYL. Early-stage invasive breast cancers: Potential role of optical tomography with US localization in assisting diagnosis: Zhu Q, Hegde PU, Ricci a Jr, et al (Univ of Connecticut, Storrs; Univ of Connecticut Health Ctr, Farmington; Hartford Hosp, CT; et al) Radiology 256:367-378, 2010. Breast Dis. 2011;22(2):151-2.

1406. Sun W, Li A, Abreo F, et al. Comparison of fine-needle aspiration cytology and core biopsy for diagnosis of breast cancer. Diagn Cytopathol. 2001 Jun;24(6):421-5. PMID: 11391825.

1407. Suzuki K, Shiraishi A, Arakawa A. Analysis of stereotactic vacuum-assisted breast biopsy for patients with segmental calcifications. Jpn J Radiol. 2009 Dec;27(10):450-4. PMID: 20035418.

1408. Svahn TM, Chakraborty DP, Ikeda D, et al. Breast tomosynthesis and digital mammography: a comparison of diagnostic accuracy. Br J Radiol. 2012 Nov;85(1019):e1074-82. PMID: 22674710.

1409. Swan JS, Ying J, Stahl J, et al. Initial development of the Temporary Utilities Index: a multiattribute system for classifying the functional health impact of diagnostic testing. Qual Life Res. 2010 Apr;19(3):401-12. PMID: 20084464.

1410. Symmans WF, Weg N, Gross J, et al. A prospective comparison of stereotaxic fine-needle aspiration versus stereotaxic core needle biopsy for the diagnosis of mammographic abnormalities. Cancer. 1999 Mar 1;85(5):1119-32. PMID: 10091797.

1411. Takei J, Tsunoda-Shimizu H, Kikuchi M, et al. Clinical implications of architectural distortion visualized by breast ultrasonography. Breast Cancer. 2009;16(2):132-5. PMID: 19048193.

1412. Tan SM, Behranwala KA, Trott PA, et al. A retrospective study comparing the individual modalities of triple assessment in the pre-operative diagnosis of invasive lobular breast carcinoma. Eur J Surg Oncol. 2002 Apr;28(3):203-8. PMID: 11944950.

1413. Taskin F, Koseoglu K, Unsal A, et al. Sclerosing adenosis of the breast: radiologic appearance and efficiency of core needle biopsy. Diagn Interv Radiol. 2011 Dec;17(4):311-6. PMID: 21328197.

1414. Taylor K, O'Keeffe S, Britton PD, et al. Ultrasound elastography as an adjuvant to conventional ultrasound in the preoperative assessment of axillary lymph nodes in suspected breast cancer: a pilot study. Clin Radiol. 2011 Nov;66(11):1064-71. PMID: 21835398.

1415. Thomassin-Naggara I, Jalaguier-Coudray A, Chopier J, et al. Current opinion on clip placement after breast biopsy: a survey of practising radiologists in France and Quebec. Clin Radiol. 2013 Jul;68(7):e378-83. PMID: 23522486.

1416. Tice JA, O'Meara ES, Weaver DL, et al. Benign breast disease, mammographic breast density, and the risk of breast cancer. J Natl Cancer Inst. 2013 Jul 17;105(14):1043-9. PMID: 23744877.

1417. Tran DQ, Wilkerson DK, Namm J, et al. Needle-localized breast biopsy for mammographic abnormalities: a community hospital experience. Am Surg. 1999 Mar;65(3):283-8. PMID: 10075310.

1418. Tsang FH, Lo JJ, Wong JL, et al. Application of image-guided biopsy for impalpable breast lesions in Chinese women. ANZ J Surg. 2003 Jan-Feb;73(1-2):23-5. PMID: 12534733.

1419. Tudorica LA, Oh KY, Roy N, et al. A feasible high spatiotemporal resolution breast DCE-MRI protocol for clinical settings. Magn Reson Imaging. 2012 Nov;30(9):1257-67. PMID: 22770687.

1420. Turner AJ, Hick PE. Inhibition of aldehyde reductase by acidic metabolites of the biogenic amines. Biochem Pharmacol. 1975 Sep 15;24(18):1731-3. PMID: 16.

1421. Uematsu T, Kasami M. Core wash cytology of breast lesions by ultrasonographically guided core needle biopsy. Breast Cancer Res Treat. 2008 May;109(2):251-3. PMID: 17616804.

1422. Uematsu T, Kasami M, Takahashi K, et al. Clip placement after an 11-gauge vacuum-assisted stereotactic breast biopsy: correlation between breast thickness and clip movement. Breast Cancer. 2012 Jan;19(1):30-6. PMID: 21274668.

1423. Ukwenya AY, Yusufu LM, Nmadu PT, et al. Delayed treatment of symptomatic breast cancer: the experience from Kaduna, Nigeria. S Afr J Surg. 2008 Nov;46(4):106-10. PMID: 19051953.

1424. Utzon-Frank N, Vejborg I, von Euler-Chelpin M, et al. Balancing sensitivity and specificity: sixteen year's of experience from the mammography screening programme in Copenhagen, Denmark. Cancer Epidemiol. 2011 Oct;35(5):393-8. PMID: 21239242.

1425. Vargas HI, Vargas MP, Gonzalez K, et al. Percutaneous excisional biopsy of palpable breast masses under ultrasound visualization. Breast J. 2006 Sep-Oct;12(5 Suppl 2):S218-22. PMID: 16959005.

1426. Verardi N, Di Leo G, Carbonaro LA, et al. Contrast-enhanced MR imaging of the breast: association between asymmetric increased breast vascularity and ipsilateral cancer in a consecutive series of 197 patients. Radiol Med. 2013 Mar;118(2):239-50. PMID: 22872456.

1427. Verenhitach BD, Elias S, Patrocinio AC, et al. Evaluation of the clinical efficacy of minimally invasive procedures for breast cancer screening at a teaching hospital. J Clin Pathol. 2011 Oct;64(10):858-61. PMID: 21666140.

1428. Verkooijen HM, Buskens E, Peeters PH, et al. Diagnosing non-palpable breast disease: short-term impact on quality of life of large-core needle biopsy versus open breast biopsy. Surg Oncol. 2002 May;10(4):177-81. PMID: 12020672.

1429. Verkooijen HM, Peeters PH, Borel Rinkes IH, et al. Risk factors for cancellation of stereotactic large core needle biopsy on a prone biopsy table. Br J Radiol. 2001 Nov;74(887):1007-12. PMID: 11709465.

1430. Verkooijen HM, Peterse JL, Schipper ME, et al. Interobserver variability between general and expert pathologists during the histopathological assessment of large-core needle and open biopsies of non-palpable breast lesions. Eur J Cancer. 2003 Oct;39(15):2187-91. PMID: 14522377.

1431. Verschuur-Maes AH, van Gils CH, van den Bosch MA, et al. Digital mammography: more microcalcifications, more columnar cell lesions without atypia. Mod Pathol. 2011 Sep;24(9):1191-7. PMID: 21572405.

1432. Vimpeli SM, Saarenmaa I, Huhtala H, et al. Large-core needle biopsy versus fine-needle aspiration biopsy in solid breast lesions: comparison of costs and diagnostic value. Acta Radiol. 2008 Oct;49(8):863-9. PMID: 18618302.

1433. Wai CJ, Al-Mubarak G, Homer MJ, et al. A modified triple test for palpable breast masses: the value of ultrasound and core needle biopsy. Ann Surg Oncol. 2013 Mar;20(3):850-5. PMID: 23104707.

1434. Waldherr C, Cerny P, Altermatt HJ, et al. Value of one-view breast tomosynthesis versus two-view mammography in diagnostic workup of women with clinical signs and symptoms and in women recalled from screening. AJR Am J Roentgenol. 2013 Jan;200(1):226-31. PMID: 23255766.

1435. Wang S, Delproposto Z, Wang H, et al. Differentiation of breast cancer from fibroadenoma with dual-echo dynamic contrast-enhanced MRI. PLoS One. 2013;8(7):e67731. PMID: 23844077.

1436. Watanabe S. [Mammographic detection of early breast cancer]. Gan No Rinsho. 1988 Aug;34(10):1378-87. PMID: 3172495.

1437. Watermann DO, Einert A, Ehritt-Braun C, et al. Experience with the Advanced Breast Biopsy Instrumentation (ABBI) system. Anticancer Res. 2002 Sep-Oct;22(5):3067-70. PMID: 12530044.

1438. Wauters CA, Sanders-Eras CT, Kooistra BW, et al. Modified core wash cytology procedure for the immediate diagnosis of core needle biopsies of breast lesions. Cancer. 2009 Oct 25;117(5):333-7. PMID: 19739241.

1439. Wauters CA, Sanders-Eras MC, de Kievit-van der Heijden IM, et al. Modified core wash cytology (CWC), an asset in the diagnostic work-up of breast lesions. Eur J Surg Oncol. 2010 Oct;36(10):957-62. PMID: 20708371.

1440. Weigel S, Biesheuvel C, Berkemeyer S, et al. Digital mammography screening: how many breast cancers are additionally detected by bilateral ultrasound examination during assessment? Eur Radiol. 2013 Mar;23(3):684-91. PMID: 23052645.

1441. Weigert J, Steenbergen S. The connecticut experiment: the role of ultrasound in the screening of women with dense breasts. Breast J. 2012 Nov-Dec;18(6):517-22. PMID: 23009208.

1442. Weismann CF, Forstner R, Prokop E, et al. Three-dimensional targeting: a new three-dimensional ultrasound technique to evaluate needle position during breast biopsy. Ultrasound Obstet Gynecol. 2000 Sep;16(4):359-64. PMID: 11169313.

1443. Westenend PJ, Sever AR, Beekman-De Volder HJ, et al. A comparison of aspiration cytology and core needle biopsy in the evaluation of breast lesions. Cancer. 2001 Apr 25;93(2):146-50. PMID: 11309781.

1444. Whang IY. Power Doppler needle-induced fremitus for breast localization. Arch Gynecol Obstet. 2008 Oct;278(4):337-40. PMID: 18283477.

1445. Williams MB, Judy PG, Gunn S, et al. Dual-modality breast tomosynthesis. Radiology. 2010 Apr;255(1):191-8. PMID: 20308457.

1446. Wishart GC, Campisi M, Boswell M, et al. The accuracy of digital infrared imaging for breast cancer detection in women undergoing breast biopsy. Eur J Surg Oncol. 2010 Jun;36(6):535-40. PMID: 20452740.

1447. Wishart GC, Campisi MS, Chapman D, et al. O-83 Digital infrared imaging for breast cancer detection in younger women undergoing breast biopsy. EJC Supplements. 2010;8(6):31-2. PMID: 2010946272. Language: English. Entry Date: 20110304. Revision Date: 20120817. Publication Type: journal article.

1448. Witek-Janusek L, Gabram S, Mathews HL. Psychologic stress, reduced NK cell activity, and cytokine dysregulation in women experiencing diagnostic breast biopsy. Psychoneuroendocrinology. 2007 Jan;32(1):22-35. PMID: 17092654.

1449. Witt A, Yavuz D, Walchetseder C, et al. Preoperative core needle biopsy as an independent risk factor for wound infection after breast surgery. Obstet Gynecol. 2003 Apr;101(4):745-50. PMID: 12681880.

1450. Wong SL, Edwards MJ, Chao C, et al. The effect of prior breast biopsy method and concurrent definitive breast procedure on success and accuracy of sentinel lymph node biopsy. Ann Surg Oncol. 2002 Apr;9(3):272-7. PMID: 11923134.

1451. Woods RW, Oliphant L, Shinki K, et al. Validation of results from knowledge discovery: mass density as a predictor of breast cancer. J Digit Imaging. 2010 Oct;23(5):554-61. PMID: 19760292.

1452. Woods RW, Sisney GS, Salkowski LR, et al. The mammographic density of a mass is a significant predictor of breast cancer. Radiology. 2011 Feb;258(2):417-25. PMID: 21177388.

1453. Woon DT, Serpell JW. Preoperative core biopsy of soft tissue tumours facilitates their surgical management: a 10-year update. ANZ J Surg. 2008 Nov;78(11):977-81. PMID: 18959696.

1454. Wu X, Chen G, Lu J, et al. Label-free detection of breast masses using multiphoton microscopy. PLoS One. 2013;8(6):e65933. PMID: 23755295.

1455. Xie HB, Salhadar A, Haara A, et al. How stereotactic core-needle biopsy affected breast fine-needle aspiration utilization: an 11-year institutional review. Diagn Cytopathol. 2004 Aug;31(2):106-10. PMID: 15282722.

1456. Yang JH, Lee SD, Nam SJ. Diagnostic utility of ABBI®(Advanced Breast Biopsy Instrumentation) for nonpalpable breast lesions in Korea. The breast journal. 2000;6(4):257-62.

1457. Yau EJ, Gutierrez RL, DeMartini WB, et al. The utility of breast MRI as a problem-solving tool. Breast J. 2011 May-Jun;17(3):273-80. PMID: 21477168.

1458. Yazici B, Sever AR, Mills P, et al. Scar formation after stereotactic vacuum-assisted core biopsy of benign breast lesions. Clin Radiol. 2006 Jul;61(7):619-24. PMID: 16784949.

1459. Yener NA, Midi A, Cubuk R, et al. Palpable lesions as a diagnostic tool in patients with thoracic pathology. Diagn Cytopathol. 2013 Jan;41(1):28-34. PMID: 21681977.

1460. Ying X, Lin Y, Xia X, et al. A comparison of mammography and ultrasound in women with breast disease: a receiver operating characteristic analysis. Breast J. 2012 Mar-Apr;18(2):130-8. PMID: 22356352.

1461. Yong WS, Chia KH, Poh WT, et al. A comparison of trucut biopsy with fine needle aspiration cytology in the diagnosis of breast cancer. Singapore Med J. 1999 Sep;40(9):587-9. PMID: 10628249.

1462. Yoon JH, Kim MH, Kim EK, et al. Interobserver variability of ultrasound elastography: how it affects the diagnosis of breast lesions. AJR Am J Roentgenol. 2011 Mar;196(3):730-6. PMID: 21343520.

1463. Youk JH, Gweon HM, Son EJ, et al. Diagnostic value of commercially available shear-wave elastography for breast cancers: integration into BI-RADS classification with subcategories of category 4. Eur Radiol. 2013 Oct;23(10):2695-704. PMID: 23652850.

1464. Zagouri F, Sergentanis TN, Gounaris A, et al. Pain in different methods of breast biopsy: emphasis on vacuum-assisted breast biopsy. Breast. 2008 Feb;17(1):71-5. PMID: 17869106.

1465. Zagouri F, Sergentanis TN, Zografos GC. Lesions too close to the chest wall: a relative contraindication for vacuum-assisted breast biopsy. AJR Am J Roentgenol. 2008 Apr;190(4):W270. PMID: 18356420.

1466. Zahid Z, Ibrahim Z, Bilal S, et al. Comparison of diagnostic accuracy of film-Screen mammography and ultrasound in breast masses. Pak. J. Med. Health Sci. 2011;5(3):433-5.

1467. Zanca F, Chakraborty DP, Van Ongeval C, et al. An improved method for simulating microcalcifications in digital mammograms. Med Phys. 2008 Sep;35(9):4012-8. PMID: 18841852.

1468. Zheng B, Lederman D, Sumkin JH, et al. A preliminary evaluation of multi-probe resonance-frequency electrical impedance based measurements of the breast. Acad Radiol. 2011 Feb;18(2):220-9. PMID: 21126888.

1469. Zheng B, Zuley ML, Sumkin JH, et al. Detection of breast abnormalities using a prototype resonance electrical impedance spectroscopy system: a preliminary study. Med Phys. 2008 Jul;35(7):3041-8. PMID: 18697526.

1470. Zhou J, Zhan W, Chang C, et al. Role of acoustic shear wave velocity measurement in characterization of breast lesions. J Ultrasound Med. 2013 Feb;32(2):285-94. PMID: 23341385.

1471. Zhu C, Burnside ES, Sisney GA, et al. Fluorescence spectroscopy: an adjunct diagnostic tool to image-guided core needle biopsy of the breast. IEEE Trans Biomed Eng. 2009 Oct;56(10):2518-28. PMID: 19272976.

1472. Zhu J, Kurihara Y, Kanemaki Y, et al. Diagnostic accuracy of high-resolution MRI using a microscopy coil for patients with presumed DCIS following mammography screening. J Magn Reson Imaging. 2007 Jan;25(1):96-103. PMID: 17154376.

1473. Zhu Q, Hegde PU, Ricci A, Jr., et al. Early-stage invasive breast cancers: potential role of optical tomography with US localization in assisting diagnosis. Radiology. 2010 Aug;256(2):367-78. PMID: 20571122.

1474. Zimmermann CJ, Sheffield KM, Duncan CB, et al. Time trends and geographic variation in use of minimally invasive breast biopsy. J Am Coll Surg. 2013 Apr;216(4):814-24; discussion 24-7. PMID: 23376029.

1475. Zimmermann N, Ohlinger R. Diagnostic value of palpation, mammography, and ultrasonography in the diagnosis of fibroadenoma: impact of breast density, patient age, ultrasonographic size, and palpability. Ultraschall Med. 2012 Dec;33(7):E151-7. PMID: 21667430.

1476. Zografos G, Koulocheri D, Liakou P, et al. Novel technology of multimodal ultrasound tomography detects breast lesions. Eur Radiol. 2013 Mar;23(3):673-83. PMID: 22983317.

1477. Zografos GC, Zagouri F, Sergentanis TN, et al. Cytokine dysregulation during vacuum-assisted breast biopsy: early phase of a complex phenomenon. Isr Med Assoc J. 2008 Mar;10(3):246. PMID: 18494247.

1478. Zonderland H, Hermans J, Van De Vijver M, et al. Triple diagnostic approach versus ultrasound-guided 18 gauge core biopsy in suspicious breast masses. The Breast. 1998;7(3):168-72.

1479. Zonderland HM, van de Vijver MJ, Visser M. [Breast lesion diagnosis: integrating pathology and radiology]. Ned Tijdschr Geneeskd. 2011;155(18):A2967.

1480. Abbate F, Bacigalupo L, Latronico A, et al. Ultrasound-guided vacuum assisted breast biopsy in the assessment of C3 breast lesions by ultrasound-guided fine needle aspiration cytology: results and costs in comparison with surgery. Breast. 2009 Apr;18(2):73-7. PMID: 19342236.

1481. Abbate F, Cassano E, Menna S, et al. Ultrasound-guided vacuum-assisted breast biopsy: Use at the European Institute of Oncology in 2010. J Ultrasound. 2011 Dec;14(4):177-81. PMID: 23397003.

1482. Abbott AM, Portschy PR, Lee C, et al. Prospective multicenter trial evaluating balloon-catheter partial-breast irradiation for ductal carcinoma in situ. Int J Radiat Oncol Biol Phys. 2013 Nov 1;87(3):494-8. PMID: 24074922.

1483. Abdsaleh S, Warnberg F, Azavedo E, et al. Comparison of core needle biopsy and surgical specimens in malignant breast lesions regarding histological features and hormone receptor expression. Histopathology. 2008 May;52(6):773-5. PMID: 18393972.

1484. Acs G, Paragh G, Chuang ST, et al. The presence of micropapillary features and retraction artifact in core needle biopsy material predicts lymph node metastasis in breast carcinoma. Am J Surg Pathol. 2009 Feb;33(2):202-10. PMID: 18987549.

1485. Adkisson CD, Vallow LA, Kowalchik K, et al. Patient age and preoperative breast MRI in women with breast cancer: biopsy and surgical implications. Ann Surg Oncol. 2011 Jun;18(6):1678-83. PMID: 21207171.

1486. Adler DD, Light RJ, Granstrom P, et al. Follow-up of benign results of stereotactic core breast biopsy. Acad Radiol. 2000 Apr;7(4):248-53. PMID: 10766097.

1487. Aftab K, Idrees R. Nipple adenoma of breast: a masquerader of malignancy. J Coll Physicians Surg Pak. 2010 Jul;20(7):472-4. PMID: 20642949.

1488. Aftab ML, Rashid A, Aslam M, et al. Clinical value of sure cut biopsy in breast masses. Pak. J. Med. Health Sci. 2010;4(1):46-8.

1489. Agarwal T, Patel B, Rajan P, et al. Core biopsy versus FNAC for palpable breast cancers. Is image guidance necessary? Eur J Cancer. 2003 Jan;39(1):52-6. PMID: 12504658.

1490. Ahmad A, Bano U, Gondal M, et al. Her-2/neu gene overexpression in breast carcinoma and its association with clinicopathological characteristics of the disease. J Coll Physicians Surg Pak. 2009 May;19(5):297-9. PMID: 19409162.

1491. Ahmadiyeh N, Stoleru MA, Raza S, et al. Management of intraductal papillomas of the breast: an analysis of 129 cases and their outcome. Ann Surg Oncol. 2009 Aug;16(8):2264-9. PMID: 19484312.

1492. Akagi T, Kinoshita T, Shien T, et al. Clinical and pathological features of intracystic papillary carcinoma of the breast. Surg Today. 2009;39(1):5-8. PMID: 19132460.

1493. Akbulut M, Zekioglu O, Kapkac M, et al. Fine needle aspiration cytology of glycogen-rich clear cell carcinoma of the breast: review of 37 cases with histologic correlation. Acta Cytol. 2008 Jan-Feb;52(1):65-71. PMID: 18323277.

1494. Al Hassan T, Delli Fraine P, El-Khoury M, et al. Accuracy of percutaneous core needle biopsy in diagnosing papillary breast lesions and potential impact of sonographic features on their management. J Clin Ultrasound. 2013 Jan;41(1):1-9. PMID: 22987609.

1495. Al Sarakbi W, Salhab M, Thomas V, et al. Is preoperative core biopsy accurate in determining the hormone receptor status in women with invasive breast cancer? Int Semin Surg Oncol. 2005 Aug 22;2:15. PMID: 16115314.

1496. Al-Janabi S, Huisman A, Willems SM, et al. Digital slide images for primary diagnostics in breast pathology: a feasibility study. Hum Pathol. 2012 Dec;43(12):2318-25. PMID: 22901465.

1497. Al-Khawari HA, Al-Manfouhi HA, Madda JP, et al. Radiologic features of granulomatous mastitis. Breast J. 2011 Nov-Dec;17(6):645-50. PMID: 21929558.

1498. Allen LR, Lago-Toro CE, Hughes JH, et al. Is there a role for MRI in the preoperative assessment of patients with DCIS? Ann Surg Oncol. 2010 Sep;17(9):2395-400. PMID: 20217259.

1499. Allison KH, Eby PR, Kohr J, et al. Atypical ductal hyperplasia on vacuum-assisted breast biopsy: suspicion for ductal carcinoma in situ can stratify patients at high risk for upgrade. Hum Pathol. 2011 Jan;42(1):41-50. PMID: 20970167.

1500. Amir E, Miller N, Geddie W, et al. Prospective study evaluating the impact of tissue confirmation of metastatic disease in patients with breast cancer. J Clin Oncol. 2012 Feb 20;30(6):587-92. PMID: 22124102.

1501. Ancona A, Capodieci M, Galiano A, et al. Vacuum-assisted biopsy diagnosis of atypical ductal hyperplasia and patient management. Radiol Med. 2011 Mar;116(2):276-91. PMID: 21225358.

1502. Andacoglu O, Kanbour-Shakir A, Teh YC, et al. Rationale of excisional biopsy after the diagnosis of benign radial scar on core biopsy: a single institutional outcome analysis. Am J Clin Oncol. 2013 Feb;36(1):7-11. PMID: 22134516.

1503. Andrade VP, Gobbi H. Accuracy of typing and grading invasive mammary carcinomas on core needle biopsy compared with the excisional specimen. Virchows Arch. 2004 Dec;445(6):597-602. PMID: 15480766.

1504. Andrews-Tang D, Diamond AB, Rogers L, et al. Diabetic Mastopathy: Adjunctive Use of Ultrasound and Utility of Core Biopsy in Diagnosis. Breast J. 2000 May;6(3):183-8. PMID: 11348362.

1505. Andrykowski MA, Carpenter JS, Studts JL, et al. Psychological impact of benign breast biopsy: a longitudinal, comparative study. Health Psychol. 2002 Sep;21(5):485-94. PMID: 12211516.

1506. Ansari B, Boughey JC, Adamczyk DL, et al. Should axillary ultrasound be used in patients with a preoperative diagnosis of ductal carcinoma in situ? Am J Surg. 2012 Sep;204(3):290-3. PMID: 22749764.

1507. Apple SK. Variability in gross and microscopic pathology reporting in excisional biopsies of breast cancer tissue. Breast J. 2006 Mar-Apr;12(2):145-9. PMID: 16509839.

1508. Apple SK, Lowe AC, Rao PN, et al. Comparison of fluorescent in situ hybridization HER-2/neu results on core needle biopsy and excisional biopsy in primary breast cancer. Mod Pathol. 2009 Sep;22(9):1151-9. PMID: 19483670.

1509. Arazi-Kleinman T, Causer PA, Nofech-Mozes S, et al. Is ductal carcinoma in situ with "possible invasion" more predictive of invasive carcinoma than pure ductal carcinoma in situ? Can Assoc Radiol J. 2012 May;63(2):146-52. PMID: 21561735.

1510. Arnedos M, Nerurkar A, Osin P, et al. Discordance between core needle biopsy (CNB) and excisional biopsy (EB) for estrogen receptor (ER), progesterone receptor (PgR) and HER2 status in early breast cancer (EBC). Ann Oncol. 2009 Dec;20(12):1948-52. PMID: 19570962.

1511. Arnould L, Roger P, Macgrogan G, et al. Accuracy of HER2 status determination on breast core-needle biopsies (immunohistochemistry, FISH, CISH and SISH vs FISH). Mod Pathol. 2012 May;25(5):675-82. PMID: 22222637.

1512. Aroner SA, Collins LC, Schnitt SJ, et al. Columnar cell lesions and subsequent breast cancer risk: a nested case-control study. Breast Cancer Res. 2010;12(4):R61. PMID: 20691043.

1513. Arora S, Menes TS, Moung C, et al. Atypical ductal hyperplasia at margin of breast biopsy--is re-excision indicated? Ann Surg Oncol. 2008 Mar;15(3):843-7. PMID: 17987337.

1514. Arora S, Moezzi M, Kim U, et al. Is surgical excision necessary for atypical ductal hyperplasia diagnosed with 8 gauge stereotactic biopsy? Breast J. 2009 Nov-Dec;15(6):673-4. PMID: 19686226.

1515. Aruga T, Suzuki E, Saji S, et al. A low number of tumor-infiltrating FOXP3-positive cells during primary systemic chemotherapy correlates with favorable anti-tumor response in patients with breast cancer. Oncol Rep. 2009 Aug;22(2):273-8. PMID: 19578766.

1516. Athanassiou E, Sioutopoulou D, Vamvakopoulos N, et al. The fat content of small primary breast cancer interferes with radiofrequency-induced thermal ablation. Eur Surg Res. 2009;42(1):54-8. PMID: 18987475.

1517. Badoual C, Maruani A, Ghorra C, et al. Pathological prognostic factors of invasive breast carcinoma in ultrasound-guided large core biopsies-correlation with subsequent surgical excisions. Breast. 2005 Feb;14(1):22-7. PMID: 15695077.

1518. Bae MS, Moon WK, Cho N, et al. Patient age and tumor size determine the cancer yield of preoperative bilateral breast MRI in women with ductal carcinoma in situ. AJR Am J Roentgenol. 2013 Sep;201(3):684-91. PMID: 23971464.

1519. Baek SE, Kim MJ, Kim EK, et al. Effect of clinical information on diagnostic performance in breast sonography. J Ultrasound Med. 2009 Oct;28(10):1349-56. PMID: 19778881.

1520. Baez E, Huber A, Vetter M, et al. Minimal invasive complete excision of benign breast tumors using a three-dimensional ultrasound-guided mammotome vacuum device. Ultrasound Obstet Gynecol. 2003 Mar;21(3):267-72. PMID: 12666222.

1521. Bagaria SP, Shamonki J, Kinnaird M, et al. The florid subtype of lobular carcinoma in situ: marker or precursor for invasive lobular carcinoma? Ann Surg Oncol. 2011 Jul;18(7):1845-51. PMID: 21287281.

1522. Bagnall MJ, Evans AJ, Wilson AR, et al. When have mammographic calcifications been adequately sampled at needle core biopsy? Clin Radiol. 2000 Jul;55(7):548-53. PMID: 10924380.

1523. Bagnall MJ, Evans AJ, Wilson AR, et al. Predicting invasion in mammographically detected microcalcification. Clin Radiol. 2001 Oct;56(10):828-32. PMID: 11895299.

1524. Bai HX, Motwani SB, Higgins SA, et al. Breast conservation therapy for ductal carcinoma in situ (DCIS): does presentation of disease affect long-term outcomes? Int J Clin Oncol. 2013 Jun 19PMID: 23780727.

1525. Bani MR, Lux MP, Heusinger K, et al. Factors correlating with reexcision after breast-conserving therapy. Eur J Surg Oncol. 2009 Jan;35(1):32-7. PMID: 18539425.

1526. Barr FE, Degnim AC, Hartmann LC, et al. Estrogen receptor expression in atypical hyperplasia: lack of association with breast cancer. Cancer Prev Res (Phila). 2011 Mar;4(3):435-44. PMID: 21209395.

1527. Barry WT, Kernagis DN, Dressman HK, et al. Intratumor heterogeneity and precision of microarray-based predictors of breast cancer biology and clinical outcome. J Clin Oncol. 2010 May 1;28(13):2198-206. PMID: 20368555.

1528. Bathen TF, Geurts B, Sitter B, et al. Feasibility of MR metabolomics for immediate analysis of resection margins during breast cancer surgery. PLoS One. 2013;8(4):e61578. PMID: 23613877.

1529. Bauer TL, Pandelidis SM, Rhoads JE, Jr. Five-year survival of 100 women with carcinoma of the breast diagnosed by screening mammography and needle-localization biopsy. J Am Coll Surg. 1994 May;178(5):427-30. PMID: 8167877.

1530. Becker AK, Gordon PB, Harrison DA, et al. Flat ductal intraepithelial neoplasia 1A diagnosed at stereotactic core needle biopsy: is excisional biopsy indicated? AJR Am J Roentgenol. 2013 Mar;200(3):682-8. PMID: 23436863.

1531. Begum SM, Jara-Lazaro AR, Thike AA, et al. Mucin extravasation in breast core biopsies--clinical significance and outcome correlation. Histopathology. 2009 Nov;55(5):609-17. PMID: 19912367.

1532. Bendifallah S, Chabbert-Buffet N, Maurin N, et al. Predictive factors for breast cancer in patients diagnosed with ductal intraepithelial neoplasia, grade 1B. Anticancer Res. 2012 Aug;32(8):3571-9. PMID: 22843948.

1533. Bendifallah S, Defert S, Chabbert-Buffet N, et al. Scoring to predict the possibility of upgrades to malignancy in atypical ductal hyperplasia diagnosed by an 11-gauge vacuum-assisted biopsy device: an external validation study. Eur J Cancer. 2012 Jan;48(1):30-6. PMID: 22100905.

1534. Bennett LE, Ghate SV, Bentley R, et al. Is surgical excision of core biopsy proven benign papillomas of the breast necessary? Acad Radiol. 2010 May;17(5):553-7. PMID: 20223685.

1535. Berg JC, Visscher DW, Vierkant RA, et al. Breast cancer risk in women with radial scars in benign breast biopsies. Breast Cancer Res Treat. 2008 Mar;108(2):167-74. PMID: 18297395.

1536. Berg WA, Madsen KS, Schilling K, et al. Breast cancer: comparative effectiveness of positron emission mammography and MR imaging in presurgical planning for the ipsilateral breast. Radiology. 2011 Jan;258(1):59-72. PMID: 21076089.

1537. Bernard JR, Jr., Vallow LA, DePeri ER, et al. In newly diagnosed breast cancer, screening MRI of the contralateral breast detects mammographically occult cancer, even in elderly women: the mayo clinic in Florida experience. Breast J. 2010 Mar-Apr;16(2):118-26. PMID: 20136645.

1538. Bianchi S, Bendinelli B, Castellano I, et al. Morphological parameters of lobular in situ neoplasia in stereotactic 11-gauge vacuum-assisted needle core biopsy do not predict the presence of malignancy on subsequent surgical excision. Histopathology. 2013 Jul;63(1):83-95. PMID: 23692123.

1539. Bianchi S, Caini S, Cattani MG, et al. Diagnostic concordance in reporting breast needle core biopsies using the B classification-A panel in Italy. Pathol Oncol Res. 2009 Dec;15(4):725-32. PMID: 19449173.

1540. Bianchi S, Giannotti E, Vanzi E, et al. Radial scar without associated atypical epithelial proliferation on image-guided 14-gauge needle core biopsy: analysis of 49 cases from a single-centre and review of the literature. Breast. 2012 Apr;21(2):159-64. PMID: 21944431.

1541. Biggar MA, Kerr KM, Erzetich LM, et al. Columnar cell change with atypia (flat epithelial atypia) on breast core biopsy-outcomes following open excision. Breast J. 2012 Nov-Dec;18(6):578-81. PMID: 23078374.

1542. Bode MK, Rissanen T. Imaging findings and accuracy of core needle biopsy in mucinous carcinoma of the breast. Acta Radiol. 2011 Mar 1;52(2):128-33. PMID: 21498339.

1543. Bode MK, Rissanen T, Apaja-Sarkkinen M. Ultrasonography-guided core needle biopsy in differential diagnosis of papillary breast tumors. Acta Radiol. 2009 Sep;50(7):722-9. PMID: 19488890.

1544. Bodian CA, lattes R, Perzin KH. The epidemiology of gross cystic disease of the breast confirmed by biopsy or by aspiration of cyst fluid. Cancer Detect Prev. 1992;16(1):7-15. PMID: 1551140.

1545. Bohling SD, Allison KH. Immunosuppressive regulatory T cells are associated with aggressive breast cancer phenotypes: a potential therapeutic target. Mod Pathol. 2008 Dec;21(12):1527-32. PMID: 18820666.

1546. Bonanni B, Puntoni M, Cazzaniga M, et al. Dual effect of metformin on breast cancer proliferation in a randomized presurgical trial. J Clin Oncol. 2012 Jul 20;30(21):2593-600. PMID: 22564993.

1547. Bonnas C, Specht K, Spleiss O, et al. Effects of cold ischemia and inflammatory tumor microenvironment on detection of PI3K/AKT and MAPK pathway activation patterns in clinical cancer samples. Int J Cancer. 2012 Oct 1;131(7):1621-32. PMID: 22213219.

1548. Bonnefoi H, Piccart M, Bogaerts J, et al. TP53 status for prediction of sensitivity to taxane versus non-taxane neoadjuvant chemotherapy in breast cancer (EORTC 10994/BIG 1-00): a randomised phase 3 trial. Lancet Oncol. 2011 Jun;12(6):527-39. PMID: 21570352.

1549. Borecky N, Rickard M. Preoperative diagnosis of carcinoma within fibroadenoma on screening mammograms. J Med Imaging Radiat Oncol. 2008 Feb;52(1):64-7. PMID: 18373829.

1550. Boughey JC, Hartmann LC, Anderson SS, et al. Evaluation of the Tyrer-Cuzick (International Breast Cancer Intervention Study) model for breast cancer risk prediction in women with atypical hyperplasia. J Clin Oncol. 2010 Aug 1;28(22):3591-6. PMID: 20606088.

1551. Boulos FI, Dupont WD, Simpson JF, et al. Histologic associations and long-term cancer risk in columnar cell lesions of the breast: a retrospective cohort and a nested case-control study. Cancer. 2008 Nov 1;113(9):2415-21. PMID: 18816618.

1552. Bowman E, Oprea G, Okoli J, et al. Pseudoangiomatous stromal hyperplasia (PASH) of the breast: a series of 24 patients. Breast J. 2012 May-Jun;18(3):242-7. PMID: 22583194.

1553. Braun M, Fountoulakis M, Papadopoulou A, et al. Down-regulation of microfilamental network-associated proteins in leukocytes of breast cancer patients: potential application to predictive diagnosis. Cancer Genomics Proteomics. 2009 Jan-Feb;6(1):31-40. PMID: 19451088.

1554. Brem RF, Ioffe M, Rapelyea JA, et al. Invasive lobular carcinoma: detection with mammography, sonography, MRI, and breast-specific gamma imaging. AJR Am J Roentgenol. 2009 Feb;192(2):379-83. PMID: 19155397.

1555. Brem RF, Shahan C, Rapleyea JA, et al. Detection of occult foci of breast cancer using breast-specific gamma imaging in women with one mammographic or clinically suspicious breast lesion. Acad Radiol. 2010 Jun;17(6):735-43. PMID: 20457416.

1556. Brennan SB, Corben A, Liberman L, et al. Papilloma diagnosed at MRI-guided vacuum-assisted breast biopsy: is surgical excision still warranted? AJR Am J Roentgenol. 2012 Oct;199(4):W512-9. PMID: 22997402.

1557. Brkljacic B, Cikara I, Ivanac G, et al. Ultrasound-guided bipolar radiofrequency ablation of breast cancer in inoperable patients: a pilot study. Ultraschall Med. 2010 Apr;31(2):156-62. PMID: 19941254.

1558. Browne EP, Punska EC, Lenington S, et al. Increased promoter methylation in exfoliated breast epithelial cells in women with a previous breast biopsy. Epigenetics. 2011 Dec;6(12):1425-35. PMID: 22139572.

1559. Bukhari MH, Akhtar ZM. Comparison of accuracy of diagnostic modalities for evaluation of breast cancer with review of literature. Diagn Cytopathol. 2009 Jun;37(6):416-24. PMID: 19217034.

1560. Bundred NJ, Cramer A, Morris J, et al. Cyclooxygenase-2 inhibition does not improve the reduction in ductal carcinoma in situ proliferation with aromatase inhibitor therapy: results of the ERISAC randomized placebo-controlled trial. Clin Cancer Res. 2010 Mar 1;16(5):1605-12. PMID: 20179229.

1561. Bunting DM, Steel JR, Holgate CS, et al. Long term follow-up and risk of breast cancer after a radial scar or complex sclerosing lesion has been identified in a benign open breast biopsy. Eur J Surg Oncol. 2011 Aug;37(8):709-13. PMID: 21684716.

1562. Burbank F. Mammographic findings after 14-gauge automated needle and 14-gauge directional, vacuum-assisted stereotactic breast biopsies. Radiology. 1997 Jul;204(1):153-6. PMID: 9205238.

1563. Burge CN, Chang HR, Apple SK. Do the histologic features and results of breast cancer biomarker studies differ between core biopsy and surgical excision specimens? Breast. 2006 Apr;15(2):167-72. PMID: 16095904.

1564. Cahill RA, Walsh D, Landers RJ, et al. Preoperative profiling of symptomatic breast cancer by diagnostic core biopsy. Ann Surg Oncol. 2006 Jan;13(1):45-51. PMID: 16378157.

1565. Calvo-Plaza I, Ugidos L, Miro C, et al. Retrospective study assessing the role of MRI in the diagnostic procedures for early breast carcinoma: a correlation of new foci in the MRI with tumor pathological features. Clin Transl Oncol. 2013 Mar;15(3):205-10. PMID: 22872518.

1566. Campbell I, Royle G, Coddington R, et al. Management of screen-detected breast cancer: audit of the first 100 cases in the Southampton and Salisbury breast screening programme. Ann R Coll Surg Engl. 1993 Jan;75(1):13-7. PMID: 8422137.

1567. Cangiarella J, Guth A, Axelrod D, et al. Is surgical excision necessary for the management of atypical lobular hyperplasia and lobular carcinoma in situ diagnosed on core needle biopsy?: a report of 38 cases and review of the literature. Arch Pathol Lab Med. 2008 Jun;132(6):979-83. PMID: 18517282.

1568. Carder PJ, Liston JC. Will the spectrum of lesions prompting a "B3" breast core biopsy increase the benign biopsy rate? J Clin Pathol. 2003 Feb;56(2):133-8. PMID: 12560393.

1569. Carder PJ, Shaaban A, Alizadeh Y, et al. Screen-detected pleomorphic lobular carcinoma in situ (PLCIS): risk of concurrent invasive malignancy following a core biopsy diagnosis. Histopathology. 2010 Sep;57(3):472-8. PMID: 20727019.

1570. Carkaci S, Lane DL, Gilcrease MZ, et al. Do all mucocele-like lesions of the breast require surgery? Clin Imaging. 2011 Mar-Apr;35(2):94-101. PMID: 21377046.

1571. Carson W, Sanchez-Forgach E, Stomper P, et al. Lobular carcinoma in situ: observation without surgery as an appropriate therapy. Ann Surg Oncol. 1994 Mar;1(2):141-6. PMID: 7834439.

1572. Cassano E, Urban LA, Pizzamiglio M, et al. Ultrasound-guided vacuum-assisted core breast biopsy: experience with 406 cases. Breast Cancer Res Treat. 2007 Mar;102(1):103-10. PMID: 16838109.

1573. Catteau X, Simon P, Noel JC. Predictors of invasive breast cancer in mammographically detected microcalcification in patients with a core biopsy diagnosis of flat epithelial atypia, atypical ductal hyperplasia or ductal carcinoma in situ and recommendations for a selective approach to sentinel lymph node biopsy. Pathol Res Pract. 2012 Apr 15;208(4):217-20. PMID: 22445178.

1574. Caughran JL, Vicini FA, Kestin LL, et al. Optimal use of re-excision in patients diagnosed with early-stage breast cancer by excisional biopsy treated with breast-conserving therapy. Ann Surg Oncol. 2009 Nov;16(11):3020-7. PMID: 19636632.

1575. Cavaliere A, Sidoni A, Scheibel M, et al. Biopathologic profile of breast cancer core biopsy: is it always a valid method? Cancer Lett. 2005 Jan 31;218(1):117-21. PMID: 15639347.

1576. Cermik TF, Mavi A, Basu S, et al. Impact of FDG PET on the preoperative staging of newly diagnosed breast cancer. Eur J Nucl Med Mol Imaging. 2008 Mar;35(3):475-83. PMID: 17957366.

1577. Chae BJ, Lee A, Song BJ, et al. Predictive factors for breast cancer in patients diagnosed atypical ductal hyperplasia at core needle biopsy. World J Surg Oncol. 2009;7:77. PMID: 19852801.

1578. Chagpar AB, Martin RC, 2nd, Hagendoorn LJ, et al. Lumpectomy margins are affected by tumor size and histologic subtype but not by biopsy technique. Am J Surg. 2004 Oct;188(4):399-402. PMID: 15474434.

1579. Chagpar AB, Scoggins CR, Sahoo S, et al. Biopsy type does not influence sentinel lymph node status. Am J Surg. 2005 Oct;190(4):551-6. PMID: 16164918.

1580. Chambon M, Orsetti B, Berthe ML, et al. Prognostic significance of TRIM24/TIF-1alpha gene expression in breast cancer. Am J Pathol. 2011 Apr;178(4):1461-9. PMID: 21435435.

1581. Chan MY, Lim S. Predictors of invasive breast cancer in ductal carcinoma in situ initially diagnosed by core biopsy. Asian J Surg. 2010 Apr;33(2):76-82. PMID: 21029943.

1582. Chang JM, Han W, Moon WK, et al. Papillary lesions initially diagnosed at ultrasound-guided vacuum-assisted breast biopsy: rate of malignancy based on subsequent surgical excision. Ann Surg Oncol. 2011 Sep;18(9):2506-14. PMID: 21369740.

1583. Chang JM, Moon WK, Cho N, et al. Risk of carcinoma after subsequent excision of benign papilloma initially diagnosed with an ultrasound (US)-guided 14-gauge core needle biopsy: a prospective observational study. Eur Radiol. 2010 May;20(5):1093-100. PMID: 19890638.

1584. Charles M, Edge SB, Winston JS, et al. Effect of stereotactic core needle biopsy on pathologic measurement of tumor size of T1 invasive breast carcinomas presenting as mammographic masses. Cancer. 2003 May 1;97(9):2137-41. PMID: 12712464.

1585. Charlot M, Seldin DC, O'Hara C, et al. Localized amyloidosis of the breast: a case series. Amyloid. 2011 Jun;18(2):72-5. PMID: 21501022.

1586. Chen J, Yao Q, Li D, et al. Neoadjuvant rh-endostatin, docetaxel and epirubicin for breast cancer: efficacy and safety in a prospective, randomized, phase II study. BMC Cancer. 2013 May 21;13(1):248. PMID: 23693018.

1587. Chen X, Sun L, Mao Y, et al. Preoperative core needle biopsy is accurate in determining molecular subtypes in invasive breast cancer. BMC Cancer. 2013;13:390. PMID: 23957561.

1588. Cheng TY, Chen CM, Lee MY, et al. Risk factors associated with conversion from nonmalignant to malignant diagnosis after surgical excision of breast papillary lesions. Ann Surg Oncol. 2009 Dec;16(12):3375-9. PMID: 19641969.

1589. Cherrington BD, Mohanan S, Diep AN, et al. Comparative analysis of peptidylarginine deiminase-2 expression in canine, feline and human mammary tumours. J Comp Pathol. 2012 Aug-Oct;147(2-3):139-46. PMID: 22520816.

1590. Cheung YC, Wan YL, Lo YF, et al. Preoperative magnetic resonance imaging evaluation for breast cancers after sonographically guided core-needle biopsy: a comparison study. Ann Surg Oncol. 2004 Aug;11(8):756-61. PMID: 15289239.

1591. Chiesa J, Ferrer C, Arnould C, et al. Autocrine proliferative effects of hGH are maintained in primary cultures of human mammary carcinoma cells. J Clin Endocrinol Metab. 2011 Sep;96(9):E1418-26. PMID: 21733992.

1592. Chin-Lenn L, Mack LA, Temple W, et al. Predictors of treatment with mastectomy, use of sentinel lymph node biopsy and upstaging to invasive cancer in patients diagnosed with breast ductal carcinoma in situ (DCIS) on core biopsy. Ann Surg Oncol. 2014 Jan;21(1):66-73. PMID: 24046105.

1593. Chintamani, Tandon M, Mishra A, et al. Sentinel lymph node biopsy using dye alone method is reliable and accurate even after neo-adjuvant chemotherapy in locally advanced breast cancer--a prospective study. World J Surg Oncol. 2011;9:19. PMID: 21396137.

1594. Chivukula M, Bhargava R, Brufsky A, et al. Clinical importance of HER2 immunohistologic heterogeneous expression in core-needle biopsies vs resection specimens for equivocal (immunohistochemical score 2+) cases. Mod Pathol. 2008 Apr;21(4):363-8. PMID: 18246053.

1595. Chivukula M, Bhargava R, Tseng G, et al. Clinicopathologic implications of "flat epithelial atypia" in core needle biopsy specimens of the breast. Am J Clin Pathol. 2009 Jun;131(6):802-8. PMID: 19461086.

1596. Chivukula M, Haynik DM, Brufsky A, et al. Pleomorphic lobular carcinoma in situ (PLCIS) on breast core needle biopsies: clinical significance and immunoprofile. Am J Surg Pathol. 2008 Nov;32(11):1721-6. PMID: 18769331.

1597. Chivukula M, Striebel JM, Ersahin C, et al. Evaluation of morphologic features to identify "basal-like phenotype" on core needle biopsies of breast. Appl Immunohistochem Mol Morphol. 2008 Oct;16(5):411-6. PMID: 18542031.

1598. Cho N, Moon WK, Chang JM, et al. Ultrasonography-guided vacuum-assisted biopsy of microcalcifications: Comparison of the diagnostic yield of calcified cores and non-calcified cores on specimen radiographs. Acta Radiol. 2010 Mar;51(2):123-7. PMID: 19912076.

1599. Cho N, Moon WK, Chang JM, et al. Sonoelastographic lesion stiffness: preoperative predictor of the presence of an invasive focus in nonpalpable DCIS diagnosed at US-guided needle biopsy. Eur Radiol. 2011 Aug;21(8):1618-27. PMID: 21400103.

1600. Choi J, Koo JS. Comparative study of histological features between core needle biopsy and surgical excision in phyllodes tumor. Pathol Int. 2012 Feb;62(2):120-6. PMID: 22243782.

1601. Choi JS, Baek HM, Kim S, et al. HR-MAS MR spectroscopy of breast cancer tissue obtained with core needle biopsy: correlation with prognostic factors. PLoS One. 2012;7(12):e51712. PMID: 23272149.

1602. Choi YJ, Ko EY, Kook S. Diagnosis of pseudoangiomatous stromal hyperplasia of the breast: ultrasonography findings and different biopsy methods. Yonsei Med J. 2008 Oct 31;49(5):757-64. PMID: 18972596.

1603. Choi YJ, Shin YD, Kang YH, et al. The Effects of Preoperative (18)F-FDG PET/CT in Breast Cancer Patients in Comparison to the Conventional Imaging Study. J Breast Cancer. 2012 Dec;15(4):441-8. PMID: 23346174.

1604. Chung J, Son EJ, Kim JA, et al. Giant phyllodes tumors of the breast: imaging findings with clinicopathological correlation in 14 cases. Clin Imaging. 2011 Mar-Apr;35(2):102-7. PMID: 21377047.

1605. Chuthapisith S, Bean BE, Cowley G, et al. Annexins in human breast cancer: Possible predictors of pathological response to neoadjuvant chemotherapy. Eur J Cancer. 2009 May;45(7):1274-81. PMID: 19171478.

1606. Ciatto S, Houssami N. Breast imaging and needle biopsy in women with clinically evident breast cancer: does combined imaging change overall diagnostic sensitivity? Breast. 2007 Aug;16(4):382-6. PMID: 17350262.

1607. Ciocchetti JM, Joy N, Staller S, et al. The effect of magnetic resonance imaging in the workup of breast cancer. Am J Surg. 2009 Dec;198(6):824-8. PMID: 19969136.

1608. Clark CJ, Wechter D. Morphea of the breast--an uncommon cause of breast erythema. Am J Surg. 2010 Jul;200(1):173-6. PMID: 20637350.

1609. Coffey JP, Hill JC. Breast sentinel node imaging with low-dose SPECT/CT. Nucl Med Commun. 2010 Feb;31(2):107-11. PMID: 19966597.

1610. Colleoni M, Viale G, Zahrieh D, et al. Expression of ER, PgR, HER1, HER2, and response: a study of preoperative chemotherapy. Ann Oncol. 2008 Mar;19(3):465-72. PMID: 17986623.

1611. Collins LC, Wang Y, Connolly JL, et al. Potential role of tissue microarrays for the study of biomarker expression in benign breast disease and normal breast tissue. Appl Immunohistochem Mol Morphol. 2009 Oct;17(5):438-41. PMID: 19363445.

1612. Connor CS, Tawfik OW, Joyce AJ, et al. A comparison of prognostic tumor markers obtained on image-guided breast biopsies and final surgical specimens. Am J Surg. 2002 Oct;184(4):322-4. PMID: 12383893.

1613. Corben AD, Abi-Raad R, Popa I, et al. Pathologic response and long-term follow-up in breast cancer patients treated with neoadjuvant chemotherapy: a comparison between classifications and their practical application. Arch Pathol Lab Med. 2013 Aug;137(8):1074-82. PMID: 23899063.

1614. Cote ML, Ruterbusch JJ, Alosh B, et al. Benign breast disease and the risk of subsequent breast cancer in African American women. Cancer Prev Res (Phila). 2012 Dec;5(12):1375-80. PMID: 23087047.

1615. Crowe JP, Patrick RJ, Rim A. The importance of preoperative breast MRI for patients newly diagnosed with breast cancer. Breast J. 2009 Jan-Feb;15(1):52-60. PMID: 19141134.

1616. Cyr AE, Novack D, Trinkaus K, et al. Are we overtreating papillomas diagnosed on core needle biopsy? Ann Surg Oncol. 2011 Apr;18(4):946-51. PMID: 21046266.

1617. da Silva BB, dos Santos AR, Pires CG, et al. Effect of raloxifene on vascular endothelial growth factor expression in breast carcinomas of postmenopausal women. Cell Prolif. 2009 Aug;42(4):506-10. PMID: 19489979.

1618. Daidone MG, Orefice S, Mastore M, et al. Comparing core needle to surgical biopsies in breast cancer for cell kinetic and ploidy studies. Breast Cancer Res Treat. 1991 Sep;19(1):33-7. PMID: 1756265.

1619. D'Alfonso T, Liu YF, Monni S, et al. Accurately assessing her-2/neu status in needle core biopsies of breast cancer patients in the era of neoadjuvant therapy: emerging questions and considerations addressed. Am J Surg Pathol. 2010 Apr;34(4):575-81. PMID: 20216378.

1620. D'Alfonso TM, Wang K, Chiu YL, et al. Pathologic upgrade rates on subsequent excision when lobular carcinoma in situ is the primary diagnosis in the needle core biopsy with special attention to the radiographic target. Arch Pathol Lab Med. 2013 Jul;137(7):927-35. PMID: 23808465.

1621. Darvishian F, Singh B, Simsir A, et al. Atypia on breast core needle biopsies: reproducibility and significance. Ann Clin Lab Sci. 2009 Summer;39(3):270-6. PMID: 19667411.

1622. Dayton A, Soot L, Wolf R, et al. Light-guided lumpectomy: first clinical experience. J Biophotonics. 2011 Oct;4(10):752-8. PMID: 21956998.

1623. de Beca FF, Rasteiro C, Correia A, et al. Improved malignancy prediction by B3 breast lesions subclassification. Ann Diagn Pathol. 2013 Oct;17(5):434-6. PMID: 23773891.

1624. de Cremoux P, Martin EC, Vincent-Salomon A, et al. Quantitative PCR analysis of c-erb B-2 (HER2/neu) gene amplification and comparison with p185(HER2/neu) protein expression in breast cancer drill biopsies. Int J Cancer. 1999 Oct 8;83(2):157-61. PMID: 10471520.

1625. De Felice C, Cipolla V, Stagnitti A, et al. The impact of presurgical magnetic resonance in early breast cancer: an observational study. Eur J Gynaecol Oncol. 2012;33(2):193-9. PMID: 22611962.

1626. Dede DS, Gumuskaya B, Guler G, et al. Evaluation of changes of biologic markers ER, PR, HER 2 and Ki-67 in breast cancer with administration of neoadjuvant dose-dense doxorubicin, cyclophosphamide followed by paclitaxel. J BUON. 2013 Jan-Mar;18(1):57-63. PMID: 23613389.

1627. DeMartini WB, Hanna L, Gatsonis C, et al. Evaluation of tissue sampling methods used for MRI-detected contralateral breast lesions in the American College of Radiology Imaging Network 6667 trial. AJR Am J Roentgenol. 2012 Sep;199(3):W386-91. PMID: 22915431.

1628. Dennis MA, Parker S, Kaske TI, et al. Incidental treatment of nipple discharge caused by benign intraductal papilloma through diagnostic Mammotome biopsy. AJR Am J Roentgenol. 2000 May;174(5):1263-8. PMID: 10789774.

1629. Deshaies I, Provencher L, Jacob S, et al. Factors associated with upgrading to malignancy at surgery of atypical ductal hyperplasia diagnosed on core biopsy. Breast. 2011 Feb;20(1):50-5. PMID: 20619647.

1630. Destounis SV, Murphy PF, Seifert PJ, et al. Management of patients diagnosed with lobular carcinoma in situ at needle core biopsy at a community-based outpatient facility. AJR Am J Roentgenol. 2012 Feb;198(2):281-7. PMID: 22268169.

1631. Dey P, Logasundaram R, Joshi K. Artificial neural network in diagnosis of lobular carcinoma of breast in fine-needle aspiration cytology. Diagn Cytopathol. 2013 Feb;41(2):102-6. PMID: 21987420.

1632. Di Loreto C, Puglisi F, Rimondi G, et al. Large core biopsy for diagnostic and prognostic evaluation of invasive breast carcinomas. Eur J Cancer. 1996 Sep;32A(10):1693-700. PMID: 8983276.

1633. Di Saverio S, Catena F, Santini D, et al. 259 Patients with DCIS of the breast applying USC/Van Nuys prognostic index: a retrospective review with long term follow up. Breast Cancer Res Treat. 2008 Jun;109(3):405-16. PMID: 17687650.

1634. Diepstraten SC, van de Ven SM, Pijnappel RM, et al. Development and evaluation of a prediction model for underestimated invasive breast cancer in women with ductal carcinoma in situ at stereotactic large core needle biopsy. PLoS One. 2013;8(10):e77826. PMID: 24147085.

1635. Dogan L, Gulcelik MA, Yuksel M, et al. Wire-guided localization biopsy to determine surgical margin status in patients with non-palpable suspicious breast lesions. Asian Pac J Cancer Prev. 2012;13(10):4989-92. PMID: 23244096.

1636. Domeyer PJ, Sergentanis TN, Zagouri F, et al. Health-related quality of life in vacuum-assisted breast biopsy: short-term effects, long-term effects and predictors. Health Qual Life Outcomes. 2010;8:11. PMID: 20102642.

1637. Domingo L, Romero A, Blanch J, et al. Clinical and radiological features of breast tumors according to history of false-positive results in mammography screening. Cancer Epidemiol. 2013 Oct;37(5):660-5. PMID: 23962702.

1638. Dominici L, Liao GS, Brock J, et al. Large needle core biopsy of atypical ductal hyperplasia: results of surgical excision. Breast J. 2012 Sep;18(5):506-8. PMID: 22897750.

1639. dos Santos LG, da Silva BB. The effect of raloxifene on telomerase expression in breast carcinoma samples from postmenopausal women. Eur J Obstet Gynecol Reprod Biol. 2011 Nov;159(1):165-7. PMID: 21741149.

1640. Douglas-Jones AG, Collett N, Morgan JM, et al. Comparison of core oestrogen receptor (ER) assay with excised tumour: intratumoral distribution of ER in breast carcinoma. J Clin Pathol. 2001 Dec;54(12):951-5. PMID: 11729216.

1641. Doyle B, Al-Mudhaffer M, Kennedy MM, et al. Sentinel lymph node biopsy in patients with a needle core biopsy diagnosis of ductal carcinoma in situ: is it justified? J Clin Pathol. 2009 Jun;62(6):534-8. PMID: 19190009.

1642. Dragun AE, Jenrette JM, Ackerman SJ, et al. Mammographic surveillance after MammoSite breast brachytherapy: analysis of architectural patterns and additional interventions. Am J Clin Oncol. 2007 Dec;30(6):574-9. PMID: 18091050.

1643. Drev P, Grazio SF, Bracko M. Tissue microarrays for routine diagnostic assessment of HER2 status in breast carcinoma. Appl Immunohistochem Mol Morphol. 2008 Mar;16(2):179-84. PMID: 18227723.

1644. Dudley DJ, Drake J, Quinlan J, et al. Beneficial effects of a combined navigator/promotora approach for Hispanic women diagnosed with breast abnormalities. Cancer Epidemiol Biomarkers Prev. 2012 Oct;21(10):1639-44. PMID: 23045538.

1645. Dunbier AK, Anderson H, Ghazoui Z, et al. Relationship between plasma estradiol levels and estrogen-responsive gene expression in estrogen receptor-positive breast cancer in postmenopausal women. J Clin Oncol. 2010 Mar 1;28(7):1161-7. PMID: 20124184.

1646. Dundar MM, Badve S, Bilgin G, et al. Computerized classification of intraductal breast lesions using histopathological images. IEEE Trans Biomed Eng. 2011 Jul;58(7):1977-84. PMID: 21296703.

1647. Dutra I, Nassif H, Page D, et al. Integrating machine learning and physician knowledge to improve the accuracy of breast biopsy. AMIA Annu Symp Proc. 2011;2011:349-55. PMID: 22195087.

1648. Eby PR, Calhoun KE, Kurland BF, et al. Preoperative and intraoperative sonographic visibility of collagen-based breast biopsy marker clips. Acad Radiol. 2010 Mar;17(3):340-7. PMID: 20042350.

1649. Eby PR, Ochsner JE, DeMartini WB, et al. Frequency and upgrade rates of atypical ductal hyperplasia diagnosed at stereotactic vacuum-assisted breast biopsy: 9-versus 11-gauge. AJR Am J Roentgenol. 2009 Jan;192(1):229-34. PMID: 19098204.

1650. Edeiken-Monroe BS, Monroe DP, Monroe BJ, et al. Metastases to intramammary lymph nodes in patients with breast cancer: sonographic findings. J Clin Ultrasound. 2008 Jun;36(5):279-85. PMID: 18366093.

1651. Edelweiss M, Corben AD, Liberman L, et al. Focal extravasated mucin in breast core needle biopsies: is surgical excision always necessary? Breast J. 2013 May-Jun;19(3):302-9. PMID: 23534893.

1652. Edwards HD, Oakley F, Koyama T, et al. The impact of tumor size in breast needle biopsy material on final pathologic size and tumor stage: a detailed analysis of 222 consecutive cases. Am J Surg Pathol. 2013 May;37(5):739-44. PMID: 23552386.

1653. Ekmekcioglu O, Aliyev A, Yilmaz S, et al. Correlation of 18F-fluorodeoxyglucose uptake with histopathological prognostic factors in breast carcinoma. Nucl Med Commun. 2013 Nov;34(11):1055-67. PMID: 24025919.

1654. El-Sayed ME, Rakha EA, Reed J, et al. Predictive value of needle core biopsy diagnoses of lesions of uncertain malignant potential (B3) in abnormalities detected by mammographic screening. Histopathology. 2008 Dec;53(6):650-7. PMID: 19076681.

1655. El-Shinawi M, Abdelwahab SF, Sobhy M, et al. Capturing and characterizing immune cells from breast tumor microenvironment: an innovative surgical approach. Ann Surg Oncol. 2010 Oct;17(10):2677-84. PMID: 20333554.

1656. El-Sibai MF, Cohen C, Nassar A, et al. Predictive markers in primary breast cancer compared with lymph node and bloodspread metastases. Int J Physiol Pathophysiol Pharmacol. 2009;1(1):57-63. PMID: 21383878.

1657. El-Tamer M, Axiotis C, Kim E, et al. Accurate prediction of the amount of in situ tumor in palpable breast cancers by core needle biopsy: implications for neoadjuvant therapy. Ann Surg Oncol. 1999 Jul-Aug;6(5):461-6. PMID: 10458684.

1658. Erggelet J, Grosse R, Holzhausen H, et al. Correlation of human epidermal growth factor receptor 2 (HER2), estrogen receptor (ER), and progesterone receptor (PR) expression as predicted by core biopsy with the immunohistochemical results of surgical breast cancer specimens. Breast Care. 2007;2(2):94-8.

1659. Erozgen F, Ersoy YE, Akaydin M, et al. Corticosteroid treatment and timing of surgery in idiopathic granulomatous mastitis confusing with breast carcinoma. Breast Cancer Res Treat. 2010 Sep;123(2):447-52. PMID: 20625813.

1660. Fan XC, Nemoto T, Blatto K, et al. Impact of presurgical breast magnetic resonance imaging (MRI) on surgical planning - a retrospective analysis from a private radiology group. Breast J. 2013 Mar-Apr;19(2):134-41. PMID: 23294216.

1661. Fancellu A, Soro D, Castiglia P, et al. Usefulness of magnetic resonance in patients with invasive cancer eligible for breast conservation: a comparative study. Clin Breast Cancer. 2014 Apr;14(2):114-21. PMID: 24321101.

1662. Farshid G, Downey P, Gill P, et al. Assessment of 1183 screen-detected, category 3B, circumscribed masses by cytology and core biopsy with long-term follow up data. Br J Cancer. 2008 Apr 8;98(7):1182-90. PMID: 18382460.

1663. Farshid G, Walker A, Battersby G, et al. Predictors of malignancy in screen-detected breast masses with indeterminate/equivocal (grade 3) imaging features. Breast. 2011 Feb;20(1):56-61. PMID: 20691591.

1664. Fatakdawala H, Xu J, Basavanhally A, et al. Expectation-maximization-driven geodesic active contour with overlap resolution (EMaGACOR): application to lymphocyte segmentation on breast cancer histopathology. IEEE Trans Biomed Eng. 2010 Jul;57(7):1676-89. PMID: 20172780.

1665. Fedewa SA, Edge SB, Stewart AK, et al. Race and ethnicity are associated with delays in breast cancer treatment (2003-2006). J Health Care Poor Underserved. 2011 Feb;22(1):128-41. PMID: 21317511.

1666. Feldman SM, Krag DN, McNally RK, et al. Limitation in gamma probe localization of the sentinel node in breast cancer patients with large excisional biopsy. J Am Coll Surg. 1999 Mar;188(3):248-54. PMID: 10065813.

1667. Ferreira M, Albarracin CT, Resetkova E. Pseudoangiomatous stromal hyperplasia tumor: a clinical, radiologic and pathologic study of 26 cases. Mod Pathol. 2008 Feb;21(2):201-7. PMID: 18084246.

1668. Fillion MM, Black EA, Hudson KB, et al. The effect of multiple wire localization in breast conservation. Am Surg. 2012 May;78(5):519-22. PMID: 22546121.

1669. Fine RE, Staren ED. Percutaneous radiofrequency-assisted excision of fibroadenomas. Am J Surg. 2006 Oct;192(4):545-7. PMID: 16978972.

1670. Flegg KM, Flaherty JJ, Bicknell AM, et al. Surgical outcomes of borderline breast lesions detected by needle biopsy in a breast screening program. World J Surg Oncol. 2010;8:78. PMID: 20822548.

1671. Forghani MN, Memar B, Jangjoo A, et al. The effect of excisional biopsy on the accuracy of sentinel lymph node mapping in early stage breast cancer: comparison with core needle biopsy. Am Surg. 2010 Nov;76(11):1232-5. PMID: 21140690.

1672. Friedman PD, Sanders LM, Menendez C, et al. Retrieval of lost microcalcifications during stereotactic vacuum-assisted core biopsy. AJR Am J Roentgenol. 2003 Jan;180(1):275-80. PMID: 12490519.

1673. Fu CY, Chen TW, Hong ZJ, et al. Papillary breast lesions diagnosed by core biopsy require complete excision. Eur J Surg Oncol. 2012 Nov;38(11):1029-35. PMID: 22959140.

1674. Fuehrer N, Hartmann L, Degnim A, et al. Atypical apocrine adenosis of the breast: long-term follow-up in 37 patients. Arch Pathol Lab Med. 2012 Feb;136(2):179-82. PMID: 22288965.

1675. Gadre SA, Perkins GH, Sahin AA, et al. Neovascularization in mucinous ductal carcinoma in situ suggests an alternative pathway for invasion. Histopathology. 2008 Nov;53(5):545-53. PMID: 18983463.

1676. Gao F, Carter G, Tseng G, et al. Clinical importance of histologic grading of lobular carcinoma in situ in breast core needle biopsy specimens: current issues and controversies. Am J Clin Pathol. 2010 May;133(5):767-71. PMID: 20395524.

1677. Garcia-Manero M, Olartecoechea B, Royo P. Different injection sites of radionuclide for sentinel lymph node detection in breast cancer: single institution experience. Eur J Obstet Gynecol Reprod Biol. 2010 Dec;153(2):185-7. PMID: 20702018.

1678. Garg S, Mohan H, Bal A, et al. A comparative analysis of core needle biopsy and fine-needle aspiration cytology in the evaluation of palpable and mammographically detected suspicious breast lesions. Diagn Cytopathol. 2007 Nov;35(11):681-9. PMID: 17924407.

1679. Garwood ER, Kumar AS, Baehner FL, et al. Fluvastatin reduces proliferation and increases apoptosis in women with high grade breast cancer. Breast Cancer Res Treat. 2010 Jan;119(1):137-44. PMID: 19728082.

1680. Gautier N, Lalonde L, Tran-Thanh D, et al. Chronic granulomatous mastitis: Imaging, pathology and management. Eur J Radiol. 2013 Apr;82(4):e165-75. PMID: 23200627.

1681. Gazic B, Pizem J, Bracko M, et al. S-phase fraction determined on fine needle aspirates is an independent prognostic factor in breast cancer - a multivariate study of 770 patients. Cytopathology. 2008 Oct;19(5):294-302. PMID: 18070112.

1682. Gemignani ML, Patil S, Seshan VE, et al. Feasibility and predictability of perioperative PET and estrogen receptor ligand in patients with invasive breast cancer. J Nucl Med. 2013 Oct;54(10):1697-702. PMID: 23970364.

1683. Gerloff A, Dittmer A, Oerlecke I, et al. Protein expression of the Ets transcription factor Elf-1 in breast cancer cells is negatively correlated with histological grading, but not with clinical outcome. Oncol Rep. 2011 Nov;26(5):1121-5. PMID: 21811762.

1684. Germano S, Kennedy S, Rani S, et al. MAGE-D4B is a novel marker of poor prognosis and potential therapeutic target involved in breast cancer tumorigenesis. Int J Cancer. 2012 May 1;130(9):1991-2002. PMID: 21618523.

1685. Gill HK, Ioffe OB, Berg WA. When is a diagnosis of sclerosing adenosis acceptable at core biopsy? Radiology. 2003 Jul;228(1):50-7. PMID: 12738875.

1686. Giskeodegard GF, Lundgren S, Sitter B, et al. Lactate and glycine-potential MR biomarkers of prognosis in estrogen receptor-positive breast cancers. NMR Biomed. 2012 Nov;25(11):1271-9. PMID: 22407957.

1687. Glazebrook KN, Reynolds C, Smith RL, et al. Adenoid cystic carcinoma of the breast. AJR Am J Roentgenol. 2010 May;194(5):1391-6. PMID: 20410430.

1688. Go EM, Chan SK, Vong JS, et al. Predictors of invasion in needle core biopsies of the breast with ductal carcinoma in situ. Mod Pathol. 2010 May;23(5):737-42. PMID: 20081814.

1689. Gobbi H, Tse G, Page DL, et al. Reactive spindle cell nodules of the breast after core biopsy or fine-needle aspiration. Am J Clin Pathol. 2000 Feb;113(2):288-94. PMID: 10664632.

1690. Godinez J, Gombos EC, Chikarmane SA, et al. Breast MRI in the evaluation of eligibility for accelerated partial breast irradiation. AJR Am J Roentgenol. 2008 Jul;191(1):272-7. PMID: 18562758.

1691. Golshan M, Fung BB, Wiley E, et al. Prediction of breast cancer size by ultrasound, mammography and core biopsy. Breast. 2004 Aug;13(4):265-71. PMID: 15325659.

1692. Goto M, Yuen S, Akazawa K, et al. The role of breast MR imaging in pre-operative determination of invasive disease for ductal carcinoma in situ diagnosed by needle biopsy. Eur Radiol. 2012 Jun;22(6):1255-64. PMID: 22205445.

1693. Gould DJ, Salmans JA, Lassinger BK, et al. Factors associated with phyllodes tumor of the breast after core needle biopsy identifies fibroepithelial neoplasm. J Surg Res. 2012 Nov;178(1):299-303. PMID: 22524977.

1694. Govindarajulu S, Narreddy S, Shere MH, et al. Preoperative mammotome biopsy of ducts beneath the nipple areola complex. Eur J Surg Oncol. 2006 May;32(4):410-2. PMID: 16516432.

1695. Grady I, Gorsuch-Rafferty H, Hadley P. Preoperative staging with magnetic resonance imaging, with confirmatory biopsy, improves surgical outcomes in women with breast cancer without increasing rates of mastectomy. Breast J. 2012 May-Jun;18(3):214-8. PMID: 22487017.

1696. Graesslin O, Antoine M, Chopier J, et al. Histology after lumpectomy in women with epithelial atypia on stereotactic vacuum-assisted breast biopsy. Eur J Surg Oncol. 2010 Feb;36(2):170-5. PMID: 19811884.

1697. Greco FA, Spigel DR, Yardley DA, et al. Molecular profiling in unknown primary cancer: accuracy of tissue of origin prediction. Oncologist. 2010;15(5):500-6. PMID: 20427384.

1698. Green S, Khalkhali I, Azizollahi E, et al. Excisional biopsy of borderline lesions after large bore vacuum-assisted core needle biopsy- is it necessary? Am Surg. 2011 Oct;77(10):1358-60. PMID: 22127088.

1699. Greer LT, Rosman M, Mylander WC, et al. Does breast tumor heterogeneity necessitate further immunohistochemical staining on surgical specimens? J Am Coll Surg. 2013 Feb;216(2):239-51. PMID: 23141136.

1700. Greif F, Sharon E, Shechtman I, et al. Carcinoma within solitary ductal papilloma of the breast. Eur J Surg Oncol. 2010 Apr;36(4):384-6. PMID: 19646841.

1701. Gresik CM, Godellas C, Aranha GV, et al. Pseudoangiomatous stromal hyperplasia of the breast: a contemporary approach to its clinical and radiologic features and ideal management. Surgery. 2010 Oct;148(4):752-7; discussion 7-8. PMID: 20708765.

1702. Grin A, O'Malley FP, Mulligan AM. Cytokeratin 5 and estrogen receptor immunohistochemistry as a useful adjunct in identifying atypical papillary lesions on breast needle core biopsy. Am J Surg Pathol. 2009 Nov;33(11):1615-23. PMID: 19675450.

1703. Groheux D, Giacchetti S, Moretti JL, et al. Correlation of high 18F-FDG uptake to clinical, pathological and biological prognostic factors in breast cancer. Eur J Nucl Med Mol Imaging. 2011 Mar;38(3):426-35. PMID: 21057787.

1704. Gunalp B, Ince S, Karacalioglu AO, et al. Clinical impact of (18)F-FDG PET/CT on initial staging and therapy planning for breast cancer. Exp Ther Med. 2012 Oct;4(4):693-8. PMID: 23170128.

1705. Gutierrez RL, DeMartini WB, Silbergeld JJ, et al. High cancer yield and positive predictive value: outcomes at a center routinely using preoperative breast MRI for staging. AJR Am J Roentgenol. 2011 Jan;196(1):W93-9. PMID: 21178040.

1706. Hahn M, Okamgba S, Scheler P, et al. Vacuum-assisted breast biopsy: a comparison of 11-gauge and 8-gauge needles in benign breast disease. World J Surg Oncol. 2008;6:51. PMID: 18489771.

1707. Haigh PI, Hansen NM, Qi K, et al. Biopsy method and excision volume do not affect success rate of subsequent sentinel lymph node dissection in breast cancer. Ann Surg Oncol. 2000 Jan-Feb;7(1):21-7. PMID: 10674444.

1708. Haj M, Loberant N, Salamon V, et al. Membranous fat necrosis of the breast: diagnosis by minimally invasive technique. Breast J. 2004 Nov-Dec;10(6):504-8. PMID: 15569206.

1709. Han JS, Molberg KH, Sarode V. Predictors of invasion and axillary lymph node metastasis in patients with a core biopsy diagnosis of ductal carcinoma in situ: an analysis of 255 cases. Breast J. 2011 May-Jun;17(3):223-9. PMID: 21545433.

1710. Hanley C, Kessaram R. Quality of diagnosis and surgical management of breast lesions in a community hospital: room for improvement? Can J Surg. 2006 Jun;49(3):185-92. PMID: 16749979.

1711. Hanley KZ, Birdsong GG, Cohen C, et al. Immunohistochemical detection of estrogen receptor, progesterone receptor, and human epidermal growth factor receptor 2 expression in breast carcinomas: comparison on cell block, needle-core, and tissue block preparations. Cancer. 2009 Aug 25;117(4):279-88. PMID: 19551847.

1712. Harada S, Mick R, Roses RE, et al. The significance of HER-2/neu receptor positivity and immunophenotype in ductal carcinoma in situ with early invasive disease. J Surg Oncol. 2011 Oct;104(5):458-65. PMID: 21557226.

1713. Haraldsdottir KH, Ivarsson K, Gotberg S, et al. Interstitial laser thermotherapy (ILT) of breast cancer. Eur J Surg Oncol. 2008 Jul;34(7):739-45. PMID: 18291614.

1714. Hargaden GC, Yeh ED, Georgian-Smith D, et al. Analysis of the mammographic and sonographic features of pseudoangiomatous stromal hyperplasia. AJR Am J Roentgenol. 2008 Aug;191(2):359-63. PMID: 18647902.

1715. Harris GC, Denley HE, Pinder SE, et al. Correlation of histologic prognostic factors in core biopsies and therapeutic excisions of invasive breast carcinoma. Am J Surg Pathol. 2003 Jan;27(1):11-5. PMID: 12502923.

1716. Harrison RL, Britton P, Warren R, et al. Can we be sure about a radiological diagnosis of fat necrosis of the breast? Clin Radiol. 2000 Feb;55(2):119-23. PMID: 10657157.

1717. Hasebe T, Tamura N, Iwasaki M, et al. Grading system for lymph vessel tumor emboli: significant outcome predictor for patients with invasive ductal carcinoma of the breast who received neoadjuvant therapy. Mod Pathol. 2010 Apr;23(4):581-92. PMID: 20118911.

1718. Hayes BD, O'Doherty A, Quinn CM. Correlation of needle core biopsy with excision histology in screen-detected B3 lesions: the Merrion Breast Screening Unit experience. J Clin Pathol. 2009 Dec;62(12):1136-40. PMID: 19946101.

1719. Hedayati E, Schedin A, Nyman H, et al. The effects of breast cancer diagnosis and surgery on cognitive functions. Acta Oncol. 2011 Oct;50(7):1027-36. PMID: 21554027.

1720. Heudel P, Cimarelli S, Montella A, et al. Value of PET-FDG in primary breast cancer based on histopathological and immunohistochemical prognostic factors. Int J Clin Oncol. 2010 Dec;15(6):588-93. PMID: 20809217.

1721. Hiraike H, Wada-Hiraike O, Nakagawa S, et al. Expression of DBC1 is associated with nuclear grade and HER2 expression in breast cancer. Exp Ther Med. 2011 Nov;2(6):1105-9. PMID: 22977628.

1722. Hoang JK, Hill P, Cawson JN. Can mammographic findings help discriminate between atypical ductal hyperplasia and ductal carcinoma in situ after needle core biopsy? Breast. 2008 Jun;17(3):282-8. PMID: 18063369.

1723. Holley SO, Appleton CM, Farria DM, et al. Pathologic outcomes of nonmalignant papillary breast lesions diagnosed at imaging-guided core needle biopsy. Radiology. 2012 Nov;265(2):379-84. PMID: 22952379.

1724. Hollingsworth AB, Stough RG. Multicentric and contralateral invasive tumors identified with pre-op MRI in patients newly diagnosed with ductal carcinoma in situ of the breast. Breast J. 2012 Sep;18(5):420-7. PMID: 22804792.

1725. Holmes DR, Silverstein MJ. A minimally invasive breast biopsy clinic: an innovative way to teach breast fellows how to perform breast ultrasound and ultrasound-guided breast procedures. Am J Surg. 2006 Oct;192(4):439-43. PMID: 16978945.

1726. Hong ZJ, Chu CH, Fan HL, et al. Factors predictive of breast cancer in open biopsy in cases with atypical ductal hyperplasia diagnosed by ultrasound-guided core needle biopsy. Eur J Surg Oncol. 2011 Sep;37(9):758-64. PMID: 21764539.

1727. Horiguchi K, Toi M, Horiguchi S, et al. Predictive value of CD24 and CD44 for neoadjuvant chemotherapy response and prognosis in primary breast cancer patients. J Med Dent Sci. 2010 Jun;57(2):165-75. PMID: 21073135.

1728. Horimoto Y, Tokuda E, Arakawa A, et al. Significance of HER2 protein examination in ductal carcinoma in situ. J Surg Res. 2011 May 15;167(2):e205-10. PMID: 20018297.

1729. Houssami N, Ambrogetti D, Marinovich ML, et al. Accuracy of a preoperative model for predicting invasive breast cancer in women with ductal carcinoma-in-situ on vacuum-assisted core needle biopsy. Ann Surg Oncol. 2011 May;18(5):1364-71. PMID: 21107741.

1730. Houssami N, Ciatto S, Ellis I, et al. Underestimation of malignancy of breast core-needle biopsy: concepts and precise overall and category-specific estimates. Cancer. 2007 Feb 1;109(3):487-95. PMID: 17186530.

1731. Hovanessian Larsen LJ, Peyvandi B, Klipfel N, et al. Granulomatous lobular mastitis: imaging, diagnosis, and treatment. AJR Am J Roentgenol. 2009 Aug;193(2):574-81. PMID: 19620458.

1732. Hsu HH, Yu JC, Hsu GC, et al. Atypical ductal hyperplasia of the breast diagnosed by ultrasonographically guided core needle biopsy. Ultraschall Med. 2012 Oct;33(5):447-54. PMID: 22161618.

1733. Huang CH, Veillard A, Roux L, et al. Time-efficient sparse analysis of histopathological whole slide images. Comput Med Imaging Graph. 2011 Oct-Dec;35(7-8):579-91. PMID: 21145705.

1734. Huang O, Chen C, Wu J, et al. Retrospective analysis of 119 Chinese noninflammatory locally advanced breast cancer cases treated with intravenous combination of vinorelbine and epirubicin as a neoadjuvant chemotherapy: a median follow-up of 63.4 months. BMC Cancer. 2009;9:375. PMID: 19845944.

1735. Huang YT, Cheung YC, Lo YF, et al. MRI findings of cancers preoperatively diagnosed as pure DCIS at core needle biopsy. Acta Radiol. 2011 Dec 1;52(10):1064-8. PMID: 21969708.

1736. Hukkinen K, Kivisaari L, Heikkila PS, et al. Unsuccessful preoperative biopsies, fine needle aspiration cytology or core needle biopsy, lead to increased costs in the diagnostic workup in breast cancer. Acta Oncol. 2008;47(6):1037-45. PMID: 18607862.

1737. Hung WK, Ying M, Chan M, et al. The impact of sentinel lymph node biopsy in patients with a core biopsy diagnosis of ductal carcinoma in situ. Breast Cancer. 2010 Oct;17(4):276-80. PMID: 19756924.

1738. Hunt RJ, Steel JR, Porter GJ, et al. Lesions of uncertain malignant potential (B3) on core biopsy in the NHS Breast Screening Programme: is the screening round relevant? Ann R Coll Surg Engl. 2012 Mar;94(2):108-11. PMID: 22391380.

1739. Ibrahim N, Bessissow A, Lalonde L, et al. Surgical outcome of biopsy-proven lobular neoplasia: is there any difference between lobular carcinoma in situ and atypical lobular hyperplasia? AJR Am J Roentgenol. 2012 Feb;198(2):288-91. PMID: 22268170.

1740. Ilic I, Randelovic P, Ilic R, et al. An approach to malignant mammary phyllodes tumors detection. Vojnosanit Pregl. 2009 Apr;66(4):277-82. PMID: 19441158.

1741. Ingegnoli A, d'Aloia C, Frattaruolo A, et al. Flat epithelial atypia and atypical ductal hyperplasia: carcinoma underestimation rate. Breast J. 2010 Jan-Feb;16(1):55-9. PMID: 19825003.

1742. Inoue S, Inoue M, Kawasaki T, et al. Six cases showing radial scar/complex sclerosing lesions of the breast detected by breast cancer screening. Breast Cancer. 2008;15(3):247-51. PMID: 18311480.

1743. Inui H, Watatani M, Hashimoto Y, et al. Hematoma-directed and ultrasound-guided breast-conserving surgery for nonpalpable breast cancer after Mammotome biopsy. Surg Today. 2008;38(3):279-82. PMID: 18307007.

1744. Irfan K, Brem RF. Surgical and mammographic follow-up of papillary lesions and atypical lobular hyperplasia diagnosed with stereotactic vacuum-assisted biopsy. Breast J. 2002 Jul-Aug;8(4):230-3. PMID: 12100116.

1745. Itakura K, Lessing J, Sakata T, et al. The impact of preoperative magnetic resonance imaging on surgical treatment and outcomes for ductal carcinoma in situ. Clin Breast Cancer. 2011 Mar;11(1):33-8. PMID: 21421520.

1746. Jackman RJ, Burbank F, Parker SH, et al. Atypical ductal hyperplasia diagnosed at stereotactic breast biopsy: improved reliability with 14-gauge, directional, vacuum-assisted biopsy. Radiology. 1997 Aug;204(2):485-8. PMID: 9240540.

1747. Jackman RJ, Marzoni FA, Jr., Nowels KW. Percutaneous removal of benign mammographic lesions: comparison of automated large-core and directional vacuum-assisted stereotactic biopsy techniques. AJR Am J Roentgenol. 1998 Nov;171(5):1325-30. PMID: 9798873.

1748. Jaffer S, Bleiweiss IJ, Nagi CS. Benign mucocele-like lesions of the breast: revisited. Mod Pathol. 2011 May;24(5):683-7. PMID: 21240257.

1749. Jaffer S, Nagi C, Bleiweiss IJ. Excision is indicated for intraductal papilloma of the breast diagnosed on core needle biopsy. Cancer. 2009 Jul 1;115(13):2837-43. PMID: 19402174.

1750. Jaka RC, Zaveri SS, Somashekhar SP, et al. Value of frozen section and primary tumor factors in determining sentinel lymph node spread in early breast carcinoma. Indian J Surg Oncol. 2010 Jan;1(1):27-36. PMID: 22930615.

1751. Jakate K, De Brot M, Goldberg F, et al. Papillary lesions of the breast: impact of breast pathology subspecialization on core biopsy and excision diagnoses. Am J Surg Pathol. 2012 Apr;36(4):544-51. PMID: 22314186.

1752. James TA, Mace JL, Virnig BA, et al. Preoperative needle biopsy improves the quality of breast cancer surgery. J Am Coll Surg. 2012 Oct;215(4):562-8. PMID: 22726895.

1753. Jimenez RE, Bongers S, Bouwman D, et al. Clinicopathologic significance of ductal carcinoma in situ in breast core needle biopsies with invasive cancer. Am J Surg Pathol. 2000 Jan;24(1):123-8. PMID: 10632496.

1754. Jones RJ, Young O, Renshaw L, et al. Src inhibitors in early breast cancer: a methodology, feasibility and variability study. Breast Cancer Res Treat. 2009 Mar;114(2):211-21. PMID: 18409068.

1755. Jorgensen TJ, Helzlsouer KJ, Clipp SC, et al. DNA repair gene variants associated with benign breast disease in high cancer risk women. Cancer Epidemiol Biomarkers Prev. 2009 Jan;18(1):346-50. PMID: 19124519.

1756. Jung SY, Kang HS, Kwon Y, et al. Risk factors for malignancy in benign papillomas of the breast on core needle biopsy. World J Surg. 2010 Feb;34(2):261-5. PMID: 19997916.

1757. Kadivar M, Monabati A, Joulaee A, et al. Epstein-Barr virus and breast cancer: lack of evidence for an association in Iranian women. Pathol Oncol Res. 2011 Sep;17(3):489-92. PMID: 21207256.

1758. Kalles V, Zografos GC, Provatopoulou X, et al. Circulating levels of endothelin-1 (ET-1) and its precursor (Big ET-1) in breast cancer early diagnosis. Tumour Biol. 2012 Aug;33(4):1231-6. PMID: 22415226.

1759. Kaneko S, Gerasimova T, Butler WM, et al. The use of FISH on breast core needle samples for the presurgical assessment of HER-2 oncogene status. Exp Mol Pathol. 2002 Aug;73(1):61-6. PMID: 12127055.

1760. Kaya H, Ragazzini T, Aribal E, et al. Her-2/neu gene amplification compared with HER-2/neu protein overexpression on ultrasound guided core-needle biopsy specimens of breast carcinoma. Pathol Oncol Res. 2001;7(4):279-83. PMID: 11882907.

1761. Keto JL, Kirstein L, Sanchez DP, et al. MRI versus breast-specific gamma imaging (BSGI) in newly diagnosed ductal cell carcinoma-in-situ: a prospective head-to-head trial. Ann Surg Oncol. 2012 Jan;19(1):249-52. PMID: 21739318.

1762. Khoumais NA, Scaranelo AM, Moshonov H, et al. Incidence of breast cancer in patients with pure flat epithelial atypia diagnosed at core-needle biopsy of the breast. Ann Surg Oncol. 2013 Jan;20(1):133-8. PMID: 23064777.

1763. Khoury T, Zakharia Y, Tan W, et al. Breast hormonal receptors test should be repeated on excisional biopsy after negative core needle biopsy. Breast J. 2011 Mar-Apr;17(2):180-6. PMID: 21306471.

1764. Khout H, Mohiuddin MK, Veeratterapillay R, et al. Breast cancer mimicking fibroadenomas in postmenopausal women. Int J Surg. 2011;9(1):2-4. PMID: 20804869.

1765. Kibil W, Hodorowicz-Zaniewska D, Popiela TJ, et al. Vacuum-assisted core biopsy in diagnosis and treatment of intraductal papillomas. Clin Breast Cancer. 2013 Apr;13(2):129-32. PMID: 23127339.

1766. Killelea BK, Gillego A, Kirstein LJ, et al. George Peters Award: How does breast-specific gamma imaging affect the management of patients with newly diagnosed breast cancer? Am J Surg. 2009 Oct;198(4):470-4. PMID: 19800450.

1767. Killelea BK, Grube BJ, Rishi M, et al. Is the use of preoperative breast MRI predictive of mastectomy? World J Surg Oncol. 2013;11:154. PMID: 23849218.

1768. Kim BS, Moon BI, Cha ES. A comparative study of breast-specific gamma imaging with the conventional imaging modality in breast cancer patients with dense breasts. Ann Nucl Med. 2012 Dec;26(10):823-9. PMID: 22922890.

1769. Kim HS, Seok JH, Cha ES, et al. Significance of nipple enhancement of Paget's disease in contrast enhanced breast MRI. Arch Gynecol Obstet. 2010 Aug;282(2):157-62. PMID: 19838723.

1770. Kim J, Han W, Go EY, et al. Validation of a scoring system for predicting malignancy in patients diagnosed with atypical ductal hyperplasia using an ultrasound-guided core needle biopsy. J Breast Cancer. 2012 Dec;15(4):407-11. PMID: 23346169.

1771. Kim J, Han W, Lee JW, et al. Factors associated with upstaging from ductal carcinoma in situ following core needle biopsy to invasive cancer in subsequent surgical excision. Breast. 2012 Oct;21(5):641-5. PMID: 22749854.

1772. Kim MJ, Kim EK, Kwak JY, et al. Sonographic surveillance for the detection of contralateral metachronous breast cancer in an Asian population. AJR Am J Roentgenol. 2009 Jan;192(1):221-8. PMID: 19098203.

1773. Kim MJ, Kim SI, Youk JH, et al. The diagnosis of non-malignant papillary lesions of the breast: comparison of ultrasound-guided automated gun biopsy and vacuum-assisted removal. Clin Radiol. 2011 Jun;66(6):530-5. PMID: 21353213.

1774. Kim SM, Kim HH, Kang DK, et al. Mucocele-like tumors of the breast as cystic lesions: sonographic-pathologic correlation. AJR Am J Roentgenol. 2011 Jun;196(6):1424-30. PMID: 21606308.

1775. Kim T, Jung EA, Song JY, et al. Prevalence of the CTNNB1 mutation genotype in surgically resected fibromatosis of the breast. Histopathology. 2012 Jan;60(2):347-56. PMID: 22211293.

1776. Kimmick GG, Cirrincione C, Duggan DB, et al. Fifteen-year median follow-up results after neoadjuvant doxorubicin, followed by mastectomy, followed by adjuvant cyclophosphamide, methotrexate, and fluorouracil (CMF) followed by radiation for stage III breast cancer: a phase II trial (CALGB 8944). Breast Cancer Res Treat. 2009 Feb;113(3):479-90. PMID: 18306034.

1777. Kinoshita T, Iwamoto E, Tsuda H, et al. Radiofrequency ablation as local therapy for early breast carcinomas. Breast Cancer. 2011 Jan;18(1):10-7. PMID: 20072824.

1778. Klimberg VS, Boneti C, Adkins LL, et al. Feasibility of percutaneous excision followed by ablation for local control in breast cancer. Ann Surg Oncol. 2011 Oct;18(11):3079-87. PMID: 21904959.

1779. Ko E, Han W, Lee JW, et al. Scoring system for predicting malignancy in patients diagnosed with atypical ductal hyperplasia at ultrasound-guided core needle biopsy. Breast Cancer Res Treat. 2008 Nov;112(1):189-95. PMID: 18060577.

1780. Ko EY, Bae YA, Kim MJ, et al. Factors affecting the efficacy of ultrasound-guided vacuum-assisted percutaneous excision for removal of benign breast lesions. J Ultrasound Med. 2008 Jan;27(1):65-73. PMID: 18096732.

1781. Koh C, Nelson JM, Cook PF. Evaluation of a patient navigation program. Clin J Oncol Nurs. 2011 Feb;15(1):41-8. PMID: 21278040.

1782. Kohr JR, Eby PR, Allison KH, et al. Risk of upgrade of atypical ductal hyperplasia after stereotactic breast biopsy: effects of number of foci and complete removal of calcifications. Radiology. 2010 Jun;255(3):723-30. PMID: 20173103.

1783. Kok KY, Telisinghe PU. Granulomatous mastitis: presentation, treatment and outcome in 43 patients. Surgeon. 2010 Aug;8(4):197-201. PMID: 20569938.

1784. Koo JS, Han K, Kim MJ, et al. Can additional immunohistochemistry staining replace the surgical excision for the diagnosis of papillary breast lesions classified as benign on 14-gage core needle biopsy? Breast Cancer Res Treat. 2013 Feb;137(3):797-806. PMID: 23292118.

1785. Koo JS, Jung W. Xanthogranulomatous mastitis: clinicopathology and pathological implications. Pathol Int. 2009 Apr;59(4):234-40. PMID: 19351366.

1786. Koo JS, Kim MJ, Kim EK, et al. Factors in the breast core needle biopsies of atypical ductal hyperplasia that can predict carcinoma in the subsequent surgical excision specimens. J. Breast Cancer. 2010;13(2):132-7.

1787. Koo JS, Kim MJ, Kim EK, et al. Comparison of immunohistochemical staining in breast papillary neoplasms of cytokeratin 5/6 and p63 in core needle biopsies and surgical excisions. Appl Immunohistochem Mol Morphol. 2012 Mar;20(2):108-15. PMID: 22553810.

1788. Kostopoulos S, Glotsos D, Cavouras D, et al. Computer-based association of the texture of expressed estrogen receptor nuclei with histologic grade using immunohistochemically-stained breast carcinomas. Anal Quant Cytol Histol. 2009 Aug;31(4):187-96. PMID: 19736866.

1789. Krainick-Strobel U, Huber B, Majer I, et al. Complete extirpation of benign breast lesions with an ultrasound-guided vacuum biopsy system. Ultrasound in obstetrics & gynecology. 2007;29(3):342-6.

1790. Kremer ME, Downs-Holmes C, Novak RD, et al. Neglecting to screen women between the ages of 40 and 49 years with mammography: what is the impact on breast cancer diagnosis? AJR Am J Roentgenol. 2012 May;198(5):1218-22. PMID: 22528917.

1791. Kryvenko ON, Chitale DA, VanEgmond EM, et al. Angiolipoma of the female breast: clinicomorphological correlation of 52 cases. Int J Surg Pathol. 2011 Feb;19(1):35-43. PMID: 21087987.

1792. Kundu UR, Guo M, Landon G, et al. Fine-needle aspiration cytology of sclerosing adenosis of the breast: a retrospective review of cytologic features in conjunction with corresponding histologic features and radiologic findings. Am J Clin Pathol. 2012 Jul;138(1):96-102. PMID: 22706864.

1793. Kunju LP, Cookingham C, Toy KA, et al. EZH2 and ALDH-1 mark breast epithelium at risk for breast cancer development. Mod Pathol. 2011 Jun;24(6):786-93. PMID: 21399615.

1794. Kurita T, Tsuchiya S, Watarai Y, et al. Roles of fine-needle aspiration and core needle biopsy in the diagnosis of breast cancer. Breast Cancer. 2012 Jan;19(1):23-9. PMID: 21298376.

1795. Kurniawan ED, Rose A, Mou A, et al. Risk factors for invasive breast cancer when core needle biopsy shows ductal carcinoma in situ. Arch Surg. 2010 Nov;145(11):1098-104. PMID: 21079099.

1796. Kurniawan ED, Wong MH, Windle I, et al. Predictors of surgical margin status in breast-conserving surgery within a breast screening program. Ann Surg Oncol. 2008 Sep;15(9):2542-9. PMID: 18618180.

1797. Kurz KD, Roy S, Saleh A, et al. MRI features of intraductal papilloma of the breast: sheep in wolf's clothing? Acta Radiol. 2011 Apr 1;52(3):264-72. PMID: 21498361.

1798. Kushwaha AC, O'Toole M, Sneige N, et al. Mammographic-pathologic correlation of apocrine metaplasia diagnosed using vacuum-assisted stereotactic core-needle biopsy: our 4-year experience. AJR Am J Roentgenol. 2003 Mar;180(3):795-8. PMID: 12591698.

1799. Kvasnovsky CL, Kesmodel SB, Gragasin JL, et al. Expansion of screening mammography in the Veterans Health Administration: implications for breast cancer treatment. JAMA Surg. 2013 Nov;148(11):999-1004. PMID: 24048217.

1800. Kwok KMK, Lui CY, Fung PYE, et al. Incidence, causes, and implications of unsuccessful calcification retrieval at stereotactic breast biopsy - 5 years' experience. J. HK Coll. Radiol. 2009;11(4):154-60.

1801. Kwok TC, Rakha EA, Lee AH, et al. Histological grading of breast cancer on needle core biopsy: the role of immunohistochemical assessment of proliferation. Histopathology. 2010 Aug;57(2):212-9. PMID: 20716163.

1802. Lacambra MD, Lam CC, Mendoza P, et al. Biopsy sampling of breast lesions: comparison of core needle- and vacuum-assisted breast biopsies. Breast Cancer Res Treat. 2012 Apr;132(3):917-23. PMID: 21698409.

1803. Lau B, Romero LM. Does preoperative magnetic resonance imaging beneficially alter surgical management of invasive lobular carcinoma? Am Surg. 2011 Oct;77(10):1368-71. PMID: 22127091.

1804. Lau K, Lui C, Tee L, et al. Role of Breast Magnetic Resonance Imaging in the Preoperative Assessment and Its Impact on Surgical Management of Patients with Newly Diagnosed Breast Cancer.

1805. Lavoue V, Roger CM, Poilblanc M, et al. Pure flat epithelial atypia (DIN 1a) on core needle biopsy: study of 60 biopsies with follow-up surgical excision. Breast Cancer Res Treat. 2011 Jan;125(1):121-6. PMID: 20945087.

1806. Law Y, Cheung PS, Lau S, et al. Impact of magnetic resonance imaging on preoperative planning for breast cancer surgery. Hong Kong Med J. 2013 Aug;19(4):294-9. PMID: 23832947.

1807. Lebeau A, Turzynski A, Braun S, et al. Reliability of human epidermal growth factor receptor 2 immunohistochemistry in breast core needle biopsies. J Clin Oncol. 2010 Jul 10;28(20):3264-70. PMID: 20498397.

1808. Lee AH, Denley HE, Pinder SE, et al. Excision biopsy findings of patients with breast needle core biopsies reported as suspicious of malignancy (B4) or lesion of uncertain malignant potential (B3). Histopathology. 2003 Apr;42(4):331-6. PMID: 12653944.

1809. Lee AH, Key HP, Bell JA, et al. Concordance of HER2 status assessed on needle core biopsy and surgical specimens of invasive carcinoma of the breast. Histopathology. 2012 May;60(6):880-4. PMID: 22320892.

1810. Lee AH, Rakha EA, Hodi Z, et al. Re-audit of revised method for assessing the mitotic component of histological grade in needle core biopsies of invasive carcinoma of the breast. Histopathology. 2012 Jun;60(7):1166-7. PMID: 22385388.

1811. Lee CH, Philpotts LE, Horvath LJ, et al. Follow-up of breast lesions diagnosed as benign with stereotactic core-needle biopsy: frequency of mammographic change and false-negative rate. Radiology. 1999 Jul;212(1):189-94. PMID: 10405741.

1812. Lee E, Wylie E, Metcalf C. Ultrasound imaging features of radial scars of the breast. Australas Radiol. 2007 Jun;51(3):240-5. PMID: 17504315.

1813. Lee JW, Han W, Ko E, et al. Sonographic lesion size of ductal carcinoma in situ as a preoperative predictor for the presence of an invasive focus. J Surg Oncol. 2008 Jul 1;98(1):15-20. PMID: 18459155.

1814. Lee KA, Zuley ML, Chivukula M, et al. Risk of malignancy when microscopic radial scars and microscopic papillomas are found at percutaneous biopsy. AJR Am J Roentgenol. 2012 Feb;198(2):W141-5. PMID: 22268203.

1815. Lee TY, Macintosh RF, Rayson D, et al. Flat epithelial atypia on breast needle core biopsy: a retrospective study with clinical-pathological correlation. Breast J. 2010 Jul-Aug;16(4):377-83. PMID: 20459431.

1816. Leidenius MH, Vironen JH, von Smitten KA, et al. The outcome of sentinel node biopsy in breast cancer patients with preoperative surgical biopsy. J Surg Oncol. 2009 Jun 1;99(7):420-3. PMID: 19350567.

1817. Lewis JL, Lee DY, Tartter PI. The significance of lobular carcinoma in situ and atypical lobular hyperplasia of the breast. Ann Surg Oncol. 2012 Dec;19(13):4124-8. PMID: 22847126.

1818. Li J, Dershaw DD, Lee CH, et al. MRI follow-up after concordant, histologically benign diagnosis of breast lesions sampled by MRI-guided biopsy. AJR Am J Roentgenol. 2009 Sep;193(3):850-5. PMID: 19696301.

1819. Li JL, Wang ZL, Su L, et al. Breast lesions with ultrasound imaging-histologic discordance at 16-gauge core needle biopsy: can re-biopsy with 10-gauge vacuum-assisted system get definitive diagnosis? Breast. 2010 Dec;19(6):446-9. PMID: 20869243.

1820. Li S, Wu J, Chen K, et al. Clinical outcomes of 1,578 Chinese patients with breast benign diseases after ultrasound-guided vacuum-assisted excision: recurrence and the risk factors. Am J Surg. 2013 Jan;205(1):39-44. PMID: 23040695.

1821. Li SP, Padhani AR, Taylor NJ, et al. Vascular characterisation of triple negative breast carcinomas using dynamic MRI. Eur Radiol. 2011 Jul;21(7):1364-73. PMID: 21258931.

1822. Li X, Deavers MT, Guo M, et al. The effect of prolonged cold ischemia time on estrogen receptor immunohistochemistry in breast cancer. Mod Pathol. 2013 Jan;26(1):71-8. PMID: 22899286.

1823. Li X, Weaver O, Desouki MM, et al. Microcalcification is an important factor in the management of breast intraductal papillomas diagnosed on core biopsy. Am J Clin Pathol. 2012 Dec;138(6):789-95. PMID: 23161711.

1824. Liberman L, Cody HS, 3rd. Percutaneous biopsy and sentinel lymphadenectomy: minimally invasive diagnosis and treatment of nonpalpable breast cancer. AJR Am J Roentgenol. 2001 Oct;177(4):887-91. PMID: 11566696.

1825. Liberman L, Cody HS, 3rd, Hill AD, et al. Sentinel lymph node biopsy after percutaneous diagnosis of nonpalpable breast cancer. Radiology. 1999 Jun;211(3):835-44. PMID: 10352613.

1826. Liberman L, Dershaw DD, Rosen PP, et al. Stereotaxic core biopsy of breast carcinoma: accuracy at predicting invasion. Radiology. 1995 Feb;194(2):379-81. PMID: 7824713.

1827. Liberman L, Morris EA, Dershaw DD, et al. MR imaging of the ipsilateral breast in women with percutaneously proven breast cancer. AJR Am J Roentgenol. 2003 Apr;180(4):901-10. PMID: 12646427.

1828. Liberman L, Zakowski MF, Avery S, et al. Complete percutaneous excision of infiltrating carcinoma at stereotactic breast biopsy: how can tumor size be assessed? AJR Am J Roentgenol. 1999 Nov;173(5):1315-22. PMID: 10541111.

1829. Lieberman S, Sella T, Maly B, et al. Breast magnetic resonance imaging characteristics in women with occult primary breast carcinoma. Isr Med Assoc J. 2008 Jun;10(6):448-52. PMID: 18669145.

1830. Lieske B, Ravichandran D, Alvi A, et al. Screen-detected breast lesions with an indeterminate (B3) core needle biopsy should be excised. Eur J Surg Oncol. 2008 Dec;34(12):1293-8. PMID: 18162359.

1831. Lieu D. Value of cytopathologist-performed ultrasound-guided fine-needle aspiration as a screening test for ultrasound-guided core-needle biopsy in nonpalpable breast masses. Diagn Cytopathol. 2009 Apr;37(4):262-9. PMID: 19217029.

1832. Lin SJ, Cawson J, Hill P, et al. Image-guided sampling reveals increased stroma and lower glandular complexity in mammographically dense breast tissue. Breast Cancer Res Treat. 2011 Jul;128(2):505-16. PMID: 21258862.

1833. Lind DS, Minter R, Steinbach B, et al. Stereotactic core biopsy reduces the reexcision rate and the cost of mammographically detected cancer. Journal of Surgical Research. 1998;78(1):23-6.

1834. Linda A, Zuiani C, Bazzocchi M, et al. Borderline breast lesions diagnosed at core needle biopsy: can magnetic resonance mammography rule out associated malignancy? Preliminary results based on 79 surgically excised lesions. Breast. 2008 Apr;17(2):125-31. PMID: 18083514.

1835. Linda A, Zuiani C, Furlan A, et al. Radial scars without atypia diagnosed at imaging-guided needle biopsy: how often is associated malignancy found at subsequent surgical excision, and do mammography and sonography predict which lesions are malignant? AJR Am J Roentgenol. 2010 Apr;194(4):1146-51. PMID: 20308524.

1836. Linda A, Zuiani C, Furlan A, et al. Nonsurgical management of high-risk lesions diagnosed at core needle biopsy: can malignancy be ruled out safely with breast MRI? AJR Am J Roentgenol. 2012 Feb;198(2):272-80. PMID: 22268168.

1837. Linda A, Zuiani C, Londero V, et al. What to do with B3 lesions at needle biopsy. Eur J Radiol. 2012 Sep;81 Suppl 1:S90-2. PMID: 23083618.

1838. Ling CM, Coffey CM, Rapelyea JA, et al. Breast-specific gamma imaging in the detection of atypical ductal hyperplasia and lobular neoplasia. Acad Radiol. 2012 Jun;19(6):661-6. PMID: 22578225.

1839. Lips EH, Mukhtar RA, Yau C, et al. Lobular histology and response to neoadjuvant chemotherapy in invasive breast cancer. Breast Cancer Res Treat. 2012 Nov;136(1):35-43. PMID: 22961065.

1840. Londero V, Zuiani C, Linda A, et al. Borderline breast lesions: comparison of malignancy underestimation rates with 14-gauge core needle biopsy versus 11-gauge vacuum-assisted device. Eur Radiol. 2011 Jun;21(6):1200-6. PMID: 21225267.

1841. Londero V, Zuiani C, Linda A, et al. High-risk breast lesions at imaging-guided needle biopsy: usefulness of MRI for treatment decision. AJR Am J Roentgenol. 2012 Aug;199(2):W240-50. PMID: 22826427.

1842. Lopes-Costa PV, dos Santos AR, dos Santos LG, et al. Evaluation of Ki-67 and Bcl-2 antigen expression in breast carcinomas of women treated with raloxifene. Cell Prolif. 2010 Apr;43(2):124-9. PMID: 20447057.

1843. Lorenzetti MA, De Matteo E, Gass H, et al. Characterization of Epstein Barr virus latency pattern in Argentine breast carcinoma. PLoS One. 2010;5(10):e13603. PMID: 21042577.

1844. Lorgis V, Algros MP, Villanueva C, et al. Discordance in early breast cancer for tumour grade, estrogen receptor, progesteron receptors and human epidermal receptor-2 status between core needle biopsy and surgical excisional primary tumour. Breast. 2011 Jun;20(3):284-7. PMID: 21288720.

1845. Lu Q, Tan EY, Ho B, et al. Surgical excision of intraductal breast papilloma diagnosed on core biopsy. ANZ J Surg. 2012 Mar;82(3):168-72. PMID: 22510128.

1846. Lyon DE, McCain NL, Walter J, et al. Cytokine comparisons between women with breast cancer and women with a negative breast biopsy. Nurs Res. 2008 Jan-Feb;57(1):51-8. PMID: 18091292.

1847. Macaskill EJ, Bartlett JM, Sabine VS, et al. The mammalian target of rapamycin inhibitor everolimus (RAD001) in early breast cancer: results of a pre-operative study. Breast Cancer Res Treat. 2011 Aug;128(3):725-34. PMID: 20941539.

1848. Macaskill EJ, Purdie CA, Jordan LB, et al. Axillary lymph node core biopsy for breast cancer metastases -- how many needle passes are enough? Clin Radiol. 2012 May;67(5):417-9. PMID: 22119100.

1849. Majewski SA, Zuley ML, Pinnamaneni N, et al. Frequency of carcinoma at secondary imaging-guided percutaneous breast biopsy performed after a high-risk pathologic result at primary biopsy. AJR Am J Roentgenol. 2013 Aug;201(2):439-47. PMID: 23883227.

1850. Manenti G, Bolacchi F, Perretta T, et al. Small breast cancers: in vivo percutaneous US-guided radiofrequency ablation with dedicated cool-tip radiofrequency system. Radiology. 2009 May;251(2):339-46. PMID: 19304918.

1851. Manfrin E, Mariotto R, Remo A, et al. Benign breast lesions at risk of developing cancer--a challenging problem in breast cancer screening programs: five years' experience of the Breast Cancer Screening Program in Verona (1999-2004). Cancer. 2009 Feb 1;115(3):499-507. PMID: 19117040.

1852. Mansoor S, Ip C, Stomper PC. Yield of Terminal Duct Lobule Units in Normal Breast Stereotactic Core Biopsy Specimens: Implications for Biomarker Studies. Breast J. 2000 Jul;6(4):220-4. PMID: 11348369.

1853. Marcotte-Bloch C, Balu-Maestro C, Chamorey E, et al. MRI for the size assessment of pure ductal carcinoma in situ (DCIS): a prospective study of 33 patients. Eur J Radiol. 2011 Mar;77(3):462-7. PMID: 19896789.

1854. Margenthaler JA, Duke D, Monsees BS, et al. Correlation between core biopsy and excisional biopsy in breast high-risk lesions. Am J Surg. 2006 Oct;192(4):534-7. PMID: 16978969.

1855. Marsden CG, Wright MJ, Pochampally R, et al. Breast tumor-initiating cells isolated from patient core biopsies for study of hormone action. Methods Mol Biol. 2009;590:363-75. PMID: 19763516.

1856. Mathew J, Crawford DJ, Lwin M, et al. Ultrasound-guided, vacuum-assisted excision in the diagnosis and treatment of clinically benign breast lesions. Ann R Coll Surg Engl. 2007 Jul;89(5):494-6. PMID: 17688722.

1857. Matos AV, Canella Ede O, Koch HA, et al. Fat necrosis in the breast after reconstruction with transverse rectus abdominis myocutaneous flap: MRI features. Eur J Radiol. 2012 Sep;81 Suppl 1:S97-8. PMID: 23083621.

1858. Maxwell AJ, Mataka G, Pearson JM. Benign papilloma diagnosed on image-guided 14 G core biopsy of the breast: effect of lesion type on likelihood of malignancy at excision. Clin Radiol. 2013 Apr;68(4):383-7. PMID: 23206431.

1859. Maxwell AJ, Pearson JM. Criteria for the safe avoidance of needle sampling in young women with solid breast masses. Clin Radiol. 2010 Mar;65(3):218-22. PMID: 20152278.

1860. McCann B, Miaskowski C, Koetters T, et al. Associations between pro- and anti-inflammatory cytokine genes and breast pain in women prior to breast cancer surgery. J Pain. 2012 May;13(5):425-37. PMID: 22515947.

1861. McCormack VA, Joffe M, van den Berg E, et al. Breast cancer receptor status and stage at diagnosis in over 1,200 consecutive public hospital patients in Soweto, South Africa: a case series. Breast Cancer Res. 2013;15(5):R84. PMID: 24041225.

1862. McGhan LJ, Pockaj BA, Wasif N, et al. Atypical ductal hyperplasia on core biopsy: an automatic trigger for excisional biopsy? Ann Surg Oncol. 2012 Oct;19(10):3264-9. PMID: 22878619.

1863. McLaughlin JM, Anderson RT, Ferketich AK, et al. Effect on survival of longer intervals between confirmed diagnosis and treatment initiation among low-income women with breast cancer. J Clin Oncol. 2012 Dec 20;30(36):4493-500. PMID: 23169521.

1864. Mehrotra R, Pandya S, Singhla M, et al. Spectrum of malignancies in Allahabad, North India: a hospital-based study. Asian Pac J Cancer Prev. 2008 Jul-Sep;9(3):525-8. PMID: 18990032.

1865. Meloni GB, Dessole S, Becchere MP, et al. Effectiveness of "core biopsy" by the mammotome device for diagnosis of inflammatory carcinoma. Clin Exp Obstet Gynecol. 1999;26(3-4):181-2. PMID: 10668149.

1866. Menes TS, Zissman S, Golan O, et al. Yield of selective magnetic resonance imaging in preoperative workup of newly diagnosed breast cancer patients planned for breast conserving surgery. Am Surg. 2012 Apr;78(4):451-5. PMID: 22472404.

1867. Merdad AA, Bahadur YA, Fawzy EE, et al. Phase II study on the use of intraoperative radiotherapy in early breast cancer. Saudi Med J. 2013 Nov;34(11):1133-8. PMID: 24252890.

1868. Mesurolle B, Sygal V, Lalonde L, et al. Sonographic and mammographic appearances of breast hemangioma. AJR Am J Roentgenol. 2008 Jul;191(1):W17-22. PMID: 18562711.

1869. Meyer JE, Smith DN, Lester SC, et al. Large-needle core biopsy: nonmalignant breast abnormalities evaluated with surgical excision or repeat core biopsy. Radiology. 1998 Mar;206(3):717-20. PMID: 9494490.

1870. Middleton LP, Price KM, Puig P, et al. Implementation of American Society of Clinical Oncology/College of American Pathologists HER2 Guideline Recommendations in a tertiary care facility increases HER2 immunohistochemistry and fluorescence in situ hybridization concordance and decreases the number of inconclusive cases. Arch Pathol Lab Med. 2009 May;133(5):775-80. PMID: 19415952.

1871. Mihalik JE, Krupka L, Davenport R, et al. The rate of imaging-histologic discordance of benign breast disease: a multidisciplinary approach to the management of discordance at a large university-based hospital. Am J Surg. 2010 Mar;199(3):319-23; discussion 23. PMID: 20226903.

1872. Miller NA, Chapman JA, Qian J, et al. Heterogeneity Between Ducts of the Same Nuclear Grade Involved by Duct Carcinoma In Situ (DCIS) of the Breast. Cancer Inform. 2010;9:209-16. PMID: 20981137.

1873. Mimmi MC, Picotti P, Corazza A, et al. High-performance metabolic marker assessment in breast cancer tissue by mass spectrometry. Clin Chem Lab Med. 2011 Feb;49(2):317-24. PMID: 21143022.

1874. Minot DM, Kipp BR, Root RM, et al. Automated cellular imaging system III for assessing HER2 status in breast cancer specimens: development of a standardized scoring method that correlates with FISH. Am J Clin Pathol. 2009 Jul;132(1):133-8. PMID: 19864244.

1875. Mittendorf EA, Arciero CA, Gutchell V, et al. Core biopsy diagnosis of ductal carcinoma in situ: an indication for sentinel lymph node biopsy. Curr Surg. 2005 Mar-Apr;62(2):253-7. PMID: 15796952.

1876. Miyake T, Shimazu K, Ohashi H, et al. Indication for sentinel lymph node biopsy for breast cancer when core biopsy shows ductal carcinoma in situ. Am J Surg. 2011 Jul;202(1):59-65. PMID: 21741518.

1877. Miyashita M, Amano G, Ishida T, et al. The clinical significance of breast MRI in the management of ductal carcinoma in situ diagnosed on needle biopsy. Jpn J Clin Oncol. 2013 Jun;43(6):654-63. PMID: 23592884.

1878. Mohammed S, Statz A, Lacross JS, et al. Granulomatous mastitis: a 10 year experience from a large inner city county hospital. J Surg Res. 2013 Sep;184(1):299-303. PMID: 23890401.

1879. Mondal HP, Roy H, Mondal P, et al. Usefulness of serum CA-15.3 in the management of benign breast lesion. J Indian Med Assoc. 2012 Apr;110(4):242-4. PMID: 23025224.

1880. Monticciolo DL. Histologic grading at breast core needle biopsy: comparison with results from the excised breast specimen. Breast J. 2005 Jan-Feb;11(1):9-14. PMID: 15647072.

1881. Moon HG, Han W, Lee JW, et al. Limitations of conventional contrast-enhanced MRI in selecting sentinel node biopsy candidates among DCIS patients. J. Breast Cancer. 2010;13(2):154-9.

1882. Morgan EA, Kozono DE, Wang Q, et al. Cutaneous radiation-associated angiosarcoma of the breast: poor prognosis in a rare secondary malignancy. Ann Surg Oncol. 2012 Nov;19(12):3801-8. PMID: 22890593.

1883. Morgan JM, Douglas-Jones AG, Gupta SK. Analysis of histological features in needle core biopsy of breast useful in preoperative distinction between fibroadenoma and phyllodes tumour. Histopathology. 2010 Mar;56(4):489-500. PMID: 20459556.

1884. Mori M, Tsunoda H, Takamoto Y, et al. MRI and ultrasound evaluation of invasive lobular carcinoma of the breast after primary systemic therapy. Breast Cancer. 2013 Aug 9PMID: 23929123.

1885. Mori N, Ota H, Mugikura S, et al. Detection of invasive components in cases of breast ductal carcinoma in situ on biopsy by using apparent diffusion coefficient MR parameters. Eur Radiol. 2013 Oct;23(10):2705-12. PMID: 23732688.

1886. Mosier AD, Keylock J, Smith DV. Benign papillomas diagnosed on large-gauge vacuum-assisted core needle biopsy which span <1.5 cm do not need surgical excision. Breast J. 2013 Nov-Dec;19(6):611-7. PMID: 24102818.

1887. Mudduwa L, Liyanage T. Immunohistochemical assessment of hormone receptor status of breast carcinoma: interobserver variation of the quick score. Indian J Med Sci. 2009 Jan;63(1):21-7. PMID: 19346635.

1888. Mulheron B, Gray RJ, Pockaj BA, et al. Is excisional biopsy indicated for patients with lobular neoplasia diagnosed on percutaneous core needle biopsy of the breast? Am J Surg. 2009 Dec;198(6):792-7. PMID: 19969131.

1889. Muller BM, Brase JC, Haufe F, et al. Comparison of the RNA-based EndoPredict multigene test between core biopsies and corresponding surgical breast cancer sections. J Clin Pathol. 2012 Jul;65(7):660-2. PMID: 22447922.

1890. Murata Y, Hamada N, Kubota K, et al. Choline by magnetic spectroscopy and dynamic contrast enhancement curve by magnetic resonance imaging in neoadjuvant chemotherapy for invasive breast cancer. Mol Med Rep. 2009 Jan-Feb;2(1):39-43. PMID: 21475788.

1891. Murray MP, Luedtke C, Liberman L, et al. Classic lobular carcinoma in situ and atypical lobular hyperplasia at percutaneous breast core biopsy: outcomes of prospective excision. Cancer. 2013 Mar 1;119(5):1073-9. PMID: 23132235.

1892. Murthy SS, Sandhya DG, Ahmed F, et al. Assessment of HER2/Neu status by fluorescence in situ hybridization in immunohistochemistry-equivocal cases of invasive ductal carcinoma and aberrant signal patterns: a study at a tertiary cancer center. Indian J Pathol Microbiol. 2011 Jul-Sep;54(3):532-8. PMID: 21934215.

1893. Muttarak M, Sangchan S, Kongmebhol P, et al. Mammographic and ultrasonographic features of invasive lobular carcinoma: A review of 16 patients. Biomed. Imaging Intervent. J. 2010;6(3).

1894. Nagi CS, O'Donnell JE, Tismenetsky M, et al. Lobular neoplasia on core needle biopsy does not require excision. Cancer. 2008 May 15;112(10):2152-8. PMID: 18348299.

1895. Nakai K, Mitomi H, Alkam Y, et al. Predictive value of MGMT, hMLH1, hMSH2 and BRCA1 protein expression for pathological complete response to neoadjuvant chemotherapy in basal-like breast cancer patients. Cancer Chemother Pharmacol. 2012 Apr;69(4):923-30. PMID: 22083523.

1896. Nakano S, Sakamoto H, Ohtsuka M, et al. Evaluation and indications of ultrasound-guided vacuum-assisted core needle breast biopsy. Breast Cancer. 2007;14(3):292-6. PMID: 17690507.

1897. Naoi Y, Kishi K, Tanei T, et al. High genomic grade index associated with poor prognosis for lymph node-negative and estrogen receptor-positive breast cancers and with good response to chemotherapy. Cancer. 2011 Feb 1;117(3):472-9. PMID: 20878674.

1898. Nayak A, Carkaci S, Gilcrease MZ, et al. Benign papillomas without atypia diagnosed on core needle biopsy: experience from a single institution and proposed criteria for excision. Clin Breast Cancer. 2013 Dec;13(6):439-49. PMID: 24119786.

1899. Neuman HB, Brogi E, Ebrahim A, et al. Desmoid tumors (fibromatoses) of the breast: a 25-year experience. Ann Surg Oncol. 2008 Jan;15(1):274-80. PMID: 17896146.

1900. Ngai JH, Zelles GW, Rumore GJ, et al. Breast biopsy techniques and adequacy of margins. Arch Surg. 1991 Nov;126(11):1343-6; discussion 6-7. PMID: 1747047.

1901. Nguyen CV, Albarracin CT, Whitman GJ, et al. Atypical ductal hyperplasia in directional vacuum-assisted biopsy of breast microcalcifications: considerations for surgical excision. Ann Surg Oncol. 2011 Mar;18(3):752-61. PMID: 20972636.

1902. Niell B, Specht M, Gerade B, et al. Is excisional biopsy required after a breast core biopsy yields lobular neoplasia? AJR Am J Roentgenol. 2012 Oct;199(4):929-35. PMID: 22997389.

1903. Niraula S, Dowling RJ, Ennis M, et al. Metformin in early breast cancer: a prospective window of opportunity neoadjuvant study. Breast Cancer Res Treat. 2012 Oct;135(3):821-30. PMID: 22933030.

1904. Nishimura R, Osako T, Okumura Y, et al. Clinical significance of Ki-67 in neoadjuvant chemotherapy for primary breast cancer as a predictor for chemosensitivity and for prognosis. Breast Cancer. 2010 Oct;17(4):269-75. PMID: 19730975.

1905. Noel JC, Buxant F, Engohan-Aloghe C. Immediate surgical resection of residual microcalcifications after a diagnosis of pure flat epithelial atypia on core biopsy: a word of caution. Surg Oncol. 2010 Dec;19(4):243-6. PMID: 19783426.

1906. Nofech-Mozes S, Holloway C, Hanna W. The role of cytokeratin 5/6 as an adjunct diagnostic tool in breast core needle biopsies. Int J Surg Pathol. 2008 Oct;16(4):399-406. PMID: 18499686.

1907. Nori J, Bazzocchi M, Boeri C, et al. Role of axillary lymph node ultrasound and large core biopsy in the preoperative assessment of patients selected for sentinel node biopsy. Radiol Med. 2005 Apr;109(4):330-44. PMID: 15883518.

1908. Noske A, Pahl S, Fallenberg E, et al. Flat epithelial atypia is a common subtype of B3 breast lesions and is associated with noninvasive cancer but not with invasive cancer in final excision histology. Hum Pathol. 2010 Apr;41(4):522-7. PMID: 20004938.

1909. O'Flynn EA, Morel JC, Gonzalez J, et al. Prediction of the presence of invasive disease from the measurement of extent of malignant microcalcification on mammography and ductal carcinoma in situ grade at core biopsy. Clin Radiol. 2009 Feb;64(2):178-83. PMID: 19103348.

1910. Ohlschlegel C, Kradolfer D, Hell M, et al. Comparison of automated and manual FISH for evaluation of HER2 gene status on breast carcinoma core biopsies. BMC Clin Pathol. 2013;13:13. PMID: 23601823.

1911. Okunade G, Green AR, Ying M, et al. Biological profile of oestrogen receptor positive primary breast cancers in the elderly and response to primary endocrine therapy. Crit Rev Oncol Hematol. 2009 Oct;72(1):76-82. PMID: 19515574.

1912. O'Neil M, Madan R, Tawfik OW, et al. Lobular carcinoma in situ/atypical lobular hyperplasia on breast needle biopsies: does it warrant surgical excisional biopsy? A study of 27 cases. Ann Diagn Pathol. 2010 Aug;14(4):251-5. PMID: 20637429.

1913. Ooi A, Inokuchi M, Harada S, et al. Gene amplification of ESR1 in breast cancers--fact or fiction? A fluorescence in situ hybridization and multiplex ligation-dependent probe amplification study. J Pathol. 2012 May;227(1):8-16. PMID: 22170254.

1914. Oran ES, Gurdal SO, Yankol Y, et al. Management of idiopathic granulomatous mastitis diagnosed by core biopsy: a retrospective multicenter study. Breast J. 2013 Jul-Aug;19(4):411-8. PMID: 23663101.

1915. Osborn G, Wilton F, Stevens G, et al. A review of needle core biopsy diagnosed radial scars in the Welsh Breast Screening Programme. Ann R Coll Surg Engl. 2011 Mar;93(2):123-6. PMID: 21073820.

1916. O'Shea AM, Rakha EA, Hodi Z, et al. Histological grade of invasive carcinoma of the breast assessed on needle core biopsy - modifications to mitotic count assessment to improve agreement with surgical specimens. Histopathology. 2011 Sep;59(3):543-8. PMID: 21906126.

1917. Ough M, Velasco J, Hieken TJ. A comparative analysis of core needle biopsy and final excision for breast cancer: histology and marker expression. Am J Surg. 2011 May;201(5):692-4. PMID: 20850706.

1918. Ozdemir A, Voyvoda NK, Gultekin S, et al. Can core biopsy be used instead of surgical biopsy in the diagnosis and prognostic factor analysis of breast carcinoma? Clin Breast Cancer. 2007 Oct;7(10):791-5. PMID: 18021481.

1919. Ozel L, Unal A, Unal E, et al. Granulomatous mastitis: is it an autoimmune disease? Diagnostic and therapeutic dilemmas. Surg Today. 2012 Aug;42(8):729-33. PMID: 22068681.

1920. Ozturk E, Akin M, Can MF, et al. Idiopathic granulomatous mastitis. Saudi Med J. 2009 Jan;30(1):45-9. PMID: 19139772.

1921. Paajanen H, Hermunen H. Does preoperative core needle biopsy increase surgical site infections in breast cancer surgery? Randomized study of antibiotic prophylaxis. Surg Infect (Larchmt). 2009 Aug;10(4):317-21. PMID: 19673597.

1922. Pachnicki JP, Czeczko NG, Tuon F, et al. Immunohistochemical evaluation of estrogen and progesterone receptors of pre and post-neoadjuvant chemotherapy for breast cancer. Rev Col Bras Cir. 2012 Apr;39(2):86-92. PMID: 22664513.

1923. Papalas JA, Wylie JD, Dash RC. Recurrence risk and margin status in granular cell tumors of the breast: a clinicopathologic study of 13 patients. Arch Pathol Lab Med. 2011 Jul;135(7):890-5. PMID: 21732779.

1924. Park HS, Kim HY, Park S, et al. A nomogram for predicting underestimation of invasiveness in ductal carcinoma in situ diagnosed by preoperative needle biopsy. Breast. 2013 Oct;22(5):869-73. PMID: 23601760.

1925. Park HS, Park S, Cho J, et al. Risk predictors of underestimation and the need for sentinel node biopsy in patients diagnosed with ductal carcinoma in situ by preoperative needle biopsy. J Surg Oncol. 2013 Mar;107(4):388-92. PMID: 23007901.

1926. Park HS, Park S, Kim JH, et al. Clinicopathologic features and outcomes of metaplastic breast carcinoma: comparison with invasive ductal carcinoma of the breast. Yonsei Med J. 2010 Nov;51(6):864-9. PMID: 20879052.

1927. Park JS, Park YM, Kim EK, et al. Sonographic findings of high-grade and non-high-grade ductal carcinoma in situ of the breast. J Ultrasound Med. 2010 Dec;29(12):1687-97. PMID: 21098839.

1928. Park KJ, Kang SH, Park DH, et al. Usefulness of thallium-201 SPECT for prediction of early progression in low-grade astrocytomas diagnosed by stereotactic biopsy. Clin Neurol Neurosurg. 2012 Apr;114(3):223-9. PMID: 22104697.

1929. Parsian S, Rahbar H, Allison KH, et al. Nonmalignant breast lesions: ADCs of benign and high-risk subtypes assessed as false-positive at dynamic enhanced MR imaging. Radiology. 2012 Dec;265(3):696-706. PMID: 23033500.

1930. Pathmanathan N, Albertini AF, Provan PJ, et al. Diagnostic evaluation of papillary lesions of the breast on core biopsy. Mod Pathol. 2010 Jul;23(7):1021-8. PMID: 20473278.

1931. Pazaitou-Panayiotou K, Chemonidou C, Poupi A, et al. Gonadotropin-releasing hormone neuropeptides and receptor in human breast cancer: correlation to poor prognosis parameters. Peptides. 2013 Apr;42:15-24. PMID: 23287110.

1932. Pediconi F, Kubik-Huch R, Chilla B, et al. Intra-individual randomised comparison of gadobutrol 1.0 M versus gadobenate dimeglumine 0.5 M in patients scheduled for preoperative breast MRI. Eur Radiol. 2013 Jan;23(1):84-92. PMID: 22797979.

1933. Pediconi F, Padula S, Dominelli V, et al. Role of breast MR imaging for predicting malignancy of histologically borderline lesions diagnosed at core needle biopsy: prospective evaluation. Radiology. 2010 Dec;257(3):653-61. PMID: 20884914.

1934. Penel N, Yazdanpanah Y, Chauvet MP, et al. Prevention of surgical site infection after breast cancer surgery by targeted prophylaxis antibiotic in patients at high risk of surgical site infection. J Surg Oncol. 2007 Aug 1;96(2):124-9. PMID: 17443747.

1935. Peres A, Barranger E, Becette V, et al. Rates of upgrade to malignancy for 271 cases of flat epithelial atypia (FEA) diagnosed by breast core biopsy. Breast Cancer Res Treat. 2012 Jun;133(2):659-66. PMID: 22042365.

1936. Perono Biacchiardi C, Brizzi D, Genta F, et al. Breast cancer preoperative staging: does contrast-enhanced magnetic resonance mammography modify surgery? Int J Breast Cancer. 2011;2011:757234. PMID: 22295233.

1937. Peters NH, van Esser S, van den Bosch MA, et al. Preoperative MRI and surgical management in patients with nonpalpable breast cancer: the MONET - randomised controlled trial. Eur J Cancer. 2011 Apr;47(6):879-86. PMID: 21195605.

1938. Petrarca CR, Brunetto AT, Duval V, et al. Survivin as a predictive biomarker of complete pathologic response to neoadjuvant chemotherapy in patients with stage II and stage III breast cancer. Clin Breast Cancer. 2011 Apr;11(2):129-34. PMID: 21569999.

1939. Pettit K, Swatske ME, Gao F, et al. The impact of breast MRI on surgical decision-making: are patients at risk for mastectomy? J Surg Oncol. 2009 Dec 1;100(7):553-8. PMID: 19757442.

1940. Picouleau E, Denis M, Lavoue V, et al. Atypical hyperplasia of the breast: the black hole of routine breast cancer screening. Anticancer Res. 2012 Dec;32(12):5441-6. PMID: 23225449.

1941. Pilewskie M, Kennedy C, Shappell C, et al. Effect of MRI on the management of ductal carcinoma in situ of the breast. Ann Surg Oncol. 2013 May;20(5):1522-9. PMID: 23224903.

1942. Pimiento JM, Lee MC, Esposito NN, et al. Role of axillary staging in women diagnosed with ductal carcinoma in situ with microinvasion. J Oncol Pract. 2011 Sep;7(5):309-13. PMID: 22211128.

1943. Pinhel IF, Macneill FA, Hills MJ, et al. Extreme loss of immunoreactive p-Akt and p-Erk1/2 during routine fixation of primary breast cancer. Breast Cancer Res. 2010;12(5):R76. PMID: 20920193.

1944. Piubello Q, Parisi A, Eccher A, et al. Flat epithelial atypia on core needle biopsy: which is the right management? Am J Surg Pathol. 2009 Jul;33(7):1078-84. PMID: 19390424.

1945. Poellinger A, Diekmann S, Dietz E, et al. In patients with DCIS: is it sufficient to histologically examine only those tissue specimens that contain microcalcifications? Eur Radiol. 2008 May;18(5):925-30. PMID: 18183402.

1946. Pohlodek K, Galbavy S, Bartosova M, et al. Semi-quantitative RT-PCR assessment of molecular markers in breast large-core needle biopsies. Neoplasma. 2004;51(6):415-21. PMID: 15640949.

1947. Polat AK, Kanbour-Shakir A, Andacoglu O, et al. Atypical hyperplasia on core biopsy: is further surgery needed? Am J Med Sci. 2012 Jul;344(1):28-31. PMID: 22205116.

1948. Polom K, Murawa D, Pawelska A, et al. Atypical lobular hyperplasia and lobular carcinoma in situ without other high-risk lesions diagnosed on vacuum-assisted core needle biopsy. The problem of excisional biopsy. Tumori. 2009 Jan-Feb;95(1):32-5. PMID: 19366053.

1949. Polom K, Murawa D, Wasiewicz J, et al. The role of sentinel node biopsy in ductal carcinoma in situ of the breast. Eur J Surg Oncol. 2009 Jan;35(1):43-7. PMID: 18723312.

1950. Porter AJ, Evans EB, Foxcroft LM, et al. Mammographic and ultrasound features of invasive lobular carcinoma of the breast. J Med Imaging Radiat Oncol. 2013.

1951. Provencher L, Jacob S, Cote G, et al. Low frequency of cancer occurrence in same breast quadrant diagnosed with lobular neoplasia at percutaneous needle biopsy. Radiology. 2012 Apr;263(1):43-52. PMID: 22344406.

1952. Puglisi F, Scalone S, Bazzocchi M, et al. Image-guided core breast biopsy: a suitable method for preoperative biological characterization of small (pT1) breast carcinomas. Cancer Lett. 1998 Nov 27;133(2):223-9. PMID: 10072173.

1953. Purdie CA, Jordan LB, McCullough JB, et al. HER2 assessment on core biopsy specimens using monoclonal antibody CB11 accurately determines HER2 status in breast carcinoma. Histopathology. 2010 May;56(6):702-7. PMID: 20546335.

1954. Purdie CA, McLean D, Stormonth E, et al. Management of in situ lobular neoplasia detected on needle core biopsy of breast. J Clin Pathol. 2010 Nov;63(11):987-93. PMID: 20972243.

1955. Radisky DC, Santisteban M, Berman HK, et al. p16(INK4a) expression and breast cancer risk in women with atypical hyperplasia. Cancer Prev Res (Phila). 2011 Dec;4(12):1953-60. PMID: 21920875.

1956. Rahusen FD, Taets van Amerongen AH, van Diest PJ, et al. Ultrasound-guided lumpectomy of nonpalpable breast cancers: A feasibility study looking at the accuracy of obtained margins. J Surg Oncol. 1999 Oct;72(2):72-6. PMID: 10518102.

1957. Railo M, Nordling S, Krogerus L, et al. Preoperative assessment of proliferative activity and hormonal receptor status in carcinoma of the breast: a comparison of needle aspiration and needle-core biopsies to the surgical specimen. Diagn Cytopathol. 1996 Sep;15(3):205-10. PMID: 8955602.

1958. Rajan S, Shaaban AM, Dall BJ, et al. New patient pathway using vacuum-assisted biopsy reduces diagnostic surgery for B3 lesions. Clin Radiol. 2012 Mar;67(3):244-9. PMID: 22014554.

1959. Rajan S, Sharma N, Dall BJ, et al. What is the significance of flat epithelial atypia and what are the management implications? J Clin Pathol. 2011 Nov;64(11):1001-4. PMID: 21725040.

1960. Rajan S, Wason AM, Carder PJ. Conservative management of screen-detected radial scars: role of mammotome excision. J Clin Pathol. 2011 Jan;64(1):65-8. PMID: 21097791.

1961. Rakha EA, El-Sayed ME, Reed J, et al. Screen-detected breast lesions with malignant needle core biopsy diagnoses and no malignancy identified in subsequent surgical excision specimens (potential false-positive diagnosis). Eur J Cancer. 2009 May;45(7):1162-7. PMID: 19121932.

1962. Rakha EA, Ho BC, Naik V, et al. Outcome of breast lesions diagnosed as lesion of uncertain malignant potential (B3) or suspicious of malignancy (B4) on needle core biopsy, including detailed review of epithelial atypia. Histopathology. 2011 Mar;58(4):626-32. PMID: 21371081.

1963. Rakha EA, Lee AH, Jenkins JA, et al. Characterization and outcome of breast needle core biopsy diagnoses of lesions of uncertain malignant potential (B3) in abnormalities detected by mammographic screening. Int J Cancer. 2011 Sep 15;129(6):1417-24. PMID: 21128240.

1964. Rakha EA, Lee AH, Reed J, et al. Screen-detected malignant breast lesions diagnosed following benign (B2) or normal (B1) needle core biopsy diagnoses. Eur J Cancer. 2010 Jul;46(10):1835-40. PMID: 20392631.

1965. Rakha EA, Shaaban AM, Haider SA, et al. Outcome of pure mucocele-like lesions diagnosed on breast core biopsy. Histopathology. 2013 May;62(6):894-8. PMID: 23402386.

1966. Reefy S, Osman H, Chao C, et al. Surgical excision for B3 breast lesions diagnosed by vacuum-assisted core biopsy. Anticancer Res. 2010 Jun;30(6):2287-90. PMID: 20651381.
1967. Reisenbichler ES, Adams AL, Hameed O. The predictive ability of a CK5/p63/CK8/18 antibody cocktail in stratifying breast papillary lesions on needle biopsy: an algorithmic approach works best. Am J Clin Pathol. 2013 Dec;140(6):767-79. PMID: 24225742.
1968. Rendi MH, Dintzis SM, Lehman CD, et al. Lobular in-situ neoplasia on breast core needle biopsy: imaging indication and pathologic extent can identify which patients require excisional biopsy. Ann Surg Oncol. 2012 Mar;19(3):914-21. PMID: 21861212.
1969. Renshaw AA. Improved reporting methods for atypia and atypical ductal hyperplasia in breast core needle biopsy specimens. Potential for interlaboratory comparisons. Am J Clin Pathol. 2001 Jul;116(1):87-91. PMID: 11447757.
1970. Renshaw AA. Predicting invasion in the excision specimen from breast core needle biopsy specimens with only ductal carcinoma in situ. Arch Pathol Lab Med. 2002 Jan;126(1):39-41. PMID: 11800645.
1971. Resetkova E, Edelweiss M, Albarracin CT, et al. Management of radial sclerosing lesions of the breast diagnosed using percutaneous vacuum-assisted core needle biopsy: recommendations for excision based on seven years' of experience at a single institution. Breast Cancer Res Treat. 2011 Jun;127(2):335-43. PMID: 18626769.
1972. Resetkova E, Khazai L, Albarracin CT, et al. Clinical and radiologic data and core needle biopsy findings should dictate management of cellular fibroepithelial tumors of the breast. Breast J. 2010 Nov-Dec;16(6):573-80. PMID: 21070433.
1973. Revelon G, Sherman ME, Gatewood OM, et al. Focal fibrosis of the breast: imaging characteristics and histopathologic correlation. Radiology. 2000 Jul;216(1):255-9. PMID: 10887257.
1974. Richard F, Segna KG, Filiberti E. Can large gauge core biopsies for high risk benign breast lesions eliminate the need for excisional biopsy: a correlation between breast biopsy and final surgical pathology. Am Surg. 2012 Aug;78(8):906-8. PMID: 22856502.
1975. Richter-Ehrenstein C, Muller S, Noske A, et al. Diagnostic accuracy and prognostic value of core biopsy in the management of breast cancer: a series of 542 patients. Int J Surg Pathol. 2009 Aug;17(4):323-6. PMID: 19029173.
1976. Richter-Ehrenstein C, Tombokan F, Fallenberg EM, et al. Intraductal papillomas of the breast: diagnosis and management of 151 patients. Breast. 2011 Dec;20(6):501-4. PMID: 21640590.
1977. Riedl O, Fitzal F, Mader N, et al. Intraoperative frozen section analysis for breast-conserving therapy in 1016 patients with breast cancer. Eur J Surg Oncol. 2009 Mar;35(3):264-70. PMID: 18706785.
1978. Rizzo M, Linebarger J, Lowe MC, et al. Management of papillary breast lesions diagnosed on core-needle biopsy: clinical pathologic and radiologic analysis of 276 cases with surgical follow-up. J Am Coll Surg. 2012 Mar;214(3):280-7. PMID: 22244207.
1979. Romero Q, Bendahl PO, Klintman M, et al. Ki67 proliferation in core biopsies versus surgical samples - a model for neo-adjuvant breast cancer studies. BMC Cancer. 2011;11:341. PMID: 21819622.
1980. Rosa M, Mohammadi A, Masood S. Lobular neoplasia displaying central necrosis: a potential diagnostic pitfall. Pathol Res Pract. 2010 Aug 15;206(8):544-9. PMID: 20359832.
1981. Ross DS, Liu YF, Pipa J, et al. The diagnostic utility of the minimal carcinoma triple stain in breast carcinomas. Am J Clin Pathol. 2013 Jan;139(1):62-70. PMID: 23270900.

1982. Roth WD, von Smitten K, Heikkila P, et al. Automated stereotactic core needle biopsy of microcalcifications with correlation to surgical biopsy. Acta Radiol. 1999 Jul;40(4):390-3. PMID: 10394866.

1983. Rotter K, Haentschel G, Koethe D, et al. Evaluation of mammographic and clinical follow-up after 755 stereotactic vacuum-assisted breast biopsies. Am J Surg. 2003 Aug;186(2):134-42. PMID: 12885605.

1984. Rouse HC, Ussher S, Kavanagh AM, et al. Examining the sensitivity of ultrasound-guided large core biopsy for invasive breast carcinoma in a population screening programme. J Med Imaging Radiat Oncol. 2013 Aug;57(4):435-43. PMID: 23870339.

1985. Ruidiaz ME, Cortes-Mateos MJ, Sandoval S, et al. Quantitative comparison of surgical margin histology following excision with traditional electrosurgery and a low-thermal-injury dissection device. J Surg Oncol. 2011 Dec;104(7):746-54. PMID: 21744349.

1986. Ryden L, Boiesen P, Jonsson PE. Assessment of microvessel density in core needle biopsy specimen in breast cancer. Anticancer Res. 2004 Jan-Feb;24(1):371-5. PMID: 15015623.

1987. Saadai P, Moezzi M, Menes T. Preoperative and intraoperative predictors of positive margins after breast-conserving surgery: a retrospective review. Breast Cancer. 2011 Jul;18(3):221-5. PMID: 21465227.

1988. Saarenmaa I, Salminen T, Geiger U, et al. Validity of radiological examinations of patients with breast cancer in different age groups in a population based study. Breast. 2001 Feb;10(1):78-81. PMID: 14965565.

1989. Sabine VS, Sims AH, Macaskill EJ, et al. Gene expression profiling of response to mTOR inhibitor everolimus in pre-operatively treated post-menopausal women with oestrogen receptor-positive breast cancer. Breast Cancer Res Treat. 2010 Jul;122(2):419-28. PMID: 20480226.

1990. Saedi HS, Nasiri MRG, Shahidsales S, et al. Comparison of hormone receptor status in primary and recurrent breast cancer. Iran. J. Cancer Prev. 2012;5(2):69-73.

1991. Sakr R, Antoine M, Barranger E, et al. Value of sentinel lymph node biopsy in breast ductal carcinoma in situ upstaged to invasive carcinoma. Breast J. 2008 Jan-Feb;14(1):55-60. PMID: 18186866.

1992. Sakr R, Rouzier R, Salem C, et al. Risk of breast cancer associated with papilloma. Eur J Surg Oncol. 2008 Dec;34(12):1304-8. PMID: 18440190.

1993. Salkowski LR, Fowler AM, Burnside ES, et al. Utility of 6-month follow-up imaging after a concordant benign breast biopsy result. Radiology. 2011 Feb;258(2):380-7. PMID: 21079199.

1994. Sancho Perez B, Hernandez Sanchez L, Noguero Meseguer R, et al. Ductal carcinoma in situ: A risk factor for mastectomy?: Carcinoma ductal in situ, factor de riesgo de mastectomia? Prog. Obstet. Ginecol. 2011;54(6):281-93.

1995. Sanger N, Effenberger KE, Riethdorf S, et al. Disseminated tumor cells in the bone marrow of patients with ductal carcinoma in situ. Int J Cancer. 2011 Nov 15;129(10):2522-6. PMID: 21207426.

1996. Sangma MB, Panda K, Dasiah S. A clinico-pathological study on benign breast diseases. J Clin Diagn Res. 2013 Mar;7(3):503-6. PMID: 23634406.

1997. Sanli Y, Kuyumcu S, Ozkan ZG, et al. Increased FDG uptake in breast cancer is associated with prognostic factors. Ann Nucl Med. 2012 May;26(4):345-50. PMID: 22359222.

1998. Santamaria G, Velasco M, Farrus B, et al. Preoperative MRI of pure intraductal breast carcinoma--a valuable adjunct to mammography in assessing cancer extent. Breast. 2008 Apr;17(2):186-94. PMID: 17964786.

1999. Saritas I. Prediction of breast cancer using artificial neural networks. J Med Syst. 2012 Oct;36(5):2901-7. PMID: 21837454.

2000. Satheesha S, Cookson VJ, Coleman LJ, et al. Response to mTOR inhibition: activity of eIF4E predicts sensitivity in cell lines and acquired changes in eIF4E regulation in breast cancer. Mol Cancer. 2011;10:19. PMID: 21320304.

2001. Sauer G, Schneiderhan-Marra N, Muche R, et al. Molecular indicators of non-sentinel node status in breast cancer determined in preoperative biopsies by multiplexed sandwich immunoassays. J Cancer Res Clin Oncol. 2011 Aug;137(8):1175-84. PMID: 21516507.

2002. Scheiden R, Sand J, Tanous AM, et al. Consequences of a National Mammography Screening Program on diagnostic procedures and tumor sizes in breast cancer. A retrospective study of 1540 cases diagnosed and histologically confirmed between 1995 and 1997. Pathol Res Pract. 2001;197(7):467-74. PMID: 11482576.

2003. Schell AM, Rosenkranz K, Lewis PJ. Role of breast MRI in the preoperative evaluation of patients with newly diagnosed breast cancer. AJR Am J Roentgenol. 2009 May;192(5):1438-44. PMID: 19380574.

2004. Schiffmann S, Sandner J, Birod K, et al. Ceramide synthases and ceramide levels are increased in breast cancer tissue. Carcinogenesis. 2009 May;30(5):745-52. PMID: 19279183.

2005. Schilling K, Narayanan D, Kalinyak JE, et al. Positron emission mammography in breast cancer presurgical planning: comparisons with magnetic resonance imaging. Eur J Nucl Med Mol Imaging. 2011 Jan;38(1):23-36. PMID: 20871992.

2006. Schneider C, Trocha S, McKinley B, et al. The use of sentinel lymph node biopsy in ductal carcinoma in situ. Am Surg. 2010 Sep;76(9):943-6. PMID: 20836339.

2007. Schoonjans JM, Brem RF. Sonographic appearance of ductal carcinoma in situ diagnosed with ultrasonographically guided large core needle biopsy: correlation with mammographic and pathologic findings. J Ultrasound Med. 2000 Jul;19(7):449-57. PMID: 10898298.

2008. Schulz S, Sinn P, Golatta M, et al. Prediction of underestimated invasiveness in patients with ductal carcinoma in situ of the breast on percutaneous biopsy as rationale for recommending concurrent sentinel lymph node biopsy. Breast. 2013 Aug;22(4):537-42. PMID: 23237921.

2009. Schwartz GF, Finkel GC, Garcia JC, et al. Subclinical ductal carcinoma in situ of the breast. Treatment by local excision and surveillance alone. Cancer. 1992 Nov 15;70(10):2468-74. PMID: 1330281.

2010. Sciallis AP, Chen B, Folpe AL. Cellular spindled histiocytic pseudotumor complicating mammary fat necrosis: a potential diagnostic pitfall. Am J Surg Pathol. 2012 Oct;36(10):1571-8. PMID: 22982900.

2011. Scoggins M, Krishnamurthy S, Santiago L, et al. Lobular carcinoma in situ of the breast: clinical, radiological, and pathological correlation. Acad Radiol. 2013 Apr;20(4):463-70. PMID: 23498988.

2012. Seferina SC, Nap M, van den Berkmortel F, et al. Reliability of receptor assessment on core needle biopsy in breast cancer patients. Tumour Biol. 2013 Apr;34(2):987-94. PMID: 23269610.

2013. Segaert I, Mottaghy F, Ceyssens S, et al. Additional value of PET-CT in staging of clinical stage IIB and III breast cancer. Breast J. 2010 Nov-Dec;16(6):617-24. PMID: 21070439.

2014. Senetta R, Campanino PP, Mariscotti G, et al. Columnar cell lesions associated with breast calcifications on vacuum-assisted core biopsies: clinical, radiographic, and histological correlations. Mod Pathol. 2009 Jun;22(6):762-9. PMID: 19287465.

2015. Seo M, Chang JM, Kim WH, et al. Columnar cell lesions without atypia initially diagnosed on breast needle biopsies: is imaging follow-up enough? AJR Am J Roentgenol. 2013 Oct;201(4):928-34. PMID: 24059386.

2016. Shah-Khan MG, Geiger XJ, Reynolds C, et al. Long-term follow-up of lobular neoplasia (atypical lobular hyperplasia/lobular carcinoma in situ) diagnosed on core needle biopsy. Ann Surg Oncol. 2012 Oct;19(10):3131-8. PMID: 22847124.

2017. Shamonki J, Chung A, Huynh KT, et al. Management of papillary lesions of the breast: can larger core needle biopsy samples identify patients who may avoid surgical excision? Ann Surg Oncol. 2013 Dec;20(13):4137-44. PMID: 23943035.

2018. Shimauchi A, Giger ML, Bhooshan N, et al. Evaluation of clinical breast MR imaging performed with prototype computer-aided diagnosis breast MR imaging workstation: reader study. Radiology. 2011 Mar;258(3):696-704. PMID: 21212365.

2019. Shimizu D, Ishikawa T, Tanabe M, et al. Preoperative endocrine therapy with goserelin acetate and tamoxifen in hormone receptor-positive premenopausal breast cancer patients. Breast Cancer. 2012 Nov 25PMID: 23184499.

2020. Shin HJ, Kim HH, Kim SM, et al. Screening-detected and symptomatic ductal carcinoma in situ: differences in the sonographic and pathologic features. AJR Am J Roentgenol. 2008 Feb;190(2):516-25. PMID: 18212241.

2021. Shouhed D, Amersi FF, Spurrier R, et al. Intraductal papillary lesions of the breast: clinical and pathological correlation. Am Surg. 2012 Oct;78(10):1161-5. PMID: 23025963.

2022. Shousha S, Peston D, Amo-Takyi B, et al. Evaluation of automated silver-enhanced in situ hybridization (SISH) for detection of HER2 gene amplification in breast carcinoma excision and core biopsy specimens. Histopathology. 2009 Jan;54(2):248-53. PMID: 19207950.

2023. Shrestha DB, Ravichandran D, Baber Y, et al. Follow-up of benign screen-detected breast lesions with suspicious preoperative needle biopsies. Eur J Surg Oncol. 2009 Feb;35(2):156-8. PMID: 18353607.

2024. Siegmann KC, Baur A, Vogel U, et al. Risk-benefit analysis of preoperative breast MRI in patients with primary breast cancer. Clin Radiol. 2009 Apr;64(4):403-13. PMID: 19264186.

2025. Silberfein EJ, Hunt KK, Broglio K, et al. Clinicopathologic factors associated with involved margins after breast-conserving surgery for invasive lobular carcinoma. Clin Breast Cancer. 2010 Feb;10(1):52-8. PMID: 20133259.

2026. Siziopikou KP, Jokich P, Cobleigh M. Pathologic findings in MRI-guided needle core biopsies of the breast in patients with newly diagnosed breast cancer. Int J Breast Cancer. 2011;2011:613285. PMID: 22332013.

2027. Skenderi F, Krakonja F, Vranic S. Infarcted fibroadenoma of the breast: report of two new cases with review of the literature. Diagn Pathol. 2013;8:38. PMID: 23445683.

2028. Sklair-Levy M, Sella T, Alweiss T, et al. Incidence and management of complex fibroadenomas. AJR Am J Roentgenol. 2008 Jan;190(1):214-8. PMID: 18094314.

2029. Smith BL, Bertagnolli M, Klein BB, et al. Evaluation of the contralateral breast. The role of biopsy at the time of treatment of primary breast cancer. Ann Surg. 1992 Jul;216(1):17-21. PMID: 1321595.

2030. Smitt MC, Horst K. Association of clinical and pathologic variables with lumpectomy surgical margin status after preoperative diagnosis or excisional biopsy of invasive breast cancer. Ann Surg Oncol. 2007 Mar;14(3):1040-4. PMID: 17203329.

2031. Sohn V, Porta R, Brown T. Flat epithelial atypia of the breast on core needle biopsy: an indication for surgical excision. Mil Med. 2011 Nov;176(11):1347-50. PMID: 22165668.

2032. Sohn VY, Causey MW, Steele SR, et al. The treatment of radial scars in the modern era--surgical excision is not required. Am Surg. 2010 May;76(5):522-5. PMID: 20506884.

2033. Sohn YM, Park SH. Comparison of sonographically guided core needle biopsy and excision in breast papillomas: clinical and sonographic features predictive of malignancy. J Ultrasound Med. 2013 Feb;32(2):303-11. PMID: 23341387.

2034. Solorzano S, Mesurolle B, Omeroglu A, et al. Flat epithelial atypia of the breast: pathological-radiological correlation. AJR Am J Roentgenol. 2011 Sep;197(3):740-6. PMID: 21862819.

2035. Son EJ, Kim EK, Youk JH, et al. Imaging-histologic discordance after sonographically guided percutaneous breast biopsy: a prospective observational study. Ultrasound Med Biol. 2011 Nov;37(11):1771-8. PMID: 21856068.

2036. Song HM, Styblo TM, Carlson GW, et al. The use of oncoplastic reduction techniques to reconstruct partial mastectomy defects in women with ductal carcinoma in situ. Breast J. 2010 Mar-Apr;16(2):141-6. PMID: 20102367.

2037. Sonnenfeld MR, Frenna TH, Weidner N, et al. Lobular carcinoma in situ: mammographic-pathologic correlation of results of needle-directed biopsy. Radiology. 1991 Nov;181(2):363-7. PMID: 1924773.

2038. Spangler ML, Zuley ML, Sumkin JH, et al. Detection and classification of calcifications on digital breast tomosynthesis and 2D digital mammography: a comparison. AJR Am J Roentgenol. 2011 Feb;196(2):320-4. PMID: 21257882.

2039. Sperber F, Blank A, Metser U, et al. Diagnosis and treatment of breast fibroadenomas by ultrasound-guided vacuum-assisted biopsy. Arch Surg. 2003 Jul;138(7):796-800. PMID: 12860764.

2040. Steffens RF, Wright HR, Hester MY, et al. Clinical, demographic, and situational factors linked to distress associated with benign breast biopsy. J Psychosoc Oncol. 2011;29(1):35-50. PMID: 21240724.

2041. Stolier A, Stone JC, Moroz K, et al. A comparison of clinical and pathologic assessments for the prediction of occult nipple involvement in nipple-sparing mastectomies. Ann Surg Oncol. 2013 Jan;20(1):128-32. PMID: 23010730.

2042. Stotter A, Walker R. Tumour markers predictive of successful treatment of breast cancer with primary endocrine therapy in patients over 70 years old: a prospective study. Crit Rev Oncol Hematol. 2010 Sep;75(3):249-56. PMID: 19969469.

2043. Striebel JM, Bhargava R, Horbinski C, et al. The equivocally amplified HER2 FISH result on breast core biopsy: indications for further sampling do affect patient management. Am J Clin Pathol. 2008 Mar;129(3):383-90. PMID: 18285260.

2044. Strien L, Leidenius M, Heikkila P. False-positive and false-negative sentinel node findings in 473 breast cancers. Hum Pathol. 2012 Nov;43(11):1940-7. PMID: 22575258.

2045. Strigel RM, Eby PR, Demartini WB, et al. Frequency, upgrade rates, and characteristics of high-risk lesions initially identified with breast MRI. AJR Am J Roentgenol. 2010 Sep;195(3):792-8. PMID: 20729462.

2046. Stuver SO, Zhu J, Simchowitz B, et al. Identifying women at risk of delayed breast cancer diagnosis. Jt Comm J Qual Patient Saf. 2011 Dec;37(12):568-75. PMID: 22235542.

2047. Subhawong AP, Subhawong TK, Khouri N, et al. Incidental minimal atypical lobular hyperplasia on core needle biopsy: correlation with findings on follow-up excision. Am J Surg Pathol. 2010 Jun;34(6):822-8. PMID: 20431477.

2048. Suh YJ, Kim MJ, Kim EK, et al. Comparison of the underestimation rate in cases with ductal carcinoma in situ at ultrasound-guided core biopsy: 14-gauge automated core-needle biopsy vs 8- or 11-gauge vacuum-assisted biopsy. Br J Radiol. 2012 Aug;85(1016):e349-56. PMID: 22422382.

2049. Sullivan ME, Khan SA, Sullu Y, et al. Lobular carcinoma in situ variants in breast cores: potential for misdiagnosis, upgrade rates at surgical excision, and practical implications. Arch Pathol Lab Med. 2010 Jul;134(7):1024-8. PMID: 20586632.

2050. Sutandyo N, Suzanna E, Haryono SJ, et al. Signaling pathways in early onset sporadic breast cancer of patients in Indonesia. Acta Med Indones. 2008 Jul;40(3):139-45. PMID: 18838752.

2051. Sutela A, Vanninen R, Sudah M, et al. Surgical specimen can be replaced by core samples in assessment of ER, PR and HER-2 for invasive breast cancer. Acta Oncol. 2008;47(1):38-46. PMID: 17851859.

2052. Sutton B, Davion S, Feldman M, et al. Mucocele-like lesions diagnosed on breast core biopsy: assessment of upgrade rate and need for surgical excision. Am J Clin Pathol. 2012 Dec;138(6):783-8. PMID: 23161710.

2053. Swapp RE, Glazebrook KN, Jones KN, et al. Management of benign intraductal solitary papilloma diagnosed on core needle biopsy. Ann Surg Oncol. 2013 Jun;20(6):1900-5. PMID: 23314624.

2054. Symmans WF, Ayers M, Clark EA, et al. Total RNA yield and microarray gene expression profiles from fine-needle aspiration biopsy and core-needle biopsy samples of breast carcinoma. Cancer. 2003 Jun 15;97(12):2960-71. PMID: 12784330.

2055. Szynglarewicz B, Matkowski R, Halon A, et al. Lobular neoplasia found on breast biopsy: marker of increased risk of malignancy or direct pre-cancerous lesion? Folia Histochem Cytobiol. 2011;49(3):417-24. PMID: 22038220.

2056. Tagaya N, Nakagawa A, Ishikawa Y, et al. Experience with ultrasonographically guided vacuum-assisted resection of benign breast tumors. Clin Radiol. 2008 Apr;63(4):396-400. PMID: 18325359.

2057. Tamaki K, Sasano H, Ishida T, et al. Comparison of core needle biopsy (CNB) and surgical specimens for accurate preoperative evaluation of ER, PgR and HER2 status of breast cancer patients. Cancer Sci. 2010 Sep;101(9):2074-9. PMID: 20557310.

2058. Tan H, Li R, Peng W, et al. Radiological and clinical features of adult non-puerperal mastitis. Br J Radiol. 2013 Apr;86(1024):20120657. PMID: 23392197.

2059. Tang SW, Parker H, Winterbottom L, et al. Early primary breast cancer in the elderly - pattern of presentation and treatment. Surg Oncol. 2011 Mar;20(1):7-12. PMID: 19679464.

2060. Taskin F, Koseoglu K, Ozbas S, et al. Sonographic features of histopathologically benign solid breast lesions that have been classified as BI-RADS 4 on sonography. J Clin Ultrasound. 2012 Jun;40(5):261-5. PMID: 22508447.

2061. Taskin F, Unsal A, Ozbas S, et al. Fibrotic lesions of the breast: radiological findings and core-neddle biopsy results. Eur J Radiol. 2011 Dec;80(3):e231-6. PMID: 21071162.

2062. Taucher S, Rudas M, Mader RM, et al. Prognostic markers in breast cancer: the reliability of HER2/neu status in core needle biopsy of 325 patients with primary breast cancer. Wien Klin Wochenschr. 2004 Jan 31;116(1-2):26-31. PMID: 15030120.

2063. Taylor D, Lazberger J, Ives A, et al. Reducing delay in the diagnosis of pregnancy-associated breast cancer: how imaging can help us. J Med Imaging Radiat Oncol. 2011 Feb;55(1):33-42. PMID: 21382187.

2064. Tebbit CL, Zhai J, Untch BR, et al. Novel tumor sampling strategies to enable microarray gene expression signatures in breast cancer: a study to determine feasibility and reproducibility in the context of clinical care. Breast Cancer Res Treat. 2009 Dec;118(3):635-43. PMID: 19224362.

2065. Teng-Swan Ho J, Tan PH, Hee SW, et al. Underestimation of malignancy of atypical ductal hyperplasia diagnosed on 11-gauge stereotactically guided Mammotome breast biopsy: an Asian breast screen experience. Breast. 2008 Aug;17(4):401-6. PMID: 18455920.

2066. Tennant SL, Evans A, Hamilton LJ, et al. Vacuum-assisted excision of breast lesions of uncertain malignant potential (B3) - an alternative to surgery in selected cases. Breast. 2008 Dec;17(6):546-9. PMID: 18829318.

2067. Tewari M, Pradhan S, Singh U, et al. Assessment of predictive markers of response to neoadjuvant chemotherapy in breast cancer. Asian J Surg. 2010 Oct;33(4):157-67. PMID: 21377101.

2068. Tfayli A, Yang J, Kojouri K, et al. Neoadjuvant therapy with celecoxib to women with early stage breast cancer. Neoplasma. 2008;55(2):122-6. PMID: 18237249.

2069. Tham TM, Iyengar KR, Taib NA, et al. Fine needle aspiration biopsy, core needle biopsy or excision biopsy to diagnose breast cancer - which is the ideal method? Asian Pac J Cancer Prev. 2009 Jan-Mar;10(1):155-8. PMID: 19469645.

2070. Thomssen C, Harbeck N, Dittmer J, et al. Feasibility of measuring the prognostic factors uPA and PAI-1 in core needle biopsy breast cancer specimens. J Natl Cancer Inst. 2009 Jul 15;101(14):1028-9. PMID: 19535782.

2071. Tohno E, Ueno E. Ultrasound (US) diagnosis of nonpalpable breast cancer. Breast Cancer. 2005;12(4):267-71. PMID: 16286906.

2072. Tomasino RM, Morello V, Gullo A, et al. Assessment of "grading" with Ki-67 and c-kit immunohistochemical expressions may be a helpful tool in management of patients with flat epithelial atypia (FEA) and columnar cell lesions (CCLs) on core breast biopsy. J Cell Physiol. 2009 Nov;221(2):343-9. PMID: 19585492.

2073. Tomasovic-Loncaric C, Milanovic R, Lambasa S, et al. Intraoperative imprint cytological assessment of the subareolar tissue of the nipple areola complex (NAC). Coll Antropol. 2010 Jun;34(2):431-5. PMID: 20698114.

2074. Tonegutti M, Girardi V, Ciatto S, et al. B3 breast lesions determined by vacuum-assisted biopsy: how to reduce the frequency of benign excision biopsies. Radiol Med. 2010 Dec;115(8):1246-57. PMID: 20852955.

2075. Trentin C, Dominelli V, Maisonneuve P, et al. Predictors of invasive breast cancer and lymph node involvement in ductal carcinoma in situ initially diagnosed by vacuum-assisted breast biopsy: experience of 733 cases. Breast. 2012 Oct;21(5):635-40. PMID: 22795363.

2076. Tsang AK, Chan SK, Lam CC, et al. Phyllodes tumours of the breast - differentiating features in core needle biopsy. Histopathology. 2011 Oct;59(4):600-8. PMID: 21916949.

2077. Tse GM, Tan PH, Lacambra MD, et al. Papillary lesions of the breast--accuracy of core biopsy. Histopathology. 2010 Mar;56(4):481-8. PMID: 20459555.

2078. Tseng HS, Chen YL, Chen ST, et al. The management of papillary lesion of the breast by core needle biopsy. Eur J Surg Oncol. 2009 Jan;35(1):21-4. PMID: 18640002.

2079. Tsuda H, Kurosumi M, Umemura S, et al. HER2 testing on core needle biopsy specimens from primary breast cancers: interobserver reproducibility and concordance with surgically resected specimens. BMC Cancer. 2010;10:534. PMID: 20925963.

2080. Tunon-de-Lara C, Giard S, Buttarelli M, et al. Sentinel node procedure is warranted in ductal carcinoma in situ with high risk of occult invasive carcinoma and microinvasive carcinoma treated by mastectomy. Breast J. 2008 Mar-Apr;14(2):135-40. PMID: 18315691.

2081. Turnbull L, Brown S, Harvey I, et al. Comparative effectiveness of MRI in breast cancer (COMICE) trial: a randomised controlled trial. Lancet. 2010 Feb 13;375(9714):563-71. PMID: 20159292.

2082. Turnbull LW, Brown SR, Olivier C, et al. Multicentre randomised controlled trial examining the cost-effectiveness of contrast-enhanced high field magnetic resonance imaging in women with primary breast cancer scheduled for wide local excision (COMICE). Health Technol Assess. 2010 Jan;14(1):1-182. PMID: 20025837.

2083. Tvrdik D, Skalova H, Dundr P, et al. Apoptosis - associated genes and their role in predicting responses to neoadjuvant breast cancer treatment. Med Sci Monit. 2012 Jan;18(1):BR60-7. PMID: 22207111.

2084. Uematsu T, Kasami M. Soft-copy reading in digital mammography of mass: diagnostic performance of a 5-megapixel cathode ray tube monitor versus a 3-megapixel liquid crystal display monitor in a diagnostic setting. Acta Radiol. 2008 Jul;49(6):623-9. PMID: 18568553.

2085. Uematsu T, Yuen S, Kasami M, et al. Comparison of magnetic resonance imaging, multidetector row computed tomography, ultrasonography, and mammography for tumor extension of breast cancer. Breast Cancer Res Treat. 2008 Dec;112(3):461-74. PMID: 18193352.

2086. Ugburo AO, Olajide TO, Fadeyibi IO, et al. Differential diagnosis and management of giant fibroadenoma: comparing excision with reduction mammoplasty incision and excision with inframammary incision. J Plast Surg Hand Surg. 2012 Oct;46(5):354-8. PMID: 22998148.

2087. Usami S, Moriya T, Amari M, et al. Reliability of prognostic factors in breast carcinoma determined by core needle biopsy. Jpn J Clin Oncol. 2007 Apr;37(4):250-5. PMID: 17485439.

2088. Usmani S, Khan HA, Al Saleh N, et al. Selective approach to radionuclide-guided sentinel lymph node biopsy in high-risk ductal carcinoma in situ of the breast. Nucl Med Commun. 2011 Nov;32(11):1084-7. PMID: 21862942.

2089. Usmani S, Khan HA, Niaz K, et al. Tc-99m-methoxy isobutyl isonitrile scintimammography: imaging postexcision biopsy for residual and multifocal breast tumor. Nucl Med Commun. 2008 Sep;29(9):826-9. PMID: 18677211.

2090. Uy GB, Laudico AV, Carnate JM, Jr., et al. Breast cancer hormone receptor assay results of core needle biopsy and modified radical mastectomy specimens from the same patients. Clin Breast Cancer. 2010 Apr;10(2):154-9. PMID: 20299318.

2091. Uzan C, Mazouni C, Ferchiou M, et al. A model to predict the risk of upgrade to malignancy at surgery in atypical breast lesions discovered on percutaneous biopsy specimens. Ann Surg Oncol. 2013 Sep;20(9):2850-7. PMID: 23702641.

2092. Uzoaru I, Morgan BR, Liu ZG, et al. Flat epithelial atypia with and without atypical ductal hyperplasia: to re-excise or not. Results of a 5-year prospective study. Virchows Arch. 2012 Oct;461(4):419-23. PMID: 22961104.

2093. Vamesu S. Angiogenesis and tumor grading in primary breast cancer patients: an analysis of 158 needle core biopsies. Rom J Morphol Embryol. 2006;47(3):251-7. PMID: 17308684.

2094. Vamesu S. Angiogenesis and ER/PR status in primary breast cancer patients: an analysis of 158 needle core biopsies. Rom J Morphol Embryol. 2007;48(1):25-31. PMID: 17502947.

2095. Vamesu S. Angiogenesis and tumor histologic type in primary breast cancer patients: an analysis of 155 needle core biopsies. Rom J Morphol Embryol. 2008;49(2):181-8. PMID: 18516324.

2096. Vamesu S. Angiogenesis and co-expressed of ER and c-erbB-2 (HER2/neu) protein in primary breast cancer patients: an analysis of 158 needle core biopsies. Rom J Morphol Embryol. 2008;49(4):469-78. PMID: 19050794.

2097. van Esser S, Peters NH, van den Bosch MA, et al. Surgical outcome of patients with core-biopsy-proven nonpalpable breast carcinoma: a large cohort follow-up study. Ann Surg Oncol. 2009 Aug;16(8):2252-8. PMID: 19437077.

2098. van Esser S, Stapper G, van Diest PJ, et al. Ultrasound-guided laser-induced thermal therapy for small palpable invasive breast carcinomas: a feasibility study. Ann Surg Oncol. 2009 Aug;16(8):2259-63. PMID: 19506958.

2099. Vandenbussche CJ, Khouri N, Sbaity E, et al. Borderline atypical ductal hyperplasia/low-grade ductal carcinoma in situ on breast needle core biopsy should be managed conservatively. Am J Surg Pathol. 2013 Jun;37(6):913-23. PMID: 23598968.

2100. Venta LA, Wiley EL, Gabriel H, et al. Imaging features of focal breast fibrosis: mammographic-pathologic correlation of noncalcified breast lesions. AJR Am J Roentgenol. 1999 Aug;173(2):309-16. PMID: 10430125.

2101. Veronesi U, Luini A, Botteri E, et al. Nonpalpable breast carcinomas: long-term evaluation of 1,258 cases. Oncologist. 2010;15(12):1248-52. PMID: 21147866.

2102. Verschuur-Maes AH, Van Diest PJ. The mucinous variant of columnar cell lesions. Histopathology. 2011 May;58(6):847-53. PMID: 21585423.

2103. Verschuur-Maes AH, Witkamp AJ, de Bruin PC, et al. Progression risk of columnar cell lesions of the breast diagnosed in core needle biopsies. Int J Cancer. 2011 Dec 1;129(11):2674-80. PMID: 21225627.

2104. Vicini FA, Kestin LL, Goldstein NS, et al. Relationship between excision volume, margin status, and tumor size with the development of local recurrence in patients with ductal carcinoma-in-situ treated with breast-conserving therapy. J Surg Oncol. 2001 Apr;76(4):245-54. PMID: 11320515.

2105. Vicini FA, Lacerna MD, Goldstein NS, et al. Ductal carcinoma in situ detected in the mammographic era: an analysis of clinical, pathologic, and treatment-related factors affecting outcome with breast-conserving therapy. Int J Radiat Oncol Biol Phys. 1997 Oct 1;39(3):627-35. PMID: 9336142.

2106. Vicini FA, Shaitelman S, Wilkinson JB, et al. Long-term impact of young age at diagnosis on treatment outcome and patterns of failure in patients with ductal carcinoma in situ treated with breast-conserving therapy. Breast J. 2013 Jul-Aug;19(4):365-73. PMID: 23815268.

2107. Vilar VS, Goldman SM, Ricci MD, et al. Analysis by MRI of residual tumor after radiofrequency ablation for early stage breast cancer. AJR Am J Roentgenol. 2012 Mar;198(3):W285-91. PMID: 22358027.

2108. Vilardell F, Novell A, Martin J, et al. Importance of assessing CK19 immunostaining in core biopsies in patients subjected to sentinel node study by OSNA. Virchows Arch. 2012 Jun;460(6):569-75. PMID: 22555942.

2109. Villa A, Tagliafico A, Chiesa F, et al. Atypical ductal hyperplasia diagnosed at 11-gauge vacuum-assisted breast biopsy performed on suspicious clustered microcalcifications: could patients without residual microcalcifications be managed conservatively? AJR Am J Roentgenol. 2011 Oct;197(4):1012-8. PMID: 21940593.

2110. von Minckwitz G, Darb-Esfahani S, Loibl S, et al. Responsiveness of adjacent ductal carcinoma in situ and changes in HER2 status after neoadjuvant chemotherapy/trastuzumab treatment in early breast cancer--results from the GeparQuattro study (GBG 40). Breast Cancer Res Treat. 2012 Apr;132(3):863-70. PMID: 21667238.

2111. Voros A, Csorgo E, Nyari T, et al. An intra- and interobserver reproducibility analysis of the Ki-67 proliferation marker assessment on core biopsies of breast cancer patients and its potential clinical implications. Pathobiology. 2013;80(3):111-8. PMID: 23258384.

2112. Wagoner MJ, Laronga C, Acs G. Extent and histologic pattern of atypical ductal hyperplasia present on core needle biopsy specimens of the breast can predict ductal carcinoma in situ in subsequent excision. Am J Clin Pathol. 2009 Jan;131(1):112-21. PMID: 19095574.

2113. Walker LC, Harris GC, Wells JE, et al. Association of chromosome band 8q22 copy number gain with high grade invasive breast carcinomas by assessment of core needle biopsies. Genes Chromosomes Cancer. 2008 May;47(5):405-17. PMID: 18273837.

2114. Walls J, Knox F, Baildam AD, et al. Can preoperative factors predict for residual malignancy after breast biopsy for invasive cancer? Ann R Coll Surg Engl. 1995 Jul;77(4):248-51. PMID: 7574313.

2115. Wang ZL, Li JL, Su L, et al. An evaluation of a 10-gauge vacuum-assisted system for ultrasound-guided excision of clinically benign breast lesions. Breast. 2009 Jun;18(3):192-6. PMID: 19446453.

2116. Wang ZL, Liu G, Li JL, et al. Breast lesions with imaging-histologic discordance during 16-gauge core needle biopsy system: would vacuum-assisted removal get significantly more definitive histologic diagnosis than vacuum-assisted biopsy? Breast J. 2011 Sep-Oct;17(5):456-61. PMID: 21762244.

2117. Wani SQ, Khan T, Wani SY, et al. Clinicoepidemiological analysis of female breast cancer patients in Kashmir. J Cancer Res Ther. 2012 Jul-Sep;8(3):389-93. PMID: 23174720.

2118. Ward ST, Jewkes AJ, Jones BG, et al. The sensitivity of needle core biopsy in combination with other investigations for the diagnosis of phyllodes tumours of the breast. Int J Surg. 2012;10(9):527-31. PMID: 22892094.

2119. Warner E, Causer PA, Wong JW, et al. Improvement in DCIS detection rates by MRI over time in a high-risk breast screening study. Breast J. 2011 Jan-Feb;17(1):9-17. PMID: 21251121.

2120. Watson P, Lieberman R, Snyder C, et al. Detecting BRCA2 protein truncation in tissue biopsies to identify breast cancers that arise in BRCA2 gene mutation carriers. J Clin Oncol. 2009 Aug 20;27(24):3894-900. PMID: 19620486.

2121. Wei S, Kragel CP, Zhang K, et al. Factors associated with residual disease after initial breast-conserving surgery for ductal carcinoma in situ. Hum Pathol. 2012 Jul;43(7):986-93. PMID: 22221704.

2122. Weigel S, Decker T, Korsching E, et al. Minimal invasive biopsy results of "uncertain malignant potential" in digital mammography screening: high prevalence but also high predictive value for malignancy. Rofo. 2011 Aug;183(8):743-8. PMID: 21506072.

2123. Whiffen A, El-Tamer M, Taback B, et al. Predictors of breast cancer development in women with atypical ductal hyperplasia and atypical lobular hyperplasia. Ann Surg Oncol. 2011 Feb;18(2):463-7. PMID: 20878246.

2124. White V, Pruden M, Kitchen P, et al. The impact of publication of Australian treatment recommendations for DCIS on clinical practice: A population-based, "before-after" study. Eur J Surg Oncol. 2010 Oct;36(10):949-56. PMID: 20724103.

2125. Whitworth PW, Simpson JF, Poller WR, et al. Definitive diagnosis for high-risk breast lesions without open surgical excision: the Intact Percutaneous Excision Trial (IPET). Ann Surg Oncol. 2011 Oct;18(11):3047-52. PMID: 21947585.

2126. Wieman SM, Landercasper J, Johnson JM, et al. Tumoral pseudoangiomatous stromal hyperplasia of the breast. Am Surg. 2008 Dec;74(12):1211-4. PMID: 19097540.

2127. Wilke LG, Ballman KV, McCall LM, et al. Adherence to the National Quality Forum (NQF) breast cancer measures within cancer clinical trials: a review from ACOSOG Z0010. Ann Surg Oncol. 2010 Aug;17(8):1989-94. PMID: 20309640.

2128. Williams RT, Yao K, Stewart AK, et al. Needle versus excisional biopsy for noninvasive and invasive breast cancer: report from the National Cancer Data Base, 2003-2008. Ann Surg Oncol. 2011 Dec;18(13):3802-10. PMID: 21630122.

2129. Wiratkapun C, Chansanti O, Wibulpolprasert B, et al. Focal fibrosis of the breast diagnosed by core needle biopsy under imaging guidance. J Med Assoc Thai. 2013 Mar;96(3):340-5. PMID: 23539939.

2130. Wiratkapun C, Keeratitragoon T, Lertsithichai P, et al. Upgrading rate of papillary breast lesions diagnosed by core-needle biopsy. Diagn Interv Radiol. 2013 Sep-Oct;19(5):371-6. PMID: 23748032.

2131. Wiratkapun C, Patanajareet P, Wibulpholprasert B, et al. Factors associated with upstaging of ductal carcinoma in situ diagnosed by core needle biopsy using imaging guidance. Jpn J Radiol. 2011 Oct;29(8):547-53. PMID: 21927996.

2132. Wisinski KB, Faerber A, Wagner S, et al. Predictors of willingness to participate in window-of-opportunity breast trials. Clin Med Res. 2013 Sep;11(3):107-12. PMID: 23580787.

2133. Wisner DJ, Hwang ES, Chang CB, et al. Features of occult invasion in biopsy-proven DCIS at breast MRI. Breast J. 2013 Nov-Dec;19(6):650-8. PMID: 24165314.

2134. Wojnar A, Bartosz Pula B, Podhorska-Okolow M, et al. Discrepancies between HER2 assessment from core needle biopsies and surgical specimens of invasive ductal breast carcinoma. Adv Clin Exp Med. 2013 Jan-Feb;22(1):27-31. PMID: 23468259.

2135. Xu HN, Tchou J, Chance B, et al. Imaging the redox states of human breast cancer core biopsies. Adv Exp Med Biol. 2013;765:343-9. PMID: 22879054.

2136. Xu ZL, Zhu XQ, Lu P, et al. Activation of tumor-infiltrating antigen presenting cells by high intensity focused ultrasound ablation of human breast cancer. Ultrasound Med Biol. 2009 Jan;35(1):50-7. PMID: 18950932.

2137. Yamaguchi R, Tanaka M, Mizushima Y, et al. Myxomatous fibroadenoma of the breast: correlation with clinicopathologic and radiologic features. Hum Pathol. 2011 Mar;42(3):419-23. PMID: 21195451.

2138. Yamaguchi R, Tanaka M, Tse GM, et al. Pure flat epithelial atypia is uncommon in subsequent breast excisions for atypical epithelial proliferation. Cancer Sci. 2012 Aug;103(8):1580-5. PMID: 22533984.

2139. Yamaguchi R, Tsuchiya S, Koshikawa T, et al. Evaluation of inadequate, indeterminate, false-negative and false-positive cases in cytological examination for breast cancer according to histological type. Diagn Pathol. 2012;7:53. PMID: 22607447.

2140. Yamashita M, Hovanessian-Larsen L, Sener SF. The role of axillary ultrasound in the detection of metastases from primary breast cancers. Am J Surg. 2013 Mar;205(3):242-4; discussion 4-5. PMID: 23369307.

2141. Yang H, Liu H, Peng W, et al. Magnetic resonance imaging of the breast in evaluating residual diseases at lumpectomy site soon after excisional biopsy. J Comput Assist Tomogr. 2012 Mar-Apr;36(2):196-9. PMID: 22446359.

2142. Yildiz-Aktas IZ, Dabbs DJ, Bhargava R. The effect of cold ischemic time on the immunohistochemical evaluation of estrogen receptor, progesterone receptor, and HER2 expression in invasive breast carcinoma. Mod Pathol. 2012 Aug;25(8):1098-105. PMID: 22460807.

2143. Yohe S, Yeh IT. "Missed" diagnoses of phyllodes tumor on breast biopsy: pathologic clues to its recognition. Int J Surg Pathol. 2008 Apr;16(2):137-42. PMID: 18417670.

2144. Yoshida M, Tsuda H, Yamamoto S, et al. Loss of heterozygosity on chromosome 16q suggests malignancy in core needle biopsy specimens of intraductal papillary breast lesions. Virchows Arch. 2012 May;460(5):497-504. PMID: 22476400.

2145. Youk JH, Jung I, Kim EK, et al. US follow-up protocol in concordant benign result after US-guided 14-gauge core needle breast biopsy. Breast Cancer Res Treat. 2012 Apr;132(3):1089-97. PMID: 22218886.

2146. Youk JH, Kim EK, Kim MJ. Atypical ductal hyperplasia diagnosed at sonographically guided 14-gauge core needle biopsy of breast mass. AJR Am J Roentgenol. 2009 Apr;192(4):1135-41. PMID: 19304725.

2147. Youk JH, Kim EK, Kim MJ, et al. Analysis of false-negative results after US-guided 14-gauge core needle breast biopsy. Eur Radiol. 2010 Apr;20(4):782-9. PMID: 19862531.

2148. Youk JH, Kim EK, Kwak JY, et al. Atypical papilloma diagnosed by sonographically guided 14-gauge core needle biopsy of breast mass. AJR Am J Roentgenol. 2010 May;194(5):1397-402. PMID: 20410431.

2149. Youk JH, Kim EK, Kwak JY, et al. Benign papilloma without atypia diagnosed at US-guided 14-gauge core-needle biopsy: clinical and US features predictive of upgrade to malignancy. Radiology. 2011 Jan;258(1):81-8. PMID: 20971773.

2150. Youk JH, Kim MJ, Son EJ, et al. US-guided vacuum-assisted percutaneous excision for management of benign papilloma without atypia diagnosed at US-guided 14-gauge core needle biopsy. Ann Surg Oncol. 2012 Mar;19(3):922-8. PMID: 21863359.

2151. Youn I, Choi SH, Moon HJ, et al. Phyllodes tumors of the breast: ultrasonographic findings and diagnostic performance of ultrasound-guided core needle biopsy. Ultrasound Med Biol. 2013 Jun;39(6):987-92. PMID: 23499344.

2152. Yu CC, Chiang KC, Kuo WL, et al. Low re-excision rate for positive margins in patients treated with ultrasound-guided breast-conserving surgery. Breast. 2013 Oct;22(5):698-702. PMID: 23333255.

2153. Yu J, Monaco SE, Onisko A, et al. A validation study of quantum dot multispectral imaging to evaluate hormone receptor status in ductal carcinoma in situ of the breast. Hum Pathol. 2013 Mar;44(3):394-401. PMID: 23039940.

2154. Yuan XM, Wang N, Ouyang T, et al. Current status of diagnosis and treatment of primary breast cancer in beijing, 2008. Chin J Cancer Res. 2011 Mar;23(1):38-42. PMID: 23467615.

2155. Zagouri F, Sergentanis TN, Nonni A, et al. Comparison of molecular markers expression in vacuum-assisted biopsies and surgical specimens of human breast carcinomas. Pathol Res Pract. 2010 Jan 15;206(1):30-3. PMID: 19836148.

2156. Zhang X, Wu X, Su P, et al. Doxorubicin influences the expression of glucosylceramide synthase in invasive ductal breast cancer. PLoS One. 2012;7(11):e48492. PMID: 23133636.

2157. Zhao C, Desouki MM, Florea A, et al. Pathologic findings of follow-up surgical excision for lobular neoplasia on breast core biopsy performed for calcification. Am J Clin Pathol. 2012 Jul;138(1):72-8. PMID: 22706860.

2158. Zheng J, Alsaadi T, Blaichman J, et al. Invasive ductal carcinoma of the breast: correlation between tumor grade determined by ultrasound-guided core biopsy and surgical pathology. AJR Am J Roentgenol. 2013 Jan;200(1):W71-4. PMID: 23255773.

2159. Zhou W, Zha X, Liu X, et al. US-guided percutaneous microwave coagulation of small breast cancers: a clinical study. Radiology. 2012 May;263(2):364-73. PMID: 22438362.

2160. Zhu Y, Li Q, Gao J, et al. Clinical features and treatment response of solid neuroendocrine breast carcinoma to adjuvant chemotherapy and endocrine therapy. Breast J. 2013 Jul-Aug;19(4):382-7. PMID: 23721399.

2161. Zito FA, Verderio P, Simone G, et al. Reproducibility in the diagnosis of needle core biopsies of non-palpable breast lesions: an international study using virtual slides published on the world-wide web. Histopathology. 2010 May;56(6):720-6. PMID: 20546337.

2162. Zografos GC, Zagouri F, Sergentanis TN, et al. Diagnosing papillary lesions using vacuum-assisted breast biopsy: should conservative or surgical management follow? Onkologie. 2008 Dec;31(12):653-6. PMID: 19060502.

2163. Zwart W, Koornstra R, Wesseling J, et al. A carrier-assisted ChIP-seq method for estrogen receptor-chromatin interactions from breast cancer core needle biopsy samples. BMC Genomics. 2013;14(1):232. PMID: 23565824.

2164. Zysk AM, Nguyen FT, Chaney EJ, et al. Clinical feasibility of microscopically-guided breast needle biopsy using a fiber-optic probe with computer-aided detection. Technol Cancer Res Treat. 2009 Oct;8(5):315-21. PMID: 19754207.

Appendix C. Sensitivity Analysis to the Exclusion of High Risk Lesions on Core Needle Biopsy That Were Confirmed to be High Risk Lesions in Subsequent Open Biopsy or Surgical Excision

Table C1. Summary estimates of test performance for alternative core-needle biopsy methods – women at average risk of cancer

Biopsy method or device	Sensitivity	Specificity
Freehand, automated	0.91 (0.80 to 0.96)	0.99 (0.97 to 1.00)
US-guided, automated	0.99 (0.98 to 0.99)	0.99 (0.98 to 1.00)
US-guided, vacuum-assisted	0.97 (0.92 to 0.99)	0.99 (0.97 to 1.00)
Stereotactically guided, automated	0.97 (0.95 to 0.98)	0.98 (0.97 to 0.99)
Stereotactically guided, vacuum-assisted	0.99 (0.98 to 0.99)	0.96 (0.94 to 0.98)
MRI-guided, automated	0.90 (0.57 to 0.99)	0.99 (0.89 to 1.00)
MRI-guided, vacuum-assisted	1.00 (0.98 to 1.00)	0.93 (0.42 to 1.00)
Multiple methods/other	0.99 (0.98 to 0.99)	0.97 (0.96 to 0.99)

CrI = credible interval; DCIS = ductal carcinoma in situ; MRI = magnetic resonance imaging; N = number; NA = not applicable; US = ultrasound

Note: All numbers are medians with 95% CrIs. 'Other' denotes one study using grid guidance and one study that did not report information on the use of vacuum assistance.

Table C2. Summary estimates of test performance for alternative core-needle biopsy methods – women at high risk of cancer

Biopsy method or device	Sensitivity (95% CrI)	Specificity (95% CrI)
Stereotactically guided, automated	0.97 (0.82, 1.00)	0.98 (0.91, 1.00)
Stereotactically guided, vacuum-assisted	0.99 (0.93, 1.00)	0.97 (0.83, 0.99)
MRI-guided, automated	0.90 (0.58, 0.98)	0.99 (0.91, 1.00)
MRI-guided, vacuum-assisted	1.00 (0.98, 1.00)	0.94 (0.52, 1.00)

CrI = credible interval; DCIS = ductal carcinoma in situ; MRI = magnetic resonance imaging; N = number; US = ultrasound

Note: All numbers are medians with 95% CrIs. No studies provided information on the test performance of freehand or US-guided biopsy methods, or the use of multiple methods in populations of women at high risk of cancer. Results are based on bivariate model with risk group as a covariate.

Appendix D. Assessment of the Strength of Evidence

Key Question	Population	Outcome	Comparison or biopsy method	Risk of Bias	Consistency	Precision	Directness	Overall Rating	Key Findings and Comments
Key Question 1: Comparative effectiveness of core-needle biopsy and open surgical biopsy	Average risk women	Test performance	Freehand	Moderate to high	Consistent	Precise	Direct (studies investigating a given technique)	Low	– Sensitivity: 0.91 (0.80 to 0.96) – Specificity: 0.98 (0.95 to 1.00)
			US-guided, automated	Moderate to high	Consistent	Precise	Direct (studies investigating a given technique)	Moderate	– Sensitivity: 0.99 (0.98 to 0.99) – Specificity: 0.97 (0.95 to 0.98)
			US-guided, automated	Moderate to high	Consistent	Precise	Direct (studies investigating a given technique)	Moderate	– Sensitivity: 0.97 (0.92 to 0.99) – Specificity: 0.98 (0.96 to 0.99)
			Stereotactically guided, automated	Moderate to high	Consistent	Precise	Direct (studies investigating a given technique)	Moderate	– Sensitivity: 0.97 (0.95 to 0.98) – Specificity: 0.97 (0.96 to 0.98)
			Stereotactically guided, automated	Moderate to high	Consistent	Precise	Direct (studies investigating a given technique)	Moderate	– Sensitivity: 0.99 (0.98 to 0.99) – Specificity: 0.92 (0.89 to 0.94)
			MRI-guided, automated	Moderate to high	Consistent	Imprecise	Direct (studies investigating a given technique)	Insufficient	– Sensitivity: 0.90 (0.57 to 0.99) – Specificity: 0.99 (0.91 to 1.00)
			MRI-guided, automated	Moderate to high	Consistent	Imprecise	Direct (studies investigating a given technique)	Insufficient	– Sensitivity: 1.00 (0.98 to 1.00) – Specificity: 0.91 (0.54 to 0.99)
	Average risk women	Comparative test performance	US-guided, automated vs. vacuum-assisted	Moderate to high	Reliance on indirect comparisons does not allow assessment of consistency (effects are not estimable within studies)	Precise	Indirect (regression based comparisons across studies)	Low	– Difference in sensitivity: 0.01 (-0.01 to 0.06) [no difference] – Difference in specificity: -0.01 (-0.03 to 0.01) [no difference]
			Stereotactically-guided, automated vs. vacuum-assisted	Moderate to high	Reliance on indirect comparisons does not allow assessment of consistency	Precise	Indirect (regression based comparisons across studies)	Low	– Difference in sensitivity: -0.02 (-0.04 to -0.01) [vacuum-assisted is better] – Difference in specificity: 0.05 (0.02 to 0.08) [automated is better]

Key Question	Population	Outcome	Comparison or biopsy method	Risk of Bias	Consistency	Precision	Directness	Overall Rating	Key Findings and Comments
			MRI-guided, automated vs. vacuum-assisted	Moderate to high	Reliance on indirect comparisons does not allow assessment of consistency (effects are not estimable within studies)	Very imprecise	Indirect (regression based comparisons across studies)	Insufficient	– Difference in sensitivity: -0.10 (-0.43 to -0.01) [vacuum-assisted is better] – Difference in specificity: 0.07 (-0.03 to 0.43) [no difference]
		DCIS underestimation	Ultrasound-guided, automated	Moderate to high	Moderately inconsistent	Imprecise	Comparisons between tests were indirect (across studies)	Low	– Average underestimation probability: 0.38 (0.26 to 0.51) [14 studies]
			Ultrasound-guided, vacuum-assisted	Moderate to high	Moderately inconsistent	Imprecise	Comparisons between tests were indirect (across studies)	Low	– Average underestimation probability: 0.09 (0.02 to 0.26) [5 studies]
			Stereotactically guided, automated	Moderate to high	Moderately inconsistent	Imprecise	Comparisons between tests were indirect (across studies)	Low	– Average underestimation probability: 0.26 (0.19 to 0.36) [18 studies]
			Stereotactically guided, vacuum-assisted	Moderate to high	Moderately inconsistent	Imprecise	Comparisons between tests were indirect (across studies)	Low	– Average underestimation probability: 0.11 (0.08 to 0.14) [34 studies]
			Other biopsy methods	Moderate to high	Moderately inconsistent	Imprecise	Comparisons between tests were indirect (across studies)	Insufficient	No available studies or few studies with small numbers of lesions.
		High risk lesion underestimation rate	Ultrasound-guided, automated	Moderate to high	Moderately inconsistent	Imprecise	Comparisons between tests were indirect (across studies)	Low	– Average underestimation probability: 0.25 (0.16 to 0.36) [21 studies]
			Ultrasound-guided, vacuum-assisted	Moderate to high	Moderately inconsistent	Imprecise	Comparisons between tests were indirect (across studies)	Low	– Average underestimation probability: 0.11 (0.02 to 0.33) [9 studies]
			Stereotactically guided, automated	Moderate to high	Moderately inconsistent	Imprecise	Comparisons between tests were	Low	– Average underestimation probability: 0.47 (0.37 to 0.58) [29 studies]

Key Question	Population	Outcome	Comparison or biopsy method	Risk of Bias	Consistency	Precision	Directness	Overall Rating	Key Findings and Comments
							indirect (across studies)		
			Stereotactically guided, vacuum-assisted	Moderate to high	Moderately inconsistent	Imprecise	Comparisons between tests were indirect (across studies)	Low	– Average underestimation probability: 0.18 (0.13 to 0.24) [40 studies]
			Other biopsy methods	Moderate to high	Moderately inconsistent	Imprecise	Comparisons between tests were indirect (across studies)	Insufficient	No available studies or few studies with small numbers of lesions.
	Women at high risk of cancer	Test performance	All biopsy methods	Moderate to high	Number and sample size of studies does not allow assessment of consistency	Imprecise	Direct (studies investigating a given technique)	Insufficient	No available studies or few studies with small numbers of lesions.
		Comparative test performance	Comparisons of biopsy methods using the same imaging guidance	Moderate to high	Number and sample size of studies does not allow assessment of consistency	Imprecise	Comparisons between tests were indirect (across studies) or not possible	Insufficient	No available studies or few studies with small numbers of lesions.
		DCIS underestimation	All biopsy methods	Moderate to high	Number and sample size of studies does not allow assessment of consistency	Imprecise	Comparisons between tests were indirect (across studies) or not possible	Insufficient	No available studies or few studies with small numbers of lesions.
		High risk lesion underestimation	All biopsy methods	Moderate to high	Number and sample size of studies does not allow assessment of consistency	Imprecise	Comparisons between tests were indirect (across studies) or not possible	Insufficient	No available studies or few studies with small numbers of lesions.
	Women at average and high risk of breast cancer	Modifiers of test performance	All biopsy methods	Moderate to high	Unclear	Imprecise	Indirect	Insufficient	– Few studies provided within sample information for each modifier of interest; meta-regression results rely on cross-study comparisons so consistency of effects cannot be assessed – Within-study (direct) evidence was sparse; between study evidence relied on indirect comparisons across studies

Key Question	Population	Outcome	Comparison or biopsy method	Risk of Bias	Consistency	Precision	Directness	Overall Rating	Key Findings and Comments
									– In meta-regression analyses CrIs were wide and extreme odds ratio values were often observed because sensitivity and specificity for all tests were very close to 1 (see Results for additional details)
Key Question 2: Adverse events of core-needle biopsy and open surgical biopsy	All patient populations	Any complications	Open vs. core-needle biopsy	NA	NA	NA	NA	Not rated	– Few studies provided information on open biopsy; comparisons of methods are indirect and based on limited empirical evidence and expert opinion – Open surgical biopsy is associated with an increased incidence of adverse events compared to core-needle biopsy
		Severe complications	Open vs. core-needle biopsy	NA	NA	NA	NA	Not rated	– Few studies provided information on open biopsy; comparisons of methods are indirect and based on limited empirical evidence and expert opinion – Open surgical biopsy is associated with an increased incidence of serious adverse events compared to core-needle biopsy
		Bleeding (any severity)	Comparisons among all core-needle biopsy methods	Moderate to high	Consistent	Imprecise	Indirect	Low	– Median %: 1.21 (25th perc. = 0.33; 75th perc. = 3.97) – Selective outcome and analysis reporting likely – Few studies reported bleeding requiring treatment; the event rate was low (<0.40 perc.) in those studies
		Bleeding events that require treatment	Comparisons among all core-needle biopsy methods	Moderate to high	Consistent	Imprecise	Indirect	Low	– Median %: 0 (25th perc. = 0; 75th perc. = 0.14) – Selective outcome and analysis reporting likely – Few studies reported bleeding requiring treatment; the event rate was low
		Hematoma formation	Comparisons among all core-needle biopsy methods	Moderate to high	Consistent	Imprecise	Indirect	Low	– Median %: 1.44 (25th perc. = 0.25; 75th perc. = 8.57) – Selective outcome and analysis reporting likely
		Infectious complications	Comparisons among all core-needle biopsy methods	Moderate to high	Consistent	Imprecise	Indirect	Low	– Median %: 0 (25th perc. = 0; 75th perc.= 0.33) – Selective outcome and analysis reporting likely
		Vasovagal reactions:	Comparisons among all core-needle	Moderate to high	Consistent	Imprecise	Indirect	Low	– Median %: 1.27 (25th perc. = 0.37; 75th perc. = 3.88)

Key Question	Population	Outcome	Comparison or biopsy method	Risk of Bias	Consistency	Precision	Directness	Overall Rating	Key Findings and Comments
			biopsy methods						– Potential for selective outcome and analysis reporting
		Pain and severe pain	Comparisons among all core-needle biopsy methods	Moderate to high	Consistent	Imprecise	Indirect	Low	25 studies of a wide variety of biopsy methods reported information about patient pain during the procedure (pain was assessed heterogeneously across studies).
		Other adverse events	Comparisons among all core-needle biopsy methods	Moderate to high	Unclear	Imprecise	Indirect	Insufficient	– Most events were reported by a single study precluding assessment of consistency – Individual studies did not provide adequate information for precise estimation of the event rate) – Only informal indirect comparisons among biopsy methods were possible – Potential for selective outcome and analysis reporting
		Modifiers of test adverse events – vasovagal reactions	Sitting upright during the biopsy procedure	Moderate to high	Unclear (few available studies; heterogeneous reporting)	Imprecise	Direct	Low	– Vasovagal reactions were more common among patients sitting during the biopsy procedure – Results were reported in few studies (11 studies; 8 from the original evidence report and 3 from this update) – Potential for selective outcome and analysis reporting
		Modifiers of test adverse events – bleeding	Vacuum-assisted versus non-vacuum assisted biopsy methods	Moderate to high	Fairly consistent	Imprecise	Indirect	Low	– Vacuum-assisted procedures were generally associated with increased rates of bleeding and hematoma formation – Bleeding events were generally uncommon – Comparisons among biopsy methods were based on informal indirect comparisons (across studies) – Potential for selective outcome and analysis reporting
		All other modifiers of adverse events	Comparisons among all core-needle biopsy methods	Moderate to high	Unclear	Imprecise (and sometimes impossible to assess due to incomplete information)	Direct	Insufficient	– Most factors assessed by a single study limiting our ability to assess consistency – Potential for selective outcome and analysis reporting. – Within-study comparisons provided direct evidence

CrI = credible interval; DCIS = ductal carcinoma in situ; NA = not applicable; perc. = percentile

www.ingramcontent.com/pod-product-compliance
Lightning Source LLC
Chambersburg PA
CBHW081722170526
45167CB00009B/3661